Adult Critical Care Medicine

Jennifer A. LaRosa
Editor

Adult Critical Care Medicine

A Clinical Casebook

Springer

Editor
Jennifer A. LaRosa
Newark
NJ
USA

ISBN 978-3-319-94423-4 ISBN 978-3-319-94424-1 (eBook)
https://doi.org/10.1007/978-3-319-94424-1

Library of Congress Control Number: 2018956149

This Springer imprint is published by the registered company Springer Nature Switzerland AG
The registered company address is: Gewerbestrasse 11, 6330 Cham, Switzerland

For the Fearsome Foursome, of course….

Buon seme dà buoni frutti.
Italian Proverb

Ní neart go cur le chéile.
Gaelic Proverb

Preface

The study of disease and the application of lifesaving interventions have undergone a meteoric rise in the mid-twentieth century. Many important events have contributed to this growth, the following three of which are noteworthy examples: (1) The polio epidemic triggered the widespread use of mechanical ventilators. (2) The standardization of transfusion and resuscitative protocols made survival from catastrophic injury possible. (3) Organ transplant became a real and sustainable possibility for those dying of single organ dysfunction. For patients with organ failure, trauma, or severe infection who would have invariably succumbed to their illness, critical care medicine offered an opportunity to change that inevitable fate.

This book is a state-of-the-art reference for many of the challenges the modern practitioner faces today. The topics covered range from organ failure and transplantation to bioethical challenges and how we die. Each chapter tells a story of a real patient. Though this book is by no means all encompassing, it aims to be broad, comprehensive, and accessible for critical care providers. It is the work of over two dozen authors from around the world with firsthand experience and expertise in their subspecialty.

Newark, NJ, USA — Jennifer A. LaRosa

Contents

Contributors

Aimee Abide, PA-C, MMSc Emory Critical Care Center, Emory Healthcare, Atlanta, GA, USA

Michael J. Apostolakos, MD University of Rochester Medical Center, Rochester, NY, USA

Christopher Begley, DO University of Rochester Medical Center, Rochester, NY, USA

Jonathan Decker, DO Newark Beth Israel Medical Center, Newark, NJ, USA

R. Phillip Dellinger, MD, MCCM Critical Care Medicine, Cooper University Health Care, Cooper Medical School of Rowan University, Camden, NJ, USA

Anthony Dinallo, MD, MPH Newark Beth Israel Medical Center, Newark, NJ, USA

Joseph W. Dooley, MD Department of Anesthesiology and Perioperative Medicine, University of Rochester School of Medicine and Dentistry, Rochester, NY, USA

Christian A. Engell, MD Rutgers University New Jersey School of Medicine, Newark, NJ, USA

Patrick Hinfey, MD Newark Beth Israel Medical Center, Newark, NJ, USA

Donald S. Houston, MD, PhD Department of Internal Medicine, Section of Medical Oncology and Haematology, University of Manitoba, Winnipeg, MB, Canada

Ryan T. Hurt, MD, PhD Division of General Internal Medicine, Mayo Clinic, Rochester, MN, USA

Leeor M. Jaffe, MD Department of Medicine, Baystate Medical Center, Springfield, MA, USA

David C. Kaufman, MD, FCCM Department of Surgery, University of Rochester School of Medicine and Dentistry, Rochester, NY, USA

Adam M. Kopelan, MD, FACS Newark Beth Israel Medical Center, Newark, NJ, USA

Michael Kouch, MD, FAAEM Critical Care Medicine, Cooper University Health Care, Cooper Medical School of Rowan University, Camden, NJ, USA

Anand Kumar, MD Section of Critical Care Medicine, Section of Infectious Diseases, University of Manitoba, Winnipeg, MB, Canada

Kim Kwai, MD UC Davis Medical Center, Sacramento, CA, USA

Jennifer A. LaRosa, MD, FCCM, FCCP Newark, NJ, USA

Heath E. Latham, MD Division of Pulmonary and Critical Care Medicine, Department of Internal Medicine, The University of Kansas Medical Center, Kansas City, KS, USA

Heather Meissen, MSN, ACNP, CCRN, FCCM, FAANP Emory Critical Care Center, Emory Healthcare, Nell Hodgson Woodruff School of Nursing, Emory University, Atlanta, GA, USA

Manpreet Mundi, MD Division of Endocrinology, Diabetes, Metabolism, and Nutrition, Mayo Clinic, Rochester, MN, USA

Jayshil Patel, MD Division of Pulmonary and Critical Care Medicine, Medical College of Wisconsin, Milwaukee, WI, USA

Lars-Kristofer N. Peterson, MD Departments of Medicine and Emergency Medicine, Division of Critical Care Medicine, Cooper University Hospital, Cooper Medical School of Rowan University, Camden, NJ, USA

Yanjie Qi, MD Division of Trauma and Acute Care Surgery, Department of Surgery, University of Rochester Medical Center, Rochester, NY, USA

Caroline M. Quill, MD Division of Pulmonary and Critical Care Medicine, University of Rochester Medical Center, Rochester, NY, USA

Priyanka Rajaram, MD Emory University School of Medicine, Department of Medicine, Atlanta, GA, USA

Debra Roberts, MD, PhD University of Rochester Medical Center, Rochester, NY, USA

Jagroop S. Saran, MD Department of Anesthesiology and Perioperative Medicine, University of Rochester School of Medicine and Dentistry, Rochester, NY, USA

Margie Hodges Shaw Division of Medical Humanities and Bioethics, University of Rochester School of Medicine and Dentistry, Rochester, NY, USA

Ram Subramanian, MD Emory University School of Medicine, Department of Medicine, Atlanta, GA, USA

Victor Tremblay Section of Critical Care Medicine, University of Manitoba, Winnipeg, MB, Canada

Julia West, MD Division of Pulmonary and Critical Care Medicine, University of Rochester Medical Center, Rochester, NY, USA

Ryan Zarychanski, MD, MSc Department of Internal Medicine, Section of Medical Oncology and Haematology, University of Manitoba, Winnipeg, MB, Canada

Department of Internal Medicine, Section of Critical Care, University of Manitoba, Winnipeg, MB, Canada

Mark Jay Zucker, MD, JD, FACC, FACP, FCCP Cardiothoracic Transplantation Programs, Newark Beth Israel Medical Center, Rutgers University – New Jersey Medical School, Newark, NJ, USA

Chapter 1
Management of Intracranial Hypertension and Status Epilepticus

Christopher Begley and Debra Roberts

Case #1: Intracranial Hypertension

A 53-year-old female arrives in the emergency department (ED) intubated and sedated accompanied by EMS. She is quickly examined by an emergency medicine resident while vitals and labwork are obtained. EMS report to the attending ED physician, who instructs the EM resident to order a STAT CT of the head without contrast.

Moments later the patient's husband arrives in the ED critical care bay and begins to relay the events of the evening. He states that the patient had been in her usual state of health throughout the day and early evening. After dinner, the patient used the bathroom and returned complaining of a "terrible stabbing" headache. When the patient's husband asked if it was a migraine coming on, she stated that it felt very different from her typical migraines and that it was the

C. Begley · D. Roberts (✉)
University of Rochester Medical Center, Rochester, NY, USA
e-mail: Christopher_begley@urmc.rochester.edu; Debra_roberts@urmc.rochester.edu

J. A. LaRosa (ed.), *Adult Critical Care Medicine*,
https://doi.org/10.1007/978-3-319-94424-1_1

worst headache of her life. She hoped it would improve with rest. While getting ready for bed, the patient complained of neck pain and then began to vomit. After several episodes of emesis, he escorted her to bed and left the room to get her some ginger ale at her request. When he returned he found her slouched over and unresponsive. He immediately called 911. Upon arrival, EMS found the patient obtunded with minimal response to noxious stimuli. Given the concern for airway compromise, she was intubated at that time and transported to the hospital.

At this point the patient is transported to CT scan for the exam. The patient's husband is asked to account for the patient's past medical history. He relates the patient has a history of hypertension, kidney disease, and migraines. Although he does not know all the details, he states that when the patient was younger, the patient had a bad infection and since that time has only "one functioning kidney." She follows with a kidney doctor and may need dialysis in the future. He thinks that her migraines have been overall well controlled over the past couple of years and rarely has a flare. He states that she is compliant with her medications for her blood pressure, but is not sure of the drug names. Other than her prescribed medications, she only takes a multivitamin and occasional over-the-counter medications for migraines. Her only surgical history is carpal tunnel release performed a few years ago. The patient is a former smoker who quit about 5 years ago when she was diagnosed with hypertension and found to have kidney disease. She occasionally drinks alcoholic beverages in social settings. He denies any illicit drug abuse. He states that both her parents are alive and knows that her father has high blood pressure and heart disease and her mother has problems with her thyroid.

The patient returns from the CT scanner to the ED, and a new set of vital signs are obtained, which are notable for blood pressure of 195/95. She is on minimal ventilator settings but is breathing over the ventilator with a respiratory rate in the mid-20s. The resident describes the physical exam findings which were notable for a right pupil dilated to 6 mm and non-reactive, with a left pupil that was 3 mm and reactive. The patient did appear to localize to noxious stimuli with question of left upper extremity decerebrate posturing (extensor posturing) on exam when sedation was paused but otherwise did not follow commands or open her eyes.

CT scan was uploaded to the system and images were reviewed, see Fig. 1.1. It revealed extensive subarachnoid hemorrhage involving the basal cisterns with extension into the bilateral Sylvian and interhemispheric fissures. Additionally, there is developing hydrocephalus with ventricular dilatation. Neurosurgery and the neurocritical care teams were consulted. As neurosurgery prepared to place an external ventricular drain (EVD) the plan was to administer hyperosmolar therapy given the concern for increase intracranial pressure (ICP). The patient was given a bolus 250 ml of 3% saline. Mannitol was avoided given her history of kidney disease. The EVD was successfully placed and revealed an ICP of 22 mmHg. Her body temperature was noted to be 38.2 °C, so an external cooling blanket was applied. The patient's sedation was increased for agitation,

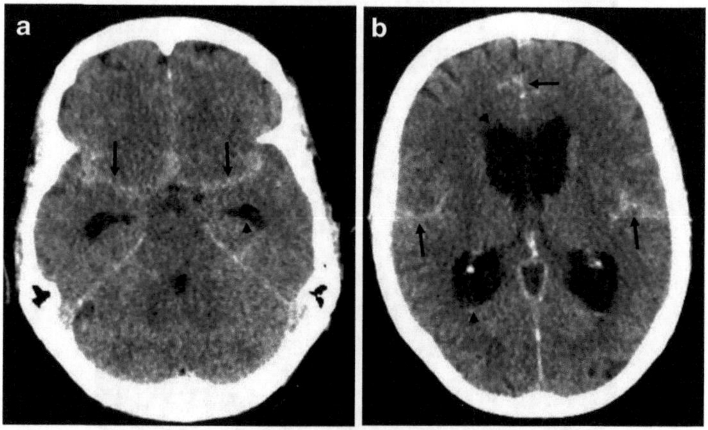

FIGURE 1.1 **a**) SAH in the lateral fissures (arrows). Dilated temporal horns of the lateral ventricles concerning for hydrocephalus (arrowheads). **b**) SAH in the Sylvian and interhemispheric fissures (arrows). Rounded lateral ventricles suggesting acute hydrocephalus (arrowheads)

and she was placed on a continuous infusion of nicardipine to lower her blood pressure to a goal systolic BP (SBP) < 160 mmHg, ensuring maintenance of her cerebral perfusion pressure (CPP) 50–70 mmHg. Shortly thereafter, her ICP improved to 14 mmHg.

CT angiography (Fig. 1.2) revealed an anterior communicating artery aneurysm without further extension of hemorrhage. The patient's ICP again began to rise, hypertonic saline was again given as bolus, and sedation was increased. Her body temperature was now 37 °C. Despite aggressive management, her neurologic exam continued to decline, and she "blew" her right pupil, which was now 7 mm, irregular and non-reactive, with the left pupil 5 mm and non-reactive. Given the persistently elevated ICP, despite CSF (cerebrospinal fluid) draining,

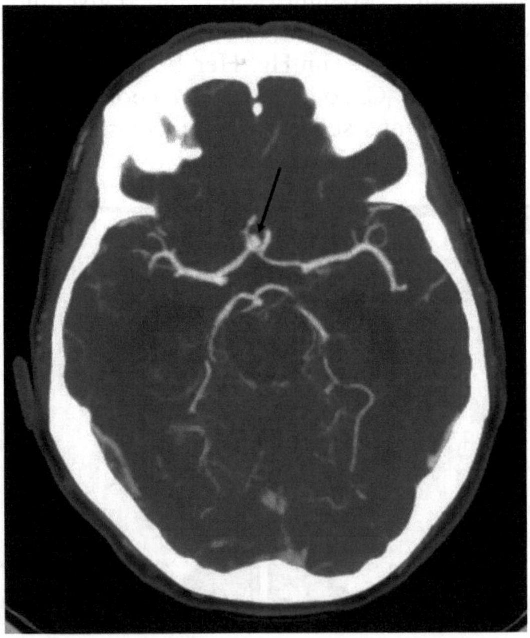

FIGURE 1.2 Brain CT angiogram with contrast demonstrating anterior communicating artery aneurysm (arrow)

sedation, normothermia, and hyperosmotic treatment, the decision was made to begin the patient on a pentobarbital infusion. She was placed on continuous EEG to titrate the pentobarbital to a burst suppression pattern which did result in reduction of her ICP. She was too sick to attempt to repair the aneurysm at this time. Hemicraniectomy was considered, but given the diffuse nature of the cerebral edema and hemorrhage, it was felt that it would be unlikely to resolve the condition. Unfortunately, the patient became increasingly hemodynamically unstable on the pentobarbital infusion and required vasopressor support. Her renal function continued to worsen which resulted in the need for renal replacement therapy. A repeat CT scan showed large hypodense regions consistent with multifocal cerebral infarctions. The patient's family decided to transition the patient to comfort measures and the patient expired.

Increased intracranial pressure (ICP) often referred to as intracranial hypertension is broadly defined as an elevated ICP measuring greater than 20 mm Hg for at least 5 min. The consequences of increased ICP are potentially devastating and may result in cerebral ischemia, infarcts, or brain herniation as a result of decreased cerebral flow; therefore, it is essential that clinicians rapidly recognize increased ICP and manage it appropriately.

The clinical presentation of a patient with elevated ICP may initially be as subtle as drowsiness or slowness in following commands, but often is more dramatic, including headache, altered mental status and level of consciousness, agitation, and nausea with or without vomiting. As ICP increases and brain herniation progresses, the patient's level of consciousness declines rapidly and they become comatose. Cranial nerve findings often begin with decreased pupil reactivity and/or anisocoria. Midbrain ischemia is evidenced by mid-size, fixed pupils. Pupils may become pinpoint at the pontine stage of herniation and finally will become large, irregular, and fixed at the medullary stage. Cough and gag will also be lost at the medullary stage. The motor portion neurologic exam will progress through stages of hemiparesis, decorticate posturing (flexor posturing), decerebrate posturing, and finally flaccid quadriplegia. The classically described Cushing triad of hypertension, bradycardia, or irregular breathing may or may not be present and is usually seen later in the course of brain herniation.

Etiologies of acute elevations of ICP may include obstructive hydrocephalus, cerebral edema, and intra- or extra-axial mass lesions. In the patient described in the case above, we are given information in the history of present illness and clinical presentation that should provide the clinician with a narrowed differential diagnosis. The patient had complained of acute onset of a severe headache which was shortly thereafter followed by neck pain and vomiting. This a classic presentation for subarachnoid hemorrhage with increased ICP and should be at the top of the differential diagnosis. One could also consider another type of spontaneous intracranial hemorrhage, such as intraparenchymal or intraventricular hemorrhage. The abruptness of the symptoms should move other potential etiologies of increased ICP further down on the differential. Brain tumors, whether metastatic or primary would be less likely unless there was an acute hemorrhage of the mass lesion. Infectious etiologies also would be less likely given the acute onset and lack of prodrome. Non-infectious neuro-inflammatory disorders may be considered, but are less likely given the presentation, as are toxic and metabolic encephalopathies for that matter. There was no description of trauma, making traumatic subdural and epidural hemorrhages very unlikely. Acute ischemic stroke should be on the differential, and the initial work-up will be very much similar, with the non-contrast CT scan being the definitive test to determine presence of hemorrhage.

In our case, the ED team's high level of suspicion for SAH leads to them ordering a non-contrasted CT of the head that revealed SAH. The appropriate teams were consulted and management was emergently initiated. Here we will focus on the management of increased ICP as the detailed management of SAH is beyond the scope of this chapter. The suspicion for elevated ICP with early brain herniation was high due to the prior complaint of headache, presence of projectile vomiting, and obtundation associated with lack of pupil reactivity. The two most commonly used types of ICP measurement devices are ventriculostomy catheters (also known as external ventricular drains or EVDs) and fiber-optic intraparenchymal monitors (colloquially called "bolts"). Each device has pros and cons, but the EVD is considered the gold standard for measuring ICP and is typically the preferred device as it can be used as a therapeutic modality to drain cerebral spinal fluid (CSF). However, in order for the EVD to give accurate ICP measurement, it must be clamped to drainage so that CSF flows only to the pressure transducer, which will prohibit drainage of the CSF at that moment. Additionally, EVDs may be technically difficult to place if the ventricles are displaced or compressed by mass lesions. Regardless of the device chosen, it is important to consider the risks as both require invasive procedures. As such, the major risks involved are bleeding and infection as each device requires a burr hole and entering into the dura. EVDs are the more invasive procedure and carry a somewhat higher risk of infection and bleeding. The risk of ventriculitis was found to be 8.1% of patients with EVD placement based on a meta-analysis [1], whereas the risk of infection with an intraparenchymal monitor has been shown to carry a risk of only 1.8% [2]. For EVDs the incidence of infection was reduced with use of catheters impregnated with antibiotics, but for each device, systemic antibiotics are typically not indicated. When placing an EVD, hemorrhages along the catheter tract are possible, but are thought to be symptomatic in less than 2.4% of cases [3]. The added advantage of draining CSF with EVD also makes for potential complications as over drainage may result in intracranial hypotension, lateral ventricle effacement, formation of subdural hematomas or hygromas, and the potential to exacerbate midline shift in the presence of hemispheric mass lesions [4].

The consequences of elevated ICP can be devastating and management must be aggressive and timely. Beyond CSF drainage, there are numerous other potential management techniques that are, in part, driven by the underlying etiology. Patients with elevated ICP are typically encephalopathic and usually require intubation and mechanical ventilation. It is important for providers to realize that in choosing ventilator settings, certain techniques may actually be detrimental in the setting of increased ICP. Hypoxia leads to further elevation of ICP; however, attempts to oxygenate with high positive end-expiratory pressure (PEEP) and large tidal volumes as well as elevated airway pressures may also lead to an increased ICP. A PEEP of 8 cmH2O or less is generally considered not to affect ICP, and much higher levels may be safely utilized if hypotension is avoided and cardiac output is maintained. If there is concern for PEEP's effect on MAP and therefore CPP, monitoring of brain tissue oxygen tension and/or cerebral blood flow (CBF) may be utilized to assist with ventilator and vasopressor/intravascular volume titration [5]. The effect of carbon dioxide on cerebral blood volume (CBV) and CBF) should be also recognized. Hypercapnea leads to cerebral vasodilation, which in turn causes increased CBV and CBF resulting in intracranial hypertension when intracranial cranial compliance is low. This physiology led to the practice of utilizing a hyperventilation strategy of mechanical ventilation. Indeed, hyperventilation does lead to cerebral vasoconstriction and decreased CBV and CBF lowering ICP, but the effect is transient, and it is now recognized that prolonged or extreme hyperventilation may result in further cerebral ischemia. Thus the use of hyperventilation to lower ICP should be limited to management of acute elevations of ICP with evidence of impending brain herniation (blown pupil(s)) while more definitive treatments are being implemented.

After placing the patient on mechanical ventilation, it is important to maintain some level of sedation and analgesia as agitation, anxiety, and pain can all result in further elevation of ICP. The sedation level may be titrated to allow for monitoring of neurologic exam. However if the patient has refractory ICP elevation, "sedation holidays" can be extremely detrimental. It may be necessary to forgo neurologic exams, focusing instead on ICP management and optimization of CPP. In these situations, monitoring the pupil exam via standard pupil checks or with the use of a pupillometer may be the best option. Proper positioning of the patient including elevating the head of the bed, midline positioning of the head, and avoiding internal jugular veins as site of central venous catheterization may facilitate adequate venous outflow and avoid additional elevation of ICP that can be easily avoided. If a patient requires a cervical collar, one should ensure that it fits properly but is not so tight as to impede venous drainage.

Cerebral perfusion pressure (CPP) is a surrogate measurement of cerebral blood flow. It is calculated by taking subtracting the ICP from the mean arterial pressure (MAP). If a patient is found to have a low CPP, then they are at greater risk of the consequences noted above. Guidelines vary as to CPP target, but in general they recommend maintaining the CCP between 50 and 80 mm Hg, with a target of about 60 mm Hg. It has been noted in patients with traumatic brain injury (TBI) that elevated CPP is detrimental and that the use of vasopressors to drive CPP greater than 80 mm Hg have been associated with increasing cerebral edema as well as lung injury [6].

Hyperosmolar therapy is utilized in the management of increased ICP by inducing an osmotic-driven fluid shift from the brain parenchyma into the plasma. This therapy can be especially beneficial when the etiology of the intracranial hypertension is secondary to cerebral edema but is less useful for intracranial hypertension associated with mass lesions. The two types of hyperosmolar therapy employed are hypertonic saline and mannitol, both of which are reasonably effective at lowering ICP [7]. Hypertonic saline ranges in concentrations from 2% to 23.4% with expectant decreased ICP effects lasting from 90 min to 4 h. Concentrations less than 7.5% may be given through peripheral IV access, but it is strongly recommended that higher concentrations be given through central access. If giving 23.4%, one should note that, in addition to requiring central venous access, the dose should be given over 5 min (typical dose is 30 mL) with close monitoring of blood pressure. Administering faster than this may result in decreased cardiac contractility. Additional caution should be taken in patients with heart failure or pulmonary edema as hypertonic saline acts as volume expander and can worsen these conditions. Given its effects as a volume expander, hypertonic saline is preferred over mannitol for ICP management in acute trauma patients who have associated hemorrhage. The decision as to whether re-dosing boluses versus bolusing and placing the patient on a continuous infusion of hypertonic saline remains controversial [8]. While on this therapy, serum electrolytes, most notably sodium must be frequently monitored. In patients who are hyponatremic at baseline, a rapid rise in serum sodium places the patient at risk of osmotic demyelination syndrome. For critically ill patients with neurological conditions, driving sodium levels to levels >160 mEq/L has been associated with worse neurologic outcomes in a retrospective analysis [9]. Furthermore, in patients whose sodium levels have been increased due to hyperosmolar therapy, caution must be taken in lowering sodium levels back down as fast of a correction may exacerbate cerebral edema and worsen intracranial hypertension.

Mannitol is the other option for hyperosmolar therapy for patients with elevated ICP. It is an osmotic diuretic excreted by the kidneys that must be avoided in patients with renal failure as drug accumulation will result in worsening cerebral edema. For this reason, the osmolar gap (measured serum osmolality – calculated serum osmolality) which detects the presence of unmeasured osmoles (such as mannitol) should be monitored in patients who are receiving multiple boluses with the goal of keeping the gap below 15 to prevent mannitol accumulation and rebound intracranial hypertension [10]. For this reason, mannitol was avoided in our patient and hypertonic saline was utilized. The dose of mannitol for increased ICP typically is 0.5–1.5 g/kg IV over 10–20 min, and effects of the diuretic last 90 min to 6 h. Unlike hypertonic saline, which may require central access at higher concentrations, mannitol can be administered through peripheral IV access with the caveat that an inline filter is required to prevent crystal formation. Potential undesired side effects, aside from those already mentioned, include hypotension, hypovolemia, and several electrolyte abnormalities through large-volume osmotic diuresis. Electrolytes and volume status should be carefully monitored and repleted as indicated.

It is well established that hyperpyrexia in patients with acute neurological insults result in prolonged hospital stay and increased mortality [11]. Additionally, fever results in vasodilation and increased cerebral metabolism, both of which may result in elevated ICP. It is therefore prudent that targeted temperature management be implemented in the care of these patients. Common techniques to accomplish this include antipyretic pharmacotherapy as well as cooling devices. The role of induced hypothermia (32–35 °C) has been explored in patients with TBI, and although decreased ICP was observed, there was no improvement in outcomes [12]. Nonetheless, inducing hypothermia may be attempted in patients with elevated ICP not responding to other therapies. In patients subjected to targeted temperature management or therapeutic hypothermia, it is imperative to monitor for shivering and aggressively treat if it occurs. Shivering, like fever, leads to increased cerebral metabolic rate and therefore may exacerbate ICP elevations. Shivering may be managed with antipyretics, opiates, propofol, or even paralytics in severe cases. The Columbia shiver protocol is often employed for the monitoring and management of shivering [13].

For patients in whom the above treatments have failed, initiation of barbiturate therapy, specifically pentobarbital, may be considered as a last-line medical treatment for their refractory intracranial hypertension. Commonly referred to as a pentobarbital coma because of the deep level of sedation and long half-life of therapy (15–50 h), this therapy decreases the cerebral metabolic rate for oxygen, which consequently results in decreased ICP [14]. In conjunction with ICP monitoring, continuous EEG is implemented to allow for pentobarbital titration to a burst suppression pattern which attempts to prevent over-sedation. Pentobarbital is typically loaded at 10 mg/kg IV followed by a continuous infusion of 1–2 mg/kg/h and then titrated based on EEG findings. Beyond the undesired loss of meaningful neurologic exam for several days, other adverse effects include hypotension and cardiac suppression which may require vasopressor support, hypothermia, predisposition to infections, and severe ileus [15].

Another potential option for the management of elevated ICP is surgical decompression. An extensive discussion of surgical decompression is beyond the scope of this chapter focusing on the medical approach in managing intracranial hypertension. What is necessary for an ICU provider to realize is that neurosurgical consultation should me made early if increased ICP is suspected as was the case with our patient.

Take-Home Points

- Increased ICP is a medical emergency with potentially devastating consequences including cerebral ischemia, herniation, and death.
- Neurosurgical consultation should be made early if intracranial hypertension is suspected for placement of ICP monitor devices and to evaluate the utility of surgical decompression.
- Initial management may include relatively simple interventions including optimizing patient positioning, sedation, fever avoidance, and minimization of potentially harmful ventilator techniques and settings.
- Hyperosmolar therapy is a staple of therapy for increased ICP, but the decision to use mannitol versus hypertonic saline should account for patient comorbidities.
- Barbiturates and induced hypothermia are potential options for refractory intracranial hypertension.

Case #2: Status Epilepticus

A 19-year-old male is brought to the emergency department by his college roommate and a friend from the nearby local university after the patient had what the roommate believes to be a seizure. The roommate describes that when he entered the dorm room the patient was on the ground with slight rhythmic jerking of his arms which would stop and then resume. They were unable to wake the patient, so they carried him to the car and drove him to the hospital. He states that he had last seen the patient about 2 h prior studying in the dorm room for a midterm exam. The roommate relates that he was aware that the patient had a seizure disorder but that up until this point in the year the patient had not had any seizures. The roommate hands the ED physician a bottle of lamotrigine, which he states the patient was very systematic in taking at the same times each day. When further questions are asked to the roommate, he is able to provide that the patient has been putting in long hours in the library and sleeping less over the last week while studying for exams. Additionally, he knows that the patient went to the student clinic a couple of days ago and was prescribed an unknown antibiotic "for a cold" and had been taking an over-the-counter medication for night cough and congestion. He denies that the patient uses illicit drugs or tobacco but admits that the patient will consume alcohol occasionally at parties but because of exams has not gone out socially in over a week. He is unaware if the patient has any other past medical or surgical history.

The patient's vital signs were notable for temperature of 38.3 °C and tachycardia with HR of 112, but otherwise unremarkable. The remainder of the physical exam's pertinent positives included bilateral left gaze deviation and a Glasgow Coma Scale (GCS) of 6. A peripheral IV was placed, and the patient was given 4 mg IV lorazepam as the ED team prepared to intubate him. Labwork and blood cultures were collected. Following administration of the lorazepam, there was no change in the patient's GCS and gaze deviation persisted.

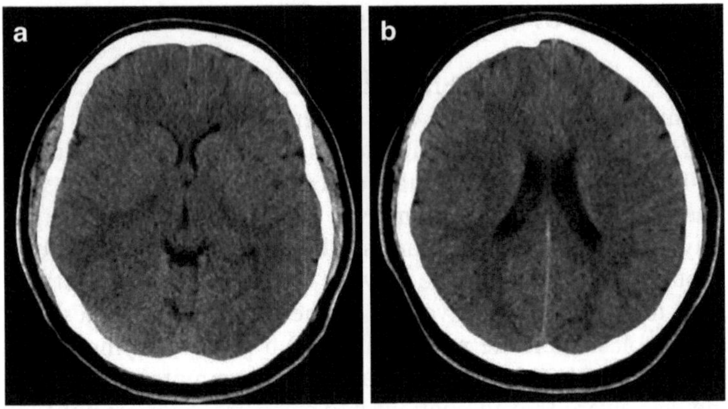

FIGURE 1.3 **a**) Normal non-contrast head CT at level of thalamus. **b**) Normal non-contrast head CT at level of lateral venticles

An additional 4 mg of lorazepam was given IV, and the team proceeded with endotracheal intubation and the patient was placed on mechanical ventilation. The patient was taken immediately to the CT scanner for STAT non-contrast CT of the head. Both the neurology team as well as the neurocritical care team were consulted. CT of the head was negative for any acute intracranial processes (Fig. 1.3). Given concern for non-convulsive status epilepticus (NCSE), fosphenytoin was given at a loading dose of 20 mg/kg. Labwork revealed a mild leukocytosis on complete blood count. A complete metabolic panel revealed a mild acute kidney injury without significant electrolyte abnormalities or liver abnormalities. An arterial blood gas after intubation revealed only a mild metabolic acidosis, due to an elevated lactate. A urine toxicology screen was negative as was an ethanol level. A continuous electroencephalogram (EEG) was ordered. Meanwhile, a lumbar puncture was performed, and cerebral spinal fluid (CSF) was sent for analysis. The patient was subsequently initiated on broad-spectrum antimicrobial coverage.

EEG showed the patient was indeed in NCSE despite having been loaded with fosphenytoin. Initial analysis of the CSF was not suggestive of infection. The patient was bolused with propofol and a continuous infusion was started. The patient's hemodynamics tolerated escalating dose of the propofol, and cessation of seizure activity was seen on EEG. He was continued on his home dose of lamotrigine and 300 mg daily of phenytoin. The patient was maintained on the propofol infusion for 24 h after seizure cessation and then gradually weaned off without recurrence of seizure activity. The patient was successfully extubated with good neurologic recovery.

Prior definitions of status epilepticus (SE) required that seizures continue or recur for greater than 30 min without a return to baseline mental status. Fortunately, recognition that prolonged time to treatment leads to an increased risk of refractory SE and puts the patient at increased risk for neurologic injury, the definition was changed to greater than 5 min of continuous seizure activity or frequently recurring seizures without returning to neurological baseline. SE may result in morbidity and mortality directly with neuronal cellular injury resulting in neuronal loss and cell death, as well as indirectly via mechanisms such as aspiration, respiratory depression or arrest, and even cardiac arrest [16]. Convulsive status epilepticus (CSE) has an estimated mortality rate upwards of 22% and while non-convulsive status epilepticus (NCSE) is approximately 18% making both conditions neurological emergencies [16, 17]. When a patient presents with generalized convulsions, the SE is easily diagnosed; unfortunately, clinical manifestations may often be elusive. Signs may be as subtle as staring spells, gaze deviation, facial twitching, abnormal behavior, or encephalopathy. Studies examining the use of continuous EEG in encephalopathic patients in medical and surgical ICUs revealed non-convulsive seizures in 10% and 16%, respectively, with up to 5% of patients found in NCSE [18, 19].

Our patient was found with rhythmic activity of the extremities, but upon arrival to the ED, the only suggestion of seizure on clinical examination was gaze deviation. The differential diagnosis of the underlying etiology associated with SE is broad. It is important for clinicians to realize that although determining the etiology may ultimately help to direct care, the initial goal is to abort the seizures; therefore treatment should not be delayed while work-up of the seizure semiology is begun.

Treatment protocols and guidelines for SE go through three- to four-phase step-wise progressions which will be described here. It should be noted that data regarding the treatment approach is based on CSE and that recommended treatment for NCSE has been extrapolated from this data. Treatment should be initiated immediately when a seizure is recognized to reduce neuronal injury and improve overall neurologic outcomes. One study found that SE patients treated within 30 min of onset with a first-line antiepileptic agent versus patients treated greater than 2 h after onset had response rates and resolution of seizures in 80% vs. 40% of patients, respectively [20]. For patients in whom blood glucose levels or alcohol consumption status is unknown, it is reasonable to give thiamine and dextrose while AEDs are being initiated.

First-line treatment for a patient with SE is a benzodiazepine. Lorazepam has been shown to be effective as this initial agent at a dose of 0.1 mg/kg, up to 4 mg IV × 2 doses, when compared to phenytoin and phenobarbital [21, 22]. Midazolam given intramuscularly (IM) at a dose of 0.2 mg/kg up to 10 mg has been shown to effectively terminate SE and may be more effective than lorazepam if the patient does not have IV access in the pre-hospital setting [23]. An additional advantage of midazolam when compared to lorazepam is that the former does not require refrigeration, which makes it an ideal option for first responders. Diazepam IV is another option, although data suggest that it may be less effective in terminating SE compared to other benzodiazepines [22]. It is important to note that dosing of benzodiazepines needs to be adequate in order to obtain SE cessation. Common side effects of this class of drugs are hypotension and respiratory suppression, so the clinician should be aware of these adverse effects; however, they should not be underdosed in order to avoid the possible requirement of intubation. In fact, it has been found that early and appropriate benzodiazepine dosing decreased the risk of respiratory failure requiring intubation which suggests that SE itself is a greater risk for respiratory failure than the side effect profile of the first-line treatment [20].

Despite the efficacy of benzodiazepines, many patients may continue with SE and will therefore require additional therapy. There are several pharmaceutical options that are in alignment with current guidelines, but most commonly administered second-line treatments consist of phenytoin and its water-soluble prodrug, fosphenytoin, as well as valproic acid. Phenytoin/fosphenytoin stabilizes neuronal membranes against hyperactivity by increasing efflux of sodium ions across cell membranes. Both are given as an IV load of 20 mg/kg (fosphenytoin is measured as phenytoin equivalents (PE)), at a maximum rate of 50 mg/min for phenytoin and 150 PE mg/min for fosphenytoin [24]. Among the side effects of phenytoin, the most significant are cardiac toxicity and hypotension. For this reason, fosphenytoin is usually the preferred agent for loading doses as these side effects are less appreciated and therefore can be loaded faster. Additionally, as phenytoin is an inducer of the cytochrome P450 system and metabolized by the liver. It may still be loaded in liver failure patients in the acute SE setting, but is less optimal for longer-term management. Typically, free and total serum levels are obtained 3 h after loading, and the patient may be given another load if levels are low. However, as SE is a neurological emergency, if seizures continue after the initial loading dose, additional therapy must be sought without delay.

Valproic acid is also commonly implemented as a second-line treatment strategy, with some data suggesting that it may actually have better efficacy when compared to phenytoin in treatment of SE [25, 26]. Valproate is thought to increase and enhance the action of GABA in the postsynaptic receptor sites. It is loaded at 20–40 mg/kg, and the dose may be given very rapidly, with rates up to 555 mg/min shown to be safe [27]. Although it lacks the cardiovascular adverse effects of phenytoin, the greatest concern when using valproate is hepatotoxicity and can cause fulminant liver failure in patients with a priori significant liver dysfunction. Further, it is a known teratogen and should therefore be avoided in pregnant patients when possible.

Another potential second-line therapy for SE is levetiracetam [28]. Despite insufficient evidence, this medication is often given in the setting of SE in addition to either phenytoin or valproate and recently has been added in the SE treatment algorithm approach by a major societal guideline [24]. The mechanism of action involves both the inhibition of voltage-dependent N-type calcium channels as well as activity at the GABA receptor. The loading dose of levetiracetam is typically 60 mg/kg IV with a maximum of 4500 mg [24]. The paucity of data reporting significant adverse events is appealing, and perhaps why it is now commonly utilized in SE.

Although less often sought as the initial choice of second-line treatments, phenobarbital is also an option for attempting to abolish SE. It also works at the GABA receptor. For SE it is loaded at 20–30 mg/kg and infused at 50–100 mg/min. Hypotension and hypoventilation are the most detrimental side effects [22].

If seizures have not been terminated despite the first- and second-line therapies described above, the patient is termed to be in refractory SE. At this point there is no clear-cut evidence in deciding therapeutic options, but continuous infusions with propofol or midazolam are implemented, with pentobarbital infusion usually reserved for super-refractory patients [24]. If the patient has not yet been intubated and placed on mechanical ventilation, the patient will require such for these therapies in order to achieve the deep level of sedation or coma typically required to abort refractory SE. All of these patients should be placed on continuous EEG if not already hooked up. The depth of sedation remains controversial, ranging from seizure suppression to burst suppression, or even full suppression of the EEG. It is also not clear what the duration of suppression at the chosen level of sedation should be. Many would recommend continuing the infusion in addition to AED therapy for at least 24 h with a maximum 72 h prior to weaning. In weaning sedation, typically it is done slowly, and if the patient has recurrent seizure activity, a different sedative, higher dose, or longer duration may be required. As noted in the discussion of increased ICP, side effects of this level of sedation are not inconsequential. Hypotension requiring vasopressors is not uncommon.

If SE continues despite titration of either propofol or midazolam, the patient is considered to have super-refractory SE and will require a pentobarbital infusion, with the goal of inducing burst suppression pattern on EEG. As with the above described infusions, the optimal duration of sedation is unknown, but the barbiturate infusion is typically continued for 24–72 h before an attempt at weaning is made. There are many side effects of barbiturate infusion including hypotension, ileus, risk of infection, and hypothermia. Hypothermia may actually be beneficial as therapeutic hypothermia has been shown to suppress seizure activity and is considered as a potential treatment in super-refractory SE [29].

Once SE is controlled, it is imperative to determine the underlying etiology. Among the most common causes of SE in a patient with known seizure disorder is discontinuation or non-adherence with antiepileptic drug (AED) therapy. Serum levels of many AEDs may be used to monitor adherence and help to titrate dosing. While these tests may assist with AED regimen titration, their utility in the acute setting is questionable as results may take several hours to days to return. Even if a patient is compliant with AED therapy, breakthrough seizures are possible. Our patient was adherent with therapy, but he was noted to have ongoing sleep deprivation while studying for exams, which likely played a role in triggering this episode of SE.

Other potential causes of SE include alcohol consumption as well as illicit, over-the-counter, and prescribed drugs. Both consumption (acute or chronic) and withdrawal of alcohol may result in seizure activity. Our patient is described as a social drinker with no recent history of consumption making this less likely, and additionally alcohol level is negative. With regards to drug ingestion, it is important to obtain urine and possibly serum toxicology screens as this may suggest the etiology. Our patient had a negative toxicology screen.

The list of over-the-counter and prescription medications that are associated with seizures is quite long. Additionally, certain AEDs interact with medications resulting in altered metabolism of the AED which may precipitate seizures. In-depth discussion is beyond this chapter but needs to be considered in all patients taking AEDs. It is noteworthy that antibiotics may decrease seizure threshold. The most common culprits are penicillins, cephalosporins, carbapenems, and metronidazole. Our patient was on an unknown antibiotic prior to presentation, which may have contributed to the onset of his SE. Furthermore, he was taking over-the-counter night cough and congestion medications, many of which include diphenhydramine which is also known to decrease seizure threshold.

Infection and sepsis are known to be associated with seizures and SE. Our patient was described to have "a cold" prior to presentation. Proper work-up was performed in the assessment of our patient when blood and CSF cultures were obtained, followed by placing the patient on broad-spectrum antimicrobials. As noted above, evaluation of antibiotic choice may be necessary in knowing that certain medications may lower seizure threshold, yet this should not prohibit use of necessary agents. Our patient did not have evidence of central nervous system infection, but meningitis and encephalitis should be considered in SE patients. While every patient does not necessarily require a lumbar puncture, it should be thoughtfully considered. Electrolyte disturbances may lead to seizure activity, with the most common being hypoglycemia, hyponatremia, hypocalcemia, and hypomagnesemia [30]. In our patient, mild acute kidney injury and a lactic acidosis were the only significant abnormalities. Lactic acidosis is a common lab finding in patients with CSE, and it will usually resolve rapidly with aborting SE and supportive care. An easy bedside or pre-hospital test that should always be performed is point-of-care glucose to evaluate for hypoglycemia which can be immediately intervened upon.

Other etiologies associated with SE include structural brain lesions including stroke, intracranial hemorrhage, traumatic brain injuries, and brain tumors. While a structural lesion seems less likely in our patient, it is important to rule out these etiologies as they may require additional urgent treatment. Obtaining an initial non-contrasted CT is adequate in most cases and will help determine the need for further imaging. In our patient, the CT of the head was unremarkable, so acute intracranial hemorrhage is ruled out, and significant trauma or large brain tumor are also unlikely in a patient with a normal head CT. If the patient has focal findings on neurologic exam and/or EEG but a normal non-contrast head CT, MRI may be considered to further evaluate for structural lesion. In patients with known seizure disorder, extensive imaging is generally not warranted.

If the seizure is thought to be secondary to mass lesion, it may be very difficult to control. Primary brain tumors as well as metastases result in vasogenic cerebral edema which can exacerbate seizures. In these situations, steroids should be considered in addition to AEDs as they may assist in seizure termination owing to reduction of edema. Dexamethasone may be used, with a 10 mg IV loading dose followed by 4 mg every 6 h, until more definitive treatment of the tumor can be performed.

Take-Home Points

- Status epilepticus is a neurological emergency that must be treated immediately in order to prevent neuron injury and apoptosis.
- Work-up for the underlying cause of SE should not delay the administration of pharmacologic therapies for treatment of seizures.
- The longer the time to first therapy administration, the more likely the SE is to be refractory.
- Fear of benzodiazepine-induced hypoventilation should not prevent therapeutic dosing of this drug class.

- First- and second-line therapies are often both required to terminate the SE.
- Current treatment guidelines were developed for CSE and treatments for NCSE have been extrapolated from these recommendations.
- Treatment of refractory SE involves deep sedation and coma; lack of data in literature makes management of this state more provider dependent.

References

1. Lozier AP, Sciacca RR, Romagnoli MF, et al. Ventriculostomy-related infections: a critical review of the literature. Neurosurgery. 2002;51:170–81.
2. Bekar A, Dogan S, Abas F, et al. Risk factors and complications of intracranial pressure monitoring with a fiberoptic device. J Clin Neurosci. 2009;16:236–40.
3. Fried HI, Nathan BR, Rowe AS, et al. The insertion and management of external ventricular devices: an evidence-based consensus statement. Neurocrit Care. 2016;24:61–81.
4. Muralidharan R. External ventricular drains: management and complications. Surg Neurol Int. 2015;6(Suppl 6):S271–4.
5. Muench E, et al. Effects of positive end-expiratory pressure on regional cerebral blood flow, intracranial pressure, and brain tissue oxygenation. Crit Care Med. 2005;33:2367–72.
6. Prabhakar H, Sandhu K, Bhagat H, et al. Current concepts of optimal cerebral perfusion pressure in traumatic brain injury. J Anaesthesiol Clin Pharmacol. 2014;30:318–27.
7. Kamel H, Navi BB, Nakagawa K, et al. Hypertonic saline versus mannitol for the treatment of elevated intracranial pressure: a meta-analysis of randomized clinical trials. Crit Care Med. 2011;39:554–9.
8. Diringer MN. New trends in hyperosmolar therapy? Curr Opin Crit Care. 2013;19:77–82.
9. Aiyagari V, Deibert E, Diringer MN. Hypernatremia in the neurologic intensive care unit: how high is too high? J Crit Care. 2006;21:163–72.

10. Garcia-Morales EJ, Cariappa R, Parvin CA, et al. Osmole gap in neurologic-neurosurgical intensive care unit: its normal value, calculation, and relationship with mannitol serum concentrations. Crit Care Med. 2004;32:986–91.
11. Greer DM, Funk SE, Reaven NL, et al. Impact of fever on outcome in patients with stroke and neurologic injury. Stroke. 2008;39:3029–35.
12. Andrews PJD, Sinclair HL, Rodriguez A, et al. Hypothermia for intracranial hypertension after traumatic brain injury. N Engl J Med. 2015;373:2403–12.
13. Choi HA, Ko SB, Presciutti M, et al. Prevention of shivering during therapeutic temperature modulation: the Columbia anti-shivering protocol. Neurocrit Care. 2011;14(3):389–94.
14. Nordstrom CH, Messeter K, Sundbarg G, et al. Cerebral blood flow, vasoreactivity, and oxygen consumption during barbiturate therapy in severe traumatic brain lesions. J Neurosurg. 1988;68:424–31.
15. Kim Y, Park S, Nam T, et al. The effect of barbiturate coma therapy for patients with severe intracranial hypertension: a 10-year experience. J Korean Neurosurg Soc. 2008;44:141–5.
16. Shneker BF, Fountain NB. Assessment of acute morbidity and mortality of non-convulsive status epilepticus. Neurology. 2003;61:1066–73.
17. DeLorenzo RJ, Hauser WA, Towne AR, et al. A prospective, population based epidemiologic study of status epilepticus in Richmond, Virginia. Neurology. 1996;46:1029–35.
18. Oddo M, Carrera E, Claassen J, et al. Continuous electroencephalography in the medical intensive care unit. Crit Care Med. 2009;37:2051–6.
19. Kurtz P, Gaspard N, Wahl AS, et al. Continuous electroencephalography in the surgical intensive care unit. Intensive Care Med. 2014;40:228–34.
20. Lowenstein DH, Alldredge BK. Status epilepticus at an urban public hospital in the 1980s. Neurology. 1993;43:483–8.
21. Alldredge BK, Gelb AM, Isaacs SM, et al. A comparison of lorazepam, diazepam and placebo for the treatment of out-of-hospital status epilepticus. N Engl J Med. 2001;345:631–7.
22. Treiman DM, Meyers PD, Walton NY, et al. A comparison of four treatments for generalized convulsive status epilepticus. Veterans affairs status epilepticus cooperative study group. N Engl J Med. 1998;339:792–8.

23. Silbergleit R, Durkalski V, Lowenstein DH, et al. Intramuscular versus intravenous therapy for prehospital status epilepticus. N Engl J Med. 2012;366:591–600.
24. Glauser T, Shinnar S, Gloss D, et al. Evidenced based guideline: treatment of convulsive status epilepticus in children and adults: report of the guideline committee of the American Epilepsy Society. Epilepsy Curr. 2016;16:48–61.
25. Gilad R, Izkovitz N, Dabby R, et al. Treatment of status epilepticus and acute repetitive seizures with i.v. valproic acid vs phenytoin. Acta Neurol Scand. 2008;118:296–300.
26. Misra UK, Kalita J, Patel R. Sodium valproate vs phenytoin in status epilepticus: a pilot study. Neurology. 2006;67:340–2.
27. Limdi NA, Faught E. The safety of rapid valproic acid infusions. Epilespia. 2000;41:1342–5.
28. Berning S, Boesebeck F, van Baalen K, et al. Intravenous levetiracetam as treatment for status epilepticus. J Neurol. 2009;256:1634–42.
29. Corry JJ, Dhar R, Murphy T, et al. Hypothermia for refractory status epilepticus. Neurocrit Care. 2008;9:189–97.
30. Nardone R, Brigo F, Trinka E. Acute symptomatic seizures caused by electrolyte disturbances. J Clin Neurol. 2016;12:21–33.

Chapter 2
Overcoming Conflicts in ICU Care of Surgical Patients

Anthony Dinallo, Jonathan Decker, and Adam M. Kopelan

Case Presentation

The patient is a 63-year-old African American male substance abuser with hypertension and a history of a myocardial infarction who presented to the emergency department with sudden onset of lower abdominal pain. The pain awoke the patient from sleep with the associated symptom of diaphoresis. At the time of presentation, the patient denied gastrointestinal or pulmonary symptoms. The patient's previous surgical history included an exploratory laparotomy with colostomy and subsequent colostomy closure related to an abdominal stab wound.

Upon presentation to the emergency department, the patient was profoundly hypotensive with an intact airway and normal sensorium. A ruptured abdominal aortic aneurysm (AAA) with diffuse aneurysmal disease of the abdominal aorta and iliac arteries was diagnosed by CT of the abdomen

A. Dinallo · J. Decker · A. M. Kopelan (✉)
Newark Beth Israel Medical Center, Newark, NJ, USA
e-mail: adam.kopelan@rwjbh.org

J. A. LaRosa (ed.), *Adult Critical Care Medicine*,
https://doi.org/10.1007/978-3-319-94424-1_2

and pelvis. The patient was taken to the operating room emergently by vascular surgery via an open approach to the abdominal aorta due to the lack of suitability for an endovascular approach. During the procedure, the left iliac vein was injured and repaired, leading to an increase in blood loss and hemodynamic instability. A bifurcated aortoiliac graft was used to repair the infrarenal aorta and iliac arteries with both internal iliac arteries ligated secondary to aneurysmal disease. Damage control was performed with the abdomen packed with laparotomy pads and temporarily closed with an open abdominal wound vacuum device (AbThera™, KCI). The patient was admitted to the medical-surgical intensive care unit (MSICU) for correction of hypothermia, acidosis, and coagulopathy. A total of 30 units of packed red blood cells and 15 units of fresh frozen plasma and platelets were used during the course of the operation.

The patient improved over the following 72 h with plans of removing abdominal packing and closure of the abdominal wall. General surgery was consulted for assistance given the complexity of the abdominal wall closure as well as the concern for ischemic colitis secondary to bilateral iliac artery ligation. Upon the planned return to the operating room, the abdominal packing was removed and an ischemic left colon was encountered. A left colectomy was performed with creation of colostomy and Hartmann's pouch; the abdomen was washed out and closed with a bridging biologic mesh (Strattice™, Lifecell) given the generalized edema of the abdominal wall and bowel. The patient was readmitted to the MSICU for postoperative management.

During the early postoperative period, the patient developed intra-abdominal sepsis with associated intra-abdominal abscesses related to a retroperitoneal cecal fistula arising from the inflammatory aneurysm sac. Because of the concerns of exposed prosthetic graft, the patient was brought back to the operating room multiple times for drainage of abscesses, removal of mesh, and debridement of the abdominal wall, with eventual exclusion of the exposed prosthetic aortic graft. As the abdomen was left open, the patient developed a traumatic enteroatmospheric fistula that required complicated wound care in order to prevent contamination of other abdominal contents.

The perioperative course was complicated by multisystem organ failure, including cardiovascular, respiratory, renal, and intestinal dysfunction. The primary MSICU intensivist team (pulmonary/critical care attending, fellows, medical residents) utilized consultations to general and vascular surgery, nephrology, infectious disease, hematology, dietary, physical therapy, enterostomal and wound care, and social work. The patient's respiratory failure required eventual tracheostomy placement, and his cardiovascular failure required hemodynamic support with vasoactive drips. His renal failure was managed with hemodialysis, while IVC filter and anticoagulation was employed for deep venous thrombosis. Additionally, parenteral nutrition was initiated and continued for intestinal failure, and complex enterostomal and wound management was utilized for integumentary failure. Extensive emotional support was provided to the patient and his family, leading to close bonds between the caregivers, the patient, and family.

Over the course of 6 months, the patient's multisystem organ failure is resolved with eventual cessation of ventilatory support, hemodialysis, and vasoactive support. Furthermore, enteral feeding was initiated, and his recovery was enhanced with physical therapy. Plans were made to repair the enteroatmospheric fistula and permanently close the abdominal wall. The abdominal wall was prepared with chemical component separation with injection of botulinum toxin into the oblique musculature. Once the patient was nearly independent, he was brought back to the operating room for the planned procedure. An extensive lysis of adhesions, three small bowel resections, and a biologic mesh-buttressed abdominal wall repair were performed. The patient was returned to the MSICU for further postoperative management.

During the early postoperative period, the patient developed a hemodynamically significant intra-abdominal bleed requiring blood transfusion. The hemorrhage was attributed to early initiation of full anticoagulation for his history of deep venous thrombosis. Given his new fevers, significant pain of distention and pressure from the hematoma, conservative measures to treat the patient failed. The patient was taken to the operating room for an abdominal washout with evacuation of hematoma complicated by a small bowel enterotomy. Postoperatively, the patient developed an intra-abdominal abscess requiring percutaneous drainage and development of enterocutaneous fistula. Further multiorgan dysfunction occurred, necessitating intensive support. An additional 3 months was required in the MSICU, leading to resolution of sepsis and multisystem dysfunction with spontaneous closure of the enterocutaneous fistula. Ultimately, the patient has fully recovered and is back to most of all of his pre-hospitalization activities.

Introduction

Several aspects of patient care that are crucial to the outcomes in intensive care unit patients have been identified in the literature. These include the relationship between surgeon and patient, communication between physicians and care teams, specialty of intensivist, conflicts in management between surgeon and intensivist, and whether the ICU is closed or open. In the following discussion, the current literature will be reviewed for each issue and how each concept applies to the care of this complex patient.

Surgeon-Patient Relationship

The surgeon-patient relationship has been built on a foundation of trust and communication. It begins with a patient's narrative of their personal and medical histories and culminates in a preoperative, operative, and postoperative treatment plan. According to anthropologist Joan Cassell, the surgeon during this time maintains a "covenantal ethic" in which they make a "promise to battle death on behalf of [their] patient" [1]. If a patient continues to trust and support a surgeon, the relationship will remain intact, and the patient's recovery will continue to be a team effort.

A surgeon has a license to inflict penetrating trauma on a patient in order to aid the body in fighting disease. Because of this awesome privilege, surgeons are trained to take full ownership of the patient and, as a result, often take successes and failures personally. Emotional distress secondary to a feeling of personal responsibility for treatment errors has been linked to surgeon burnout and suicidal ideation in some cases [2, 3]. In fact, surgeons are less likely to consider withdrawing life support after an operation when an error was directly implicated in an undesirable outcome [4]. The emotional repercussions of a poor outcome on a surgeon can strain the surgeon-patient relationship on multiple levels. This increases the importance of communication between a patient and his or her surgeon. It is crucial to discuss potential complications of surgery and goals of care early.

Communication

Communication between surgeon and intensivist has a significant impact on the quality of patient care, and failures in communication are a common cause of medical errors [5–8]. It is imperative that the surgeon and intensivist collaborate throughout the patient's course in the ICU to optimize the care of the patient [9]. Strategies that improve this relationship consist of informing the ICU team preoperatively if the patient requires ICU admission and contacting the ICU immediately postoperative for a full debriefing about the procedure – including a discussion of concerns that the surgeon feels are germane to the outcome of the patient. As such, operative observation by ICU staff foster a better understanding of surgical procedures and the patient's disease process as well as anticipating potential complications that may require rescue [9]. Throughout the postoperative course, the surgery team and ICU staff need to discuss the goals of care frequently, and the daily plan needs to be communicated every morning [10]. Haas et al. have shown that one-on-one communication was the most favored mode for quality communication with teams preferring text messaging, email, or other direct messaging communication technology. These modes were preferred over written notes as the means of inter-team communication [11]. The most common factors causing conflict among ICU teams include communication gaps, personal animosity, and mistrust; to mitigate conflicts, cooperation is crucial, and the aforementioned informal communication tactics foster better interdepartmental relationships [12].

Surgical vs. Medical Intensivist

As the elderly population continues to increase, it is anticipated that there will be a 46% shortage of intensivists by 2030. The gravity of these statistics is highlighted by the fact that 54,000 lives could be saved annually if adequate intensivist staffing could be immediately and effectively implemented [13]. Currently, only 3% of US critical care is provided by a surgical intensivist [13]. This trend is anticipated to continue to decrease as only 50% of surgical critical care training programs fill all of their positions. Therefore, it is imperative that medically trained intensivists are prepared to care for surgical patients. The surgical patient does have similar needs to that of a nonsurgical patient requiring critical care services (i.e., invasive monitoring, nutrition, treatment of shock, and ventilator management). A surgeon managing surgical ICU patients has been shown to have its advantages. As the surgeon already has knowledge of surgical diseases and understands the principles of the specific operation, communication is likely more efficient and effective between the operative and critical care surgeon. There have been some studies that suggest that surgical critical care patients cared for by surgical intensivists have better outcomes than patients cared for by other intensivists. This is especially true in surgeon-led care for trauma patients [14]. It has not been shown, however, that the specialty of the intensivist effects the postoperative survival of a non-trauma patient [15]. These results have been attributed to the fact that all ICU patients require similar care that is not entirely unique to surgical patients. In all likelihood, postoperative mortality in non-trauma patients cared for in a medical, surgical, or mixed ICU are not affected by the type of intensivist managing the patient [12].

Conflict Between Surgeon and Intensivist

Strong evidence supports that closed ICUs decrease mortality and improve resource utilization as compared to open-model ICUs. Conflicts, however, arise between surgeons and intensivists in 60% of closed units and 41% of open units [11]. Inherent to their training, surgeons and intensivists have different perspectives on patient ownership and scope of practice. Surgeons, in general, adhere to a preoperative contract that motivates them to be a patient advocate during the postoperative period. The intensivist views a patient with limited functional status who requires abundant resources and considers how to adequately distribute these limited resources to optimize outcomes for all patients in the ICU. Understanding these different perspectives can allow for more direct communication regarding specific goals of care.

Given the increased public and financial scrutiny surrounding patient experience, the importance of effective communication between healthcare providers must be valued at a premium as it has been shown to be tied to patient experience [16]. According to Haas et al., lack of familiarity with colleagues is a major barrier to good communication. Having a good rapport between surgical and medical colleagues, communicating through informal rather than formal systems (i.e., texting or face-to-face vs. charting), and avoiding assumptions about others' values or understandings based on professional stereotypes lead to better patient care and satisfaction.

It is well recognized that surgeons have a special relationship with their patients, but it is crucial that surgeons recognize the unique perspectives of their colleagues. Intensivist-led ICUs challenge a surgeon's mentality that they have a "covenant to cure" [17] and are "entirely accountable for the outcomes of their patients" [18], but collaboration is much more effective than maintaining an ego. Surgeons can still maintain responsibility of a patient's care, but the ability to be humble and recognize the mortality benefits of a closed ICU model is imperative. Many of these conflicts are related to the emotional intelligence of the practitioners caring for the patient. The Society of Critical Care Medicine recognizes the importance of emotional intelligence on the culture of care in the ICU and the effect it can have on patient outcomes [19]. Emotional intelligence training and the impact it may have on patient care is an emerging area of clinical interest.

Closed vs. Open ICU

Patient's survival is greatly impacted by high-quality supportive care postoperatively. Surgical critical care can be grouped into two broadly defined categories: an "open" ICU and a "closed" ICU [14]. In the former group, the surgeon is primarily responsible for postoperative care in the ICU, where the unit serves as a location for advanced monitoring and organ support. This method meets the principles of the American College of Surgeons in which surgeons are responsible for postoperative care of their patients. The surgeon concomitantly takes care of his/her critically ill patients while continuing with clinical obligations outside the ICU. The latter group is defined as an intensivist model of critical care delivery. The responsibility for delivery of intensive care is assumed by critical care physicians certified in one of the boarded specialties (i.e., internal medicine, anesthesiology, or surgery). In this model, the physician should have no other clinical care duties outside the ICU and is always available to the critically ill patient.

The literature has shown reductions in hospital mortality by 30–40% in patients cared for in closed- or intensivist-model ICUs compared with an open unit. The closed ICU model has also been shown to decrease medical errors, decrease duration of mechanical ventilation, decrease length of stay, decrease readmission rates, and improve patient satisfaction [20]. The Leapfrog Group, a consortium representing 130 employers and 65 Fortune 500 companies that purchase healthcare for their employees, has made ICU physician staffing an important quality indicator for its beneficiaries as a result of this data [20]. Intensivists can be board certified in different backgrounds including pulmonary/critical care, general surgery, and anesthesia and can staff several different types of ICUs (e.g., medical, surgical, mixed, cardiac, neurosurgery, etc.). Although the literature has reported better outcomes in a closed unit, it is uncertain whether specialized ICUs are needed for all types of patients [21].

Discussion

Conflict resolution through effective communication was one the most important factors in the successful recovery of this patient. The patient had a prolonged hospital stay, a complex, variable treatment plan with multiple trips to the operating room, multiple care teams, and a changing clinical course which all relied on successful collaboration. The hopes of a recovery were often thwarted by clinical setbacks and overall deconditioning. However, the patient and the surgeon remained in constant communication throughout his ICU stay, fulfilling the implied contract between them. Naturally, the patient and his family became annoyed and depressed from time to time, but both the surgeon and intensivists helped provide psychosocial support. With growing emphasis placed on autonomy, the patient and his family were involved in every decision during his recovery.

Our patient was primarily cared for by four pulmonary/critical care intensivists and their fellows with significant input from the surgeon and surgical residents in a closed ICU model. The intensivists had no other clinical care duties outside the ICU, and they would alternate on a weekly basis. Liberal use of HIPAA compliant texting throughout the day and face-to-face conversations between members of the surgical team and critical care team allowed the most informed decisions to be made daily.

One disadvantage of a closed ICU is the potential for inadequate patient handoff between intensivists. Critical information can be missed if the surgeon is not involved with the handoff. In an open ICU model, wherein the surgeon is the primary physician, this would typically not be a problem unless participating in a temporary coverage model as the surgeon rarely signs out the care of their patient. On the days where the ICU team would switch intensivists, personal communication between the surgeon and intensivist was mandatory. The intensivists and surgical team had agreed upon defined roles in this case which made for a more smooth transition of care. The technical aspects surrounding the abdominal wound and enterocutaneous fistula were solely managed by the surgery team, while ventilator, fluid, and vasoactive pressor management were provided by the critical care team. This was made possible because of a strong, trusting relationship built upon a foundation of effective communication.

Failures to exchange information appropriately can have disastrous consequences. After one of the patient's many operations, the medical team initiated anticoagulation which likely contributed to the patient's subsequent hemorrhage and need for an additional operation, which resulted in another enterocutaneous fistula. The surgeon wanted the anticoagulation to be held longer due to bleeding in the operating room, but this was not adequately communicated to the medical team. Despite an otherwise open and forthcoming relationship with the medical team, lapses in the transfer of information occurred; it is our duty to the patient, however, to prevent these instances from occurring frequently.

One of our patient's primary problems surrounded the surgical disease of an enterocutaneous fistula. Enteral fistulas are a vexing problem for both patients and surgeons. The complex issues of when to provide enteral or parenteral nutrition, the best way to control the fistula and provide skin protection, as well as the decision of when to operate are mostly in the purview of the surgeon. Enteral fistulas are commonly caused by events that occurred in an operation. These complications often evoke the nature of the "covenant to cure" between the surgeon and the patient. It is likely that a surgical intensivist would innately understand this problem more thoroughly than an intensivist from another discipline and perhaps offer a different treatment plan.

In our case, the ICU team planned to feed the patient enterally for the humoral benefits and to avoid line sepsis or hepatic dysfunction related to parenteral nutrition. A main priority of the ICU team is to avoid central line associated bloodstream infections (CLABSI) given its association with overall ICU and hospital quality. The surgeon firmly believed that an enteral feeding plan would have prevented spontaneous closure of the fistula, which in turn would mandate operative intervention. Given the high risk of operative complications, avoidance of additional surgery was a critical component to uphold his "covenant to cure." After much discussion, the two teams accepted both issues as equally important resulting in a carefully negotiated settlement of when to enterally feed the patient.

The surgeon and intensivist can have different perspectives on patient care as highlighted in this case. Surgeons, in general, feel they must adhere to an unspoken contract to advocate on behalf of their patient throughout their hospital course both pre- and postoperatively. Frequently, the intensivist must take into consideration the role of resource allocation, which may come at odds with the surgeon's contract with the patient. This patient was transferred out of the ICU earlier than the surgeon preferred as the patient would receive a decrease in level of care on a medical-surgical floor rather than the ICU. Because of this, there was concern that the patient's recovery would be stunted. Regardless of the surgeon's preference, the intensivists downgraded the patient, and, ultimately, he did well. Despite the different perspectives, the surgeon and intensivists understood one another, and their collaboration led to the patient's recovery.

Regardless of the strategy, the goal for both surgeons and intensivists remains the same – focus on what is best for the patient. Creating a team with the surgeon and intensivists, surgical and medical residents, the patient, and his family that focused on the patient's recovery was the keystone to his successful discharge home. While the literature suggests that cohesive relationships built on a foundation of open communication between all members of healthcare teams are a requisite for optimal care of the intensive care patient, further investigation of the impact that emotional intelligence training has on patient outcomes is needed.

References

1. Cassell J, Buchman TG, Streat S, Stewart RM. Surgeons, intensivists, and the covenant of care: administrative models and values affecting care at the end of life–updated. Crit Care Med. 2003;31(5):1551–7.
2. Shanafelt TD, Balch CM, Dyrbye L, et al. Special report: suicidal ideation among American surgeons. Arch Surg. 2011;146(1):54–62.
3. Shanafelt TD, Balch CM, Bechamps G, et al. Burnout and medical errors among American surgeons. Ann Surg. 2010;251(6):995–1000.
4. Schwarze ML, Redmann AJ, Brasel KJ, Alexander GC. The role of surgeon error in withdrawal of postoperative life support. Ann Surg. 2012;256(1):10–5.
5. Proctor ML, Pasotre Jm Gerstle JT, et al. Incidence of medical error and adverse outcomes on a pediatric general surgery service. J Pediatr Surg. 2003;38:1361–5.
6. Haller G, Myles PS, Taffé P, et al. Rate of undesirable events at beginning of academic year: retrospective cohort study. BMJ. 2009;339:b3974.

7. Reader T, Flin R, Lauche K, et al. Non-technical skills in the intensive care unit. Br J Anaesth. 2006;96:551–9.
8. Reader TW, Flin R, Cuthbertson BH. Communication skills and error in the intensive care unit. Curr Opin Crit Care. 2007;13:732–6.
9. Sur MD, Angelos P. Ethical issues in surgical critical care: the complexity of interpersonal relationships in the surgical intensive care unit. J Intensive Care Med. 2016;31:442–50.
10. Luchette FA. Surgical critical care workforce – are all intensivists created equal? JAMA Surg. 2013;148:674.
11. Hass B, et al. "It's parallel universes": an analysis of communication between surgeons and intensivists. Crit Care Med. 2015;43:2147–54.
12. Lee J, Eng B, Iqbal S, et al. Medicine versus surgery/anesthesiology intensivists: a retrospective review and comparison of outcomes in a mixed medical-surgical-trauma ICU. Can J Surg. 2013;56:275–9.
13. Sarani B, Toevs C, Mayglothling J, et al. The burden of the U.S. crisis in the surgical critical care workforce and workflow. Am Surg. 2015;81:19–22.
14. Nathens AB, Rivara FP, MacKenzie EJ, et al. The impact of an intensivist-model ICU on trauma-related mortality. Ann Surg. 2006;244(4):545–54.
15. Matsushima K, Goldwasser ER, Schaefer EW, et al. The impact of intensivists' base specialty of training on care process and outcomes of critically ill trauma patients. J Surg Res. 2013;184:577–81.
16. Chow A, Mayer EK, Darzi AW, et al. Patient-reported outcome measures: the importance of patient satisfaction in surgery. Surgery. 2009;146:435–43.
17. Penkoske PA, Buchman TG. The relationships between the surgeon and the intensivist in the surgical intensive care unit. Surg Clin North Am. 2006;86:1351–7.
18. Buchman TG, Cassell J, Ray SE, et al. Who should manage the dying patient? Rescue, shame, and the surgical ICU dilemma. J Am Coll Surg. 2002;194:665–73.
19. Procaccini DE, Connors C. Emotional intelligence in critical care medicine. SCCM.org. Archives 1 Feb 2015; Webpage.
20. Gasperino J. The leapfrog initiative for intensive care unit staffing and its impact on intensive care unit performance: a review. Health Policy. 2011;102:223–8.
21. Diringer MN, Edwards DF. Admission to a neurologic/neurosurgical intensive care unit is associated with reduced mortality after intracerebral hemorrhage. Crit Care Med. 2001;29:635–40.

Chapter 3
Perioperative Management of the Heart Transplant and Mechanical Circulatory Support Device Patient

Mark Jay Zucker and Leeor M. Jaffe

Key Points and Future Aims

- The number of patients undergoing heart transplantation or implantation of a mechanical circulatory support system is increasing and will soon exceed 10,000 patients annually in the United States.
- The basic post-operative critical care management of these patients must be understood by all intensivists

M. J. Zucker (✉)
Cardiothoracic Transplantation Program, Newark Beth Israel Medical Center, Rutgers University – New Jersey Medical School, Newark, NJ, USA
e-mail: Mark.Zucker@RWJBH.ORG

L. M. Jaffe
Department of Medicine,
Baystate Medical Center, Springfield, MA, USA

J. A. LaRosa (ed.), *Adult Critical Care Medicine*,
https://doi.org/10.1007/978-3-319-94424-1_3

as complications in these patients are common and may present in an atypical manner.
- Perioperative management is uniquely challenging, and the explanation for any unexpected change in clinical state needs to be identified rapidly and addressed effectively to avoid morbidity and mortality.
- At present, much of the knowledge in this field is based on empiric observations and expert experience. The development of evidence-based treatment plans and protocols that may lead to more standardized critical care management and better overall outcomes is ongoing.

Introduction

Heart transplant recipients and mechanical circulatory support device patients are among the most challenging cases encountered by the cardiac intensivist. Whereas the former have unique issues ranging from cardiac denervation and primary graft dysfunction to side effects of immunosuppression, the latter have parallel "pumps" with often unpredictable responses to alterations in preload, afterload, and contractility. As a result, standard post-operative medical interventions do not necessarily result in the expected responses in either population. Understanding the unique concepts related to the perioperative management of these patients is critical to ensuring good outcomes and avoiding foreseeable pitfalls.

[Note that many of the recommendations and suggestions in this chapter are based upon empiric observations and experience.]

Case Presentation

A 67-year-old large hypertensive African-American male with a 10-year history of diabetes mellitus, chronic systolic heart failure due to coronary artery disease (with an ejection fraction of 0.10), severe mitral regurgitation (MR), mild aortic insufficiency (AI), and stage 3 chronic kidney disease was listed for transplantation due to progressive clinical deterioration and the need for continuous intravenous milrinone as an outpatient. He eventually presented to the medical center for worsening dyspnea on exertion, edema, and abdominal bloating with right upper quadrant discomfort and early satiety.

Upon arrival at the medical center, the blood pressure (BP) was 88/59 mmHg with a heart rate of 100 bpm. A pulmonary artery catheter was placed, and the right atrial (RA) pressure was 18 mmHg with a pulmonary artery (PA) pressure of 38/26 mmHg and a pulmonary capillary wedge pressure (PCWP) of 25 mmHg. The cardiac index (CI) was calculated to be 1.4 l/m/m2 using the Fick equation. The sodium was 129 mEq/dl, and the creatinine was 1.9 mg/dl. After discussion with the team, it was determined that the patient required urgent placement of a circulatory support device. Various options were entertained recognizing that identification of a donor organ in the short term was unlikely (due to the patient's size), and he was therefore taken for implantation of a durable centrifugal left ventricular assist device (LVAD).

Initial Considerations

The experienced heart failure clinician and/or cardiac intensivist will immediately note preoperative areas of concern:

1. The presence of a markedly elevated right atrial pressure (central venous pressure (CVP)) suggests that the patient is quite fluid overloaded. This places the patient not only at high risk of perioperative morbidity, mortality, and renal dysfunction but also at higher risk of post-LVAD right heart failure [1, 2].
2. The patient's hemodynamics are notable for two other validated predictors of right ventricular (RV) failure after LVAD insertion. First, the CVP/PCWP ratio is 0.72. A ratio of greater than 0.63 has been shown to be predictive of RV failure [3]. Second, despite the elevated PCWP, the patient's RV is generating a relatively low systolic pressure of

38 mmHg, and the calculated RV stroke work index is reduced at 6.05 (normal 7.9–9.7) [4].
3. With a diastolic BP of 59 mmHg and an assumed LV end diastolic pressure of 25 mmHg (using the wedge pressure as a surrogate), the pressure gradient across the valve during diastole is only 34 mmHg as compared to a pressure gradient in a healthy individual of over 70 mmHg. Despite the low gradient, there is already mild aortic insufficiency.
4. The baseline creatinine prior to surgical intervention is elevated. How much of the elevation is attributable to poor forward flow (type 1 cardiorenal syndrome) versus how much is due to intrinsic renal dysfunction or chronic post-capillary renal congestion (type 2 cardiorenal syndrome) is unclear at this time but may become an issue later [5].

Implantation of the durable centrifugal pump proceeded uneventfully. An echocardiogram performed after device insertion demonstrated mild RV distention, but overall function of the right ventricle was considered to be "borderline adequate." Bleeding concerns were relatively few, and the patient was transferred to the cardiothoracic ICU for further management. Initial BP was 86/82 mmHg by arterial line with a heart rate of 86 bpm on vasopressin two units per hour, norepinephrine 2 mcg/kg/min, and dobutamine 5 mcg/kg/min. The RA pressure was 14 mmHg and PA pressure 36/22 mmHg. The ventilator was set to a PRVC mode with a FiO2 of 0.70. The extremities were cool and edematous.

Approximately 4 hours later, the BP fell to 68/66 mmHg, and the right atrial pressure rose to 19 mmHg. The pump flow decreased to 3.2 lpm as compared to 4.1 lpm upon arrival in the unit. The urine output decreased to 20 cc per hour from 50 cc per hour. Chest tube drainage was 475 ml since arrival but was slowing. The repeat hemoglobin was 7.2 mg/dl and creatinine 2.6 mg/dl.

Post-operative Considerations

At this point, a number of issues have developed including anemia, hypotension, and worsening renal function. Each needs to be assessed and addressed.

1. The anemia is most likely due to intraoperative and early post-operative blood loss. Since the patient is a heart transplant candidate, administration of blood products should be limited to the extent possible in order to avoid subsequent allosensitization which might complicate the identification of an immunologically compatible donor [6]. Nonetheless, the hemoglobin should probably not be allowed to drift much lower than 7 mg/dl. If blood products are required, the use of leukodepleted and perhaps washed and irradiated products should be entertained, although there is a paucity of data to support this practice [7].
2. The etiology of the worsening renal function remains unclear, but the possibility of poor forward flow, even with an LVAD, must be entertained and investigated.
3. The worsening RA pressure coupled with tenuous preoperative state of the RV and the echo finding of mild RV distension and hypokinesis suggest that failure of the unsupported RV may be contributing to the poor forward flow. Potential etiologies include tamponade, changes in septal geometry due to LV unloading, primary RV dysfunction, and secondary RV dysfunction (due to an elevated pulmonary vascular resistance or coronary disease involving the right coronary artery). A transesophageal echocardiogram in addition to continuous invasive hemodynamic monitoring may provide additional insight. In particular, a TEE will help the physician assess the position of the interventricular septum and adjust LVAD RPM to ensure that the septum is midline.

The other challenge at this time is to decide whether to administer volume (including blood) to an already distended right ventricle or to administer diuretics. Both approaches are problematic. In the presence of a normally functioning LVAD, BP and forward flow are down because left-sided filling pressures are presumably down. Thus, the administration of volume would ordinarily be the proper intervention. However, additional volume may further distend the right ventricle making the need for a temporary right ventricular assist device more likely.

Arguably, the treatment of choice at this moment would be to increase inotropes (to address any primary RV myocardial dysfunction) and perhaps introduce nitric oxide (to reduce RV afterload if there is evidence of an elevated pulmonary vascular resistance) [8]. As well, the introduction of isoproterenol to increase the heart rate or reprogramming the implanted ICD to atrial pace at 95–100 bpm might be of some incremental value, although the role of a faster heart rate in an LVAD patient is less well established than it is in a transplant patient [9].

After the dobutamine was doubled and isoproterenol added, the heart rate rose to 96 bpm, and hemodynamics improved sufficiently to permit the transfusion of two units of packed red blood cells (PRBC). On post-operative day number 1, the right atrial pressure was 14 mmHg, and the patient was successfully extubated, although he remained on fairly high doses of pressors and inotropes.

Thirty-six hours after leaving the OR, intravenous anticoagulation was started with heparin at 500 units per hour with instructions to up-titrate to a target PTT of 60 s. Oral warfarin was begun as well. Pressors and then inotropes were weaned over the next 3–4 days, and he was transferred to the step-down unit.

Anticoagulation Considerations

Heparin or a derivative of heparin is often administered preoperatively to minimize the risk of intraventricular thrombus formation. Regardless of whether heparin was infusing preoperatively or not, it is normally administered in a fairly high dose during LVAD implantation. Once the LVAD has been successfully implanted and the flow generated by the device shown to be adequate, protamine is administered to reverse the effects of heparin.

During the early post-implant period, bleeding precludes the introduction of heparin or warfarin. At some point, however, anticoagulation must be started. Some centers proceed directly to vitamin K antagonists, while others bridge with unfractionated heparin [10]. The use of direct oral anticoagulants such as apixaban and rivaroxaban is not recommended [11]. Even with appropriate anticoagulation and acceptable pump output, device thrombosis can still occur.

The following should be considered with respect to the preoperative evaluation and post-operative management of all patients who are being anticoagulated early after surgery irrespective of whether that surgery is VAD placement or transplantation:

1. The increased use of heparin prior to placement of a mechanical circulatory support device (or prior to transplantation) has resulted in an increase in the frequency of heparin-induced thrombocytopenia [12]. The diagnosis of HIT is made by the clinical history, timing/duration of heparin exposure, and measurement of antibodies to the Hep/PF4 complex and confirmed by a serotonin release assay [13]. All thrombocytopenia, however, is not HIT. Antibiotics, proton pump inhibitors, and pump-related consumption can all reduce platelet number. This is particularly true in the patient in whom an intra-aortic balloon pump was in place preoperatively.
2. In some instances, patients do not have HIT but are known to be hypercoagulable for other reasons such as antiphospholipid antibody syndrome, prothrombin gene mutations, and MTHFR mutations. These patients may be at an increased risk for pump thrombosis and need to be more aggressively anticoagulated and closely monitored [14].
3. Patients with prior hematologic conditions that place them at a high risk for bleeding or clotting such as idiopathic thrombocytopenic purpura, factor V Leiden, and elevated factor VIII have significantly higher rates of early morbidity and mortality and require particularly close monitoring [15].

The patient was discharged to home on post-operative day number 22. LVAD parameters were all within normal limits at that time although pump output was slightly high at 6.9 lpm (normal 4–6 lpm). An echocardiogram obtained prior to discharge revealed mild RV distention and hypokinesis and mild to moderate aortic insufficiency with a mean arterial pressure of 85 mmHg. Serum creatinine was 1.8 mg/dl.

Additional Considerations

On first glance, the situation appears to be fairly stable. The BP is at target. The function of the right ventricle appears adequate. However, the unexpectedly high pump output cannot be ignored. As noted, there was preoperative mild AI with a pressure gradient during diastole of 34 mmHg. Ordinarily, after LVAD placement, one can generally assume that the LV has been decompressed and that the LVEDP is nearly normal. Therefore, with a mean arterial pressure usually in the range of 85 mmHg, the pressure gradient across the valve is now 65–70 mmHg, nearly double to what it was preoperatively. Moreover, whereas the pressure gradient across the aortic valve in the non-LVAD patient is solely during diastole, in the LVAD patient (in whom aortic flow is continuous), there remains a pressure gradient even during systole. In addition, the LVAD inflow creates suction in the LV which can further contribute to the insufficiency [16]. The visible manifestation of this regurgitant flow is an increased calculated pump output as blood from the pump enters the ascending aorta and leaks back into the left ventricle creating a circulatory loop. This limits the effective forward flow and can ultimately lead to organ malperfusion and increased left ventricular diastolic pressures [17].

Four months after discharge, the patient develops recurrent shortness of breath and dyspnea. He is seen at the mechanical circulatory support clinic and admitted for further evaluation. Upon admission, device interrogation reveals consistently elevated pump output and power. Measurement of serum LDH reveals no significant change from baseline. An echocardiogram again demonstrates mild RV distention and hypokinesis but now reveals moderate to severe aortic insufficiency. Prior to making any changes to the LVAD settings a PA catheter is placed. The RA pressure was 13 mmHg, PA pressure 44/25 mmHg, and PCWP was 23 mmHg. The mixed venous saturation was 48%, and the estimated Fick CI was 1.8 lpm/m2. The LVAD RPM was increased, but no change was noted in the mixed venous saturation. The case was presented to the team for further recommendations.

Post-readmission Considerations

The stable LDH suggests that there is no pump thrombosis [18]. Hence, the logical conclusion is that the aortic insufficiency has become a significant problem. This is a well-known phenomenon in LVAD recipients and one that does not have an easy solution [16]. There are multiple reports describing the results of either replacing or oversewing the aortic valve. Outcomes have been mixed, and most surgeons are unenthusiastic about either approach [19]. For this reason, the best intervention for this problem in a transplant candidate is to proceed directly to transplantation assuming that the patient can be adequately supported during the waiting period.

As a result of the discussion with the team, it is agreed that transplantation represents the proper next step. Lab work is sent for immunologic assessment, and the patient is allosensitized to multiple HLA antigens. Nevertheless, the antibody titers are relatively low, and it is decided that no preoperative desensitization therapy is needed. After 3 weeks in the cardiac care unit, a donor heart from a 42-year-old motor vehicle accident victim is identified. The patient has one donor-specific antibody which is thought to not represent a contraindication to proceeding, and he was taken to the operating room for LVAD explantation and cardiac transplantation approximately 6 months after placement of the LVAD. The international normalized ratio (INR) at the time of transplantation was normal since anticoagulation had been maintained with heparin and aspirin.

The intraoperative course was challenging. Dense adhesions were present making dissection difficult. The donor heart was implanted after an ischemic time of 4 h. Diffuse bleeding was noted by the surgical team which did not respond well to standard measures including protamine. A massive transfusion protocol was initiated, and over eight units of packed red cells were administered in the operating room in addition to platelets, fresh frozen plasma, and cryoprecipitate. Left ventricular function was adequate although not hyperdynamic. Right ventricular function, however, was poor. Two amps (20 mcg) of liothyronine were administered in addition to milrinone 0.5 mcg/kg/min, dobutamine 5 mcg/kg/min, epinephrine 0.05 mcg/kg/min, and vasopressin two units per hour. After 7 h in the operating room, the patient was transferred to the cardiothoracic ICU.

Upon arriving in the ICU, the BP was 85/53 mmHg with a pulse of 105 bpm. The right atrial pressure was 18 mmHg, pulmonary artery pressure 37/21 mmHg, and CI 2.5 lpm/m2. Drips were as described above. Urine output was 90 ml per hour, and chest tube drainage was significant at 200 per hour. The donor was known to be cytomegalovirus positive and the recipient cytomegalovirus negative; therefore, prophylactic intravenous ganciclovir was ordered to begin on post-operative day number 2.

Posttransplant Considerations

Although there are significant differences in the management of heart transplant recipients as compared with the management of patients after routine cardiac surgery, there are similarities, as well. The great majority of patients are extubated on the first post-operative day. Although monitoring lines and Foley catheters are discontinued expeditiously, inotropic agents are withdrawn a bit more slowly due to the risk of late right heart dysfunction [20]. Line removal, as with all post-operative patients, is critically important in order to reduce the chances of a nosocomial infection induced by either indwelling catheters or monitoring devices.

The above comments notwithstanding, there are a number of issues associated with heart transplant recipients that need to be specifically addressed:

1. *Right Heart Failure* – For multiple reasons including the presence of preoperatively elevated pulmonary vascular resistance (not infrequency exacerbated by intraoperative bleeding and the need for large amounts of blood products), the recently prolonged cold time and ischemic time, and the loss of sympathetic innervation, RV dysfunction has become a common post-operative challenge seen in these patients. Transplant registry data demonstrate that despite advances in perioperative management, RV dysfunction accounts for 50% of all cardiac complications and 19% of all early deaths [21]. The following management points should be considered:

   A. As noted previously, a distinction needs to be made between right heart failure secondary to primary myocardial right heart dysfunction (as a result of ischemia, primary graft dysfunction, or an air embolus down the right coronary artery) and right heart dysfunction due to an increased afterload (as a result of a chronically elevated pulmonary vascular resistance). In the first case, therapy is primarily directed toward improving contractility of the ventricle. In the second case, therapy is directed toward both reducing ventricular afterload and improving contractility.
   B. The presence of normal pulmonary artery pressures does not rule out right ventricular dysfunction. Attention needs to be focused on the pulmonary artery (PA) pulse pressure (PAS-PAD) and the central venous pressure (CVP). Normally, in the perioperative period, the CVP should be less than 10–12 mmHg and the systolic PA pressure greater than 30–35 mmHg with a PA pulse pressure of at least 10–12 mmHg. A low PA pulse pressure and high CVP are often the first clue that the RV is struggling.

C. The donor right ventricle is frequently hypokinetic in the immediate post-operative period for the reasons noted previously. Contractility can be improved with isoproterenol at 2–4 mcg/min or with milrinone and/or dobutamine [22]. Of the two agents, milrinone may be the more effective medication, but it does cause more hypotension [23]. As such, the recommended loading dose of milrinone is not normally given. In the presence of renal insufficiency, the maintenance dose of milrinone will need to be decreased. Dobutamine may cause tachycardia which, in and of itself, is not necessarily a problem for reasons described below.

D. Empiric observations have suggested that intravenous T3 hormone (liothyronine) may also be used to improve cardiac contractility [24, 25]. The initial dosage is 0.2 mcg/kg administered as a bolus over 1 min. The use of dosages as high as 3 mcg/kg has been reported. A follow-up intravenous drip of 20–30 mcg over 24 h may be considered but is generally not needed. Thyroid hormone may increase myocardial oxygen demand ($MVO_{2)}$ and may also increase atrial and ventricular arrhythmias.

E. For patients with increased RV afterload, nitroprusside can be used to lower pulmonary pressures and perhaps improve right heart function, but it may exacerbate intrapulmonary shunting and worsen hypoxemia [26]. Secondary hypoxic pulmonary vasoconstriction may in turn further worsen right ventricular function. For this reason, nitroprusside is not normally used in the post-operative period.

F. Inhaled prostacyclins – epoprostenol (Veletri and Flolan) are used at many centers to reduce pulmonary resistance. However, both have alkaline pH values and may not be ideal for inhalation in certain patients. For this reason, nitric oxide (NO) remains the intervention of choice for afterload-mediated RV dysfunction. Unfortunately, the cost of the medication is substantial, and many medical centers are reluctant to use or even acquire this agent. Although NO is most effective when RV dysfunction is secondary to an increased pulmonary vascular resistance as compared to intrinsic RV myocardial dysfunction, distinguishing between the two etiologies is difficult. In fact, most of the time, both etiologies play a role. Thus, NO is often used in all cases of RV dysfunction.

G. Regardless of the etiology of the right heart dysfunction. In the early post-operative period, maintaining the heart rate at approximately 100–110/min by either isoproterenol infusion or atrial pacing (if wires were placed) may be beneficial. This is particularly relevant in situations where the donor heart is a bit undersized. Heart rates up to 120 bpm are acceptable. Note that isoproterenol was commonly needed in the past when atrial-atrial anastomoses were performed (which resulted in sinus node dysfunction). Isoproterenol is less commonly needed now that the bicaval technique is used. In fact, in such patients, isoproterenol may result in a marked tachycardia, and caution is advised.

H. In addition to inotropes or afterload-reducing agents, gentle diuresis should always be considered, but an echocardiogram should first be obtained to rule out tamponade. The challenge with administering diuretics is that in the presence of RV failure the systemic BP may be low due an inadequate filling volume. Thus, diuretics alone almost never adequately address the problem.

I. Oral sildenafil was the first phosphodiesterase 5 (PDE-5) inhibitor used in patients with RV dysfunction due to pulmonary hypertension. It has proven to be quite an effective medication. Moreover, in addition to its pulmonary vasodilating effects, there are reports that it also increases contractility of the RV probably due to PDE-3 inhibition, as well [27]. However, not all studies have confirmed this finding [28].

J. In certain circumstances, simply opening the sternum may be sufficient to address the RV dysfunction [29].

2. *Hemodynamic Considerations* – In general, the first 24–48 h is centered on right heart function, hemodynamic stability, and bleeding. All of these problems come together to create one of the more common posttransplant issues – hypotension. The following should be taken into account when addressing this issue:

   A. A *stable* systolic BP of >90–95 mmHg (or mean BP greater than 65–70 mmHg) is generally acceptable in the first 24 h post-operatively. Do not push fluids unless the CVP is <5–7 mmHg and even then only if the systolic BP is <85 mmHg.
   B. Persistent hypotension responsive to volume suggests intrathoracic bleeding. Chest tubes can clot, and the absence of bleeding from a chest tube can be misleading. If hypotension is unexplained or unresponsive to standard interventions, recheck the chest x-ray, rule out a pneumothorax, and consider transesophageal echocardiography.
   C. Vasoplegia defined as an inability to maintain a BP despite reasonable doses of vasopressors is being seen increasingly frequently possibly due to the increased number of patients undergoing cardiopulmonary bypass including those undergoing heart transplantation after medium- to long-term support with an LVAD [29, 30]. The reasons for this are not clear. Methylene blue (1.5 mg/kg IV over 20 min (up to a maximum of 40 mg)) may be of some value in treating this condition if the patient does not respond to standard vasopressors [31]. Preoperative amiodarone has been reported to be associated with hypotension that may be less responsive to pressors although this remains controversial [32–34].
   D. For the better part of the past 15 years, vasopressin was the pressor of choice for hypotension. As compared to norepinephrine, vasopressin does not cause tachycardia, increases renal blood flow and urine output (not seen with norepinephrine), and is effective even in the presence of hypoxia and/or acidosis. Unfortunately, the

cost of the medication increased significantly in 2014. In view of this, many centers advise introducing norepinephrine first or if the patient has been started on vasopressin attempt an early transition to norepinephrine. The role of intravenous angiotensin II has not been studied in this patient population.

3. *Post-operative Bleeding* – With respect to bleeding, a number of pre-op considerations as well as post-op complications must be entertained.

   A. The target hemoglobin is 8 gm/dl during the first 36 h. In selected stable, non-bleeding patients, the hemoglobin may be allowed to drift as low as 7.0–7.5 gm/dl after the first 36–48 h.
   B. In the past, preoperative, intraoperative, and immediate post-operative use of 5–10 gm of aminocaproic acid (Amicar) was used to reduce the incidence of bleeding by interfering with the fibrinolytic pathway, particularly in patients undergoing a second or third intrathoracic procedure. It is no longer routinely used but could represent an option for patients with considerable bleeding.
   C. An activated clotting time (ACT) can be checked more quickly than a partial thromboplastin time (PTT), but they don't always correlate.
   D. As a general rule, if the INR is 1.6 or less, the bleeding will probably not be corrected with fresh frozen plasma (FFP) alone.
   E. The use of cell saver blood (autologous blood transfusion) may involve more heparin use and may worsen coagulopathy. Additional protamine can be used to mitigate this effect.
   F. Blood replacement therapy should be performed in accordance with the hospital's center-specific massive transfusion protocol recommending the administration of a fixed ratio of PRBC to FFP to platelets.

      [Experience gleaned from trauma units and the military has taught us that blood components should be replaced in a proper proportion. Guidelines differ with regard to the ideal ratio, but in general, it seems that a 1:1:1 ratio of PRBC to FFP to platelets is simple and effective [35]. Isotonic crystalloid should not be used to replace volume as it causes dilutional coagulopathy. Low fibrinogen concentrations can be addressed with cryoprecipitate if the level is less than 150 mg/dl.]

G. For persistent bleeding, the use of recombinant factor (rFactor) VIIa may be considered. rFactor VIIa in the presence of tissue factor will convert factors IX and X to factors IXa and Xa, respectively. Factor Xa will then convert prothrombin to thrombin which will convert fibrinogen to fibrin thereby forming a hemostatic plug. The surgical dose (which is much lower than the hemophilia dose) is 10 mcg/kg delivered as a bolus, and a second dose may be required [36].

H. Each institution will define what level of continued bleeding in the chest tubes justifies a return to the operating room. However, in general, more than 300 ml over 3 h or 400 ml over 4 h is probably an indication to return to the OR unless the bleeding appears to be slowing or there is a diffuse coagulopathy in which case the coagulopathy needs to be treated first.

4. *Renal Insufficiency* – Transplant recipients seem to be at increased risk for post-operative renal insufficiency due in part to the preoperative, low-output, diuretic-dependent state of the kidney which may be exacerbated by cardiopulmonary bypass and the use of multiple nephrotoxic medications including antibiotics and calcineurin inhibitors such as cyclosporine and tacrolimus [37].

A. Decreased urine output may be an early indication of cardiac tamponade or right heart failure.

B. Early hemodialysis or continuous renal replacement therapy (CRRT) can be quite effective in preventing right heart distention and hyperkalemia in patients with renal dysfunction, anuria, or significant oliguria.

C. Intravenous ganciclovir and acyclovir may cause crystalluria and secondary renal damage. Hydration and alkalinization of the urine may be of some benefit. The infusion rate should be fairly slow.

5. *Fever and Leukocytosis* – With respect to fever and leukocytosis, the following should be remembered:

   A. A fever up to 101°F during the first 24–36 h is not unusual. After that, however, a fever of 101°F or greater should prompt a search for a cause. Of note, dexmedetomidine, a sedative, can cause fever (as well as hypotension, hypertension, nausea, and bradycardia).
   B. Immunosuppressant medications such as anti-thymocyte globulin can cause fevers.
   C. It is difficult to differentiate leukocytosis from ubiquitous steroid use from a leukocytosis triggered by infection or other inflammatory process. Empiric experience suggests that the white blood cell (WBC) count does not usually rise above the low 20,000 s from steroids alone. Any white count higher than that probably warrants further evaluation.
   D. It is not uncommon for the WBC count to increase, decrease, and then increase again approximately 7 days after transplant. This may simply reflect a stress reaction.

6. *Hematologic Abnormalities* – Multiple cytopenias can develop after heart transplantation from a number of etiologies.

   A. Leukopenia is most often drug related but can be secondary to severe infection and sepsis. Induction immunotherapy may lead to depressed WBC counts. Drugs commonly used after transplant such as mycophenolate mofetil, ganciclovir, and valganciclovir can also lower WBC counts.
   B. Anemia in the acute post-operative period is most often related to blood loss; however, renal dysfunction, vitamin or mineral deficiency, drug effects, and infections (especially viral) can result in prolonged anemia.
   C. Thrombocytopenia is relatively common after heart transplant and may be due to cardiopulmonary bypass

and the use of heparin products in the operating room. The medications noted above as causes of leukopenia can also cause thrombocytopenia.

D. Pancytopenia post-operatively can be related to bone marrow suppression from medications, infection, or other highly inflammatory state. Pancytopenia should prompt a timely and careful investigation and may require bone marrow biopsy [38].

On the evening of the second post-operative day, the nurse reported that despite only a slight reduction in the intravenous medications, the BP had fallen to 84/58 mmHg, and the heart rate had fallen to 68 bpm. A 12-lead confirmed the loss of sinus rhythm and the appearance of a junctional tachycardia. The patient was asymptomatic. The medical team initiated atrial pacing at a rate of 100 bpm. Three hours later, the nurse called and informed the on-call physician that the patient had developed atrial fibrillation with a rapid ventricular response of 138 bpm and requested directions.

Posttransplant Arrhythmias

Arrhythmias are not uncommon in all post-cardiac surgery patients, but their management in the transplant population may be a bit different:

1. Bradycardia in a transplant recipient cannot be treated with atropine due to vagal denervation of the allograft, and tachycardia including supraventricular tachycardias will not respond to vagal interventions.
2. Atrial pacing and/or isoproterenol remains the treatment of choice for bradycardia.
3. Atrial fibrillation and atrial flutter are common in the first couple weeks after surgery and probably do not indicate allograft rejection. New-onset atrial fibrillation beyond this period is concerning for rejection and/or allograft dysfunction and should prompt further evaluation including imaging and endomyocardial biopsy [39].

4. Digoxin will not terminate atrial fibrillation in transplant recipients.
5. The agent of choice for management of atrial fibrillation and/or atrial flutter is amiodarone (minimal interaction with immunosuppressive agents); however, use of prophylactic amiodarone is not generally encouraged [40]. Be aware that amiodarone boluses may cause mild, transient hypotension.
6. The use of atrial overdrive pacing to terminate atrial flutter is not advised although the arrhythmia can sometimes be terminated in this way.
7. Intravenous verapamil or diltiazem is not usually the first choice of therapy but may be used cautiously for rate control of atrial flutter in selected patients.

After two boluses with intravenous amiodarone, the atrial fibrillation resolves, and the monitor reveals atrial pacing at a rate of 100 bpm. The following morning, an echocardiogram is obtained to assess allograft function. The right ventricle was mildly dilated and hypokinetic. Left ventricular function was likewise hypokinetic with an EF of 0.40–0.45 as compared to 0.50–0.55 in the operating room at the time of transfer to the CT ICU. The intravenous medications were left at the same dose. Serum troponin level was coming down as is normally noted in the post-operative period. The findings were discussed with the team. Concern was expressed about the significance of the donor-specific antibody.

Allograft Dysfunction

One common risk affecting all transplant recipients is primary graft dysfunction (PGF) which reportedly accounts for about 40% of the early (<30 day) mortality [41]. Only recently has a definition been proposed for PGF [42]. A full description of the various subtypes is beyond the scope of this chapter. However, in most cases, the following are present:

1. Severe systolic dysfunction of one or both ventricles by direct observation in the operating room or by echocardiography during the first 24 h after transplantation
2. Severe hemodynamic compromise (SBP < 90 mmHg and/or CI < 2.2 lpm/m^2) lasting for more than 1 h and requiring at least two intravenous inotropes at high dose or mechanical circulatory support
3. The absence of any other immunologic, technical, hematologic, or pulmonary vascular cause for hemodynamic compromise

According to the definition above, the patient was not experiencing primary graft dysfunction since myocardial contractility was not severely decreased and the episode was not recognized during the first 24 h. The most likely explanation in this scenario is delayed recovery of the allograft due to a prolonged ischemic time and the somewhat advanced age of the donor (40 years old). The most prudent course of action would be watchful waiting and frequent reassessment. The decreasing troponin levels are reassuring but non-specific [43]. Hence, the matter of allograft rejection remains a consideration. An endomyocardial biopsy at post-op day number 3 would likely demonstrate diffuse ischemic injury but no cellular rejection. Studies to identify antibody-mediated rejection will be hard to interpret as they are often abnormal during the first few post-operative weeks. Therefore, if there is true concern about rejection from the known donor-specific antibody, the use of intravenous immunoglobulin with or without plasmapheresis might be worth considering. The use of high-dose steroids or rituximab at this time would be premature and inappropriate without confirmatory evidence of antibody-mediated rejection.

An echocardiogram is repeated on post-operative day number 5. Right and left ventricular functions are normal. The drips are slowly weaned off. Despite the introduction of the calcineurin inhibitor the serum creatinine actually decreased to 1.4 mg/dl. The first endomyocardial biopsy on post-operative day 7 revealed no evidence of cellular rejection but classical ischemic changes. The second endomyocardial biopsy on post-operative day 14 revealed no evidence of cellular or antibody-mediated rejection, and the patient was discharged home. All heart transplant patients are encouraged to enroll in a cardiac rehab program and return to work at 6–8 weeks post-operatively.

Conclusion

In the 1980s and 1990s, many of the problems described in this hypothetical scenario proved insurmountable. Fortunately, refinements in patient selection, surgical technique, and myocardial preservation in association with effective antibacterial and antiviral agents, nitric oxide, and left and right ventricular assist devices have resulted in better overall survival rates. The most significant change, however, in the care of mechanical circulatory support and transplant recipients however arguably came with the introduction of defined management protocols applied by well-educated teams and the understanding that early recognition and early intervention are critical to ensure acceptable outcomes.

Today, over 90% of heart transplant recipients are alive at 1 year, and more than 50% are still alive after 13 years. As a result, heart transplantation is now the recognized treatment of choice for patients with end-stage heart failure.

References

1. Stein A, de Souza LV, Belettini CR, Menegazzo WR, Viégas JR, Costa Pereira EM, Eick R, Araújo L, Consolim-Colombo F, Irigoyen MC. Fluid overload and changes in serum creatinine after cardiac surgery: predictors of mortality and longer intensive care stay. A prospective cohort study. Crit Care. 2012;16(3):R99.
2. Dang NC, Topkara VK, Mercando M, Kay J, Kruger KH, Aboodi MS, Oz MC, Naka Y. Right heart failure after left ventricular assist device implantation in patients with chronic congestive heart failure. J Heart Lung Transplant. 2006;25(1):1–6.

3. Kormos RL, Teuteberg JJ, Pagani FD, Russell SD, John R, Miller LW, Massey T, Milano CA, Moazami N, Sundareswaran KS, Farrar DJ, HeartMate II Clinical Investigators. Right ventricular failure in patients with the HeartMate II continuous-flow left ventricular assist device: incidence, risk factors, and effect on outcomes. J Thorac Cardiovasc Surg. 2010;139(5):1316–24.
4. Fukamachi K, McCarthy PM, Smedira NG, Vargo RL, Starling RC, Young JB. Preoperative risk factors for right ventricular failure after implantable left ventricular assist device insertion. Ann Thorac Surg. 1999;68(6):2181–4.
5. Ronco C, Haapio M, House AA, Anavekar N, Bellomo R. Cardiorenal syndrome. J Am Coll Cardiol. 2008;52(19):1527–39. https://doi.org/10.1016/j.jacc.2008.07.051.
6. McKenna DH Jr, Eastlund T, Segall M, Noreen HJ, Park S. HLA alloimmunization in patients requiring ventricular assist device support. J Heart Lung Transplant. 2002;21(11):1218–24.
7. Drakos SG, Stringham JC, Long JW, Gilbert EM, Fuller TC, Campbell BK, Horne BD, Hagan ME, Nelson KE, Lindblom JM, Meldrum PA, Carlson JF, Moore SA, Kfoury AG, Renlund DG. Prevalence and risks of allosensitization in HeartMate left ventricular assist device recipients: the impact of leukofiltered cellular blood product transfusions. J Thorac Cardiovasc Surg. 2007;133(6):1612–9.
8. Potapov E, Meyer D, Swaminathan M, Ramsay M, El Banayosy A, Diehl C, Veynovich B, Gregoric ID, Kukucka M, Gromann TW, Marczin N, Chittuluru K, Baldassarre JS, Zucker MJ, Hetzer R. Inhaled nitric oxide after left ventricular assist device implantation: a prospective, randomized, double-blind, multicenter, placebo-controlled trial. J Heart Lung Transplant. 2011;30:870–8.
9. Lahm T, McCaslin CA, Wozniak TC, Ghumman W, Fadl YY, Obeidat OS, Schwab K, Meldrum DR. Medical and surgical treatment of acute right ventricular failure. J Am Coll Cardiol. 2010;56(18):1435–46.
10. Slaughter MS, Naka Y, John R, Boyle A, Conte JV, Russell SD, Aaronson KD, Sundareswaran KS, Farrar DJ, Pagani FD. Post-operative heparin may not be required for transitioning patients with a HeartMate II left ventricular assist system to long-term warfarin therapy. J Heart Lung Transplant. 2010;29(6):616–24.
11. Feldman D, Pamboukian SV, Teuteberg JJ, Birks E, Lietz K, Moore SA, Morgan JA, Arabia F, Bauman ME, Buchholz HW, Deng M, Dickstein ML, El-Banayosy A, Elliot T, Goldstein DJ, Grady KL, Jones K, Hryniewicz K, John R, Kaan A,

Kusne S, Loebe M, Massicotte MP, Moazami N, Mohacsi P, Mooney M, Nelson T, Pagani F, Perry W, Potapov EV, Eduardo Rame J, Russell SD, Sorensen EN, Sun B, Strueber M, Mangi AA, Petty MG, Rogers J, International Society for Heart and Lung Transplantation. The 2013 International Society for Heart and Lung Transplantation Guidelines for mechanical circulatory support: executive summary. J Heart Lung Transplant. 2013;32(2):157–87.

12. Koster A, Huebler S, Potapov E, Meyer O, Jurmann M, Weng Y, Pasic M, Drews T, Kuppe H, Loebe M, Hetzer R. Impact of heparin-induced thrombocytopenia on outcome in patients with ventricular assist device support: single-institution experience in 358 consecutive patients. Ann Thorac Surg. 2007;83(1):72–6.
13. Schenk S, El-Banayosy A, Morshuis M, Arusoglu L, Eichler P, Lubenow N, Tenderich G, Koerfer R, Greinacher A, Prohaska W. IgG classification of anti-PF4/heparin antibodies to identify patients with heparin-induced thrombocytopenia during mechanical circulatory support. J Thromb Haemost. 2007;5(2):235–41. Epub 2006 Oct 31.
14. Alvarez P, Cordero-Reyes AM, Uribe C, De Hoyos P, Martinez D, Bhimaraj A, Trachtenberg BH, Ashrith G, Torre-Amione G, Loebe M, Amione-Guerra J, Rice L, Estep JD. Acquired and hereditary hypercoagulable states in patients with continuous flow left ventricular assist devices: prevalence and thrombotic complications. J Card Fail. 2016;22(7):501–11.
15. Fried J, Levin AP, Mody KM, Garan AR, Yuzefpolsakaya M, Takayama H, Diuguid DL, Naka Y, Jorde U, Uriel N. Prior hematologic conditions carry a high morbidity and mortality in patients supported with continuous-flow left ventricular assist devices. J Heart Lung Transplant. 2014;33(11):1119–25.
16. Cowger J, Pagani FD, Haft JW, Romano MA, Aaronson KD, Kolias TJ. The development of aortic insufficiency in left ventricular assist device-supported patients. Circ Heart Fail. 2010;3(6):668–74.
17. Holtz J, Teuteberg J. Management of aortic insufficiency in the continuous flow left ventricular assist device population. Curr Heart Fail Rep. 2014;11(1):103–10.
18. Cowger JA, Romano MA, Shah P, Shah N, Mehta V, Haft JW, Aaronson KD, Pagani FD. Hemolysis: a harbinger of adverse outcome after left ventricular assist device implant. J Heart Lung Transplant. 2014;33(1):35–43.

19. Rao V, Slater JP, Edwards NM, Naka Y, Oz MC. Surgical management of valvular disease in patients requiring left ventricular assist device support. Ann Thorac Surg. 2001;71(5):1448–53.
20. Stobierska-Dzierzek B, Awad H, Michler RE. The evolving management of acute right-sided heart failure in cardiac transplant recipients. J Am Coll Cardiol. 2001;38(4):923–31.
21. Hosenpud JD, Bennett LE, Keck BM, Boucek MM, Novick RJ. The Registry of the International Society for Heart and Lung Transplantation: seventeenth official report-2000. J Heart Lung Transplant. 2000;19(10):909–31.
22. Mentzer RM, Alegre CA, Nolan SP. The effects of dopamine and isoproterenol on the pulmonary circulation. J Thorac Cardiovasc Surg. 1976;71(6):807–14.
23. Chen EP, Bittner HB, Davis RD, Van Trigt P. Hemodynamic and inotropic effects of milrinone after heart transplantation in the setting of recipient pulmonary hypertension. J Heart Lung Transplant. 1998;17(7):669–78.
24. Jeevanandam V. Triiodothyronine: spectrum of use in heart transplantation. Thyroid. 1997;7(1):139–45.
25. Visweswaran G, Gidea C, Baran D, Cohen M, Zucker M. Acute left ventricular dysfunction complicating pregnancy on ECMO: tri-iodothyronine to the rescue with real time transesophageal echocardiography. J Cardiol Cases. 2016;13:33–6.
26. Bencowitz HZ, LeWinter MM, Wagner PD. Effect of sodium nitroprusside on ventilation-perfusion mismatching in heart failure. J Am Coll Cardiol. 1984;4(5):918–22.
27. Bonet LA, Guillén RV, Lázaro IS, de la Fuente C, Osseyran F, Dolz LM, Hernández MM, Sanz MP, Otero MR, Sanz AS. Intravenous sildenafil in right ventricular dysfunction with pulmonary hypertension following a heart transplant. Heart Int. 2014;9(1):22–5.
28. Fernandes AM, Andrade AC, Barroso ND, Borges IC, Carvalho-Andrade D, Rodrigues Junior ES, Guimarães LC, Durães AR, Borges SM, Aras JR. The immediate effect of sildenafil on right ventricular function in patients with heart failure measured by cardiac magnetic resonance: a randomized control trial. PLoS One. 2015;10(3):e0119623.
29. van Vessem ME, Palmen M, Couperus LE, Mertens B, Berendsen RR, Tops LF, Verwey HF, de Jonge E, Klautz RJ, Schalij MJ, Beeres SL. Incidence and predictors of vasoplegia after heart failure surgery. Eur J Cardiothorac Surg. 2017;51(3):532–8.

30. Levin MA, Lin HM, Castillo JG, Adams DH, Reich DL, Fischer GW. Early on-cardiopulmonary bypass hypotension and other factors associated with vasoplegic syndrome. Circulation. 2009;120(17):1664–71.
31. Abdelazim R, Salah D, Labib HA, El Midany A. Methylene blue compared to norepinephrine in the management of vasoplegic syndrome in pediatric patients after cardiopulmonary bypass: a randomized controlled study. Egypt J Anaesth. 2016;32:269–75.
32. Mets B, Michler RE, Delphin ED, Oz MC, Landry DW. Refractory vasodilation after cardiopulmonary bypass for heart transplantation in recipients on combined amiodarone and angiotensin-converting enzyme inhibitor therapy: a role for vasopressin administration. J Cardiothorac Vasc Anesth. 1998;12(3):326–9.
33. Shieh JP, Chu CC, Chen JY, Chen YH, Yeh FC, Hsing CH. Acute fatal vasoplegia and asystole induced by intravenous amiodarone after cardiopulmonary bypass in a patient with preoperative cardiogenic shock. Acta Anaesthesiol Sin. 1999;37(4):205–10.
34. Cooper LB, Mentz RJ, Edwards LB, Wilk AR, Rogers JG, Patel CB, Milano CA, Hernandez AF, Stehlik J, Lund LH. Amiodarone use in patients listed for heart transplant is associated with increased 1-year post-transplant mortality. J Heart Lung Transplant. 2017;36(2):202–10.
35. Malone DL, Hess JR, Fingerhut A. Massive transfusion practices around the globe and a suggestion for a common massive transfusion protocol. J Trauma. 2006;60(6 Suppl):S91–6.
36. Andersen ND, Bhattacharya SD, Williams JB, Fosbol EL, Lockhart EL, Patel MG, Gaca JG, Welsby IJ, Hughes GC. Intraoperative use of low-dose recombinant activated factor VII during thoracic aortic operations. Ann Thoracic Surg. 2012;93:1921–9.
37. Thakar CV, Arrigain S, Worley S, Yared JP, Paganini EP. A clinical score to predict acute renal failure after cardiac surgery. J Am Soc Nephrol. 2005;16(1):162–8.
38. Smith EP. Hematologic disorders after solid organ transplantation. Hematology Am Soc Hematol Educ Program. 2010;2010:281–6.
39. Pavri BB, O'Nunain SS, Newell JB, Ruskin JN, William G. Prevalence and prognostic significance of atrial arrhythmias after orthotopic cardiac transplantation. J Am Coll Cardiol. 1995;25(7):1673–80.

40. Lushaj EB, Dhingra R, Chindhy S, Akhter S, Kohmoto T, Ulschmid S, Osaki S, Badami A, Lozonschi L. To use or not to use? Amiodarone before heart transplantation. Surgery. 2017;161(5):1273–8.
41. Cosío Carmena MD, Gómez Bueno M, Almenar L, Delgado JF, Arizón JM, González Vilchez F, Crespo-Leiro MG, Mirabet S, Roig E, Pérez Villa F, Fernández-Yañez JF, Lambert JL, Manito N, Fuente L, Sanz Julve ML, Pascual D, Rábago G, Millán I, Alonso-Pulpón LA, Segovia J. Primary graft failure after heart transplantation: characteristics in a contemporary cohort and performance of the RADIAL risk score. J Heart Lung Transplant. 2013;32(12):1187–95.
42. Kobashigawa J, Zuckermann A, Macdonald P, Leprince P, Esmailian F, Luu M, Mancini D, Patel J, Razi R, Reichenspurner H, Russell S, Segovia J, Smedira N, Stehlik J, Wagner F, Consensus Conference Participants. Report from a consensus conference on primary graft dysfunction after cardiac transplantation. J Heart Lung Transplant. 2014;33(4):327–40.
43. Dengler TJ, Zimmermann R, Braun K, Müller-Bardorff M, Zehelein J, Sack FU, Schnabel PA, Kübler W, Katus HA. Elevated serum concentrations of cardiac troponin T in acute allograft rejection after human heart transplantation. J Am Coll Cardiol. 1998;32(2):405–12.

Chapter 4
Damage Control in the Trauma ICU

Yanjie Qi

Objectives

1. Brief description of trauma critical care in the emergency room.
2. Examine the decisions and course of damage control surgery and the challenges of treating multisystem trauma patients.
3. Discuss damage control resuscitation of a trauma patient, including treatment of hypothermia, acidosis, and coagulopathy.
4. Discuss management of an open abdomen.

Y. Qi
Division of Trauma and Acute Care Surgery, Department of Surgery, University of Rochester Medical Center, Rochester, NY, USA
e-mail: yanjie_qi@urmc.rochester.edu

J. A. LaRosa (ed.), *Adult Critical Care Medicine*,
https://doi.org/10.1007/978-3-319-94424-1_4

Prehospital Course

The patient is a 59-year-old male who presented to the emergency department after a motor vehicle accident. Prehospital providers reported that the patient was a restrained driver, and airbag deployment was noted. There was prolonged extrication time (>60 min) due to steering wheel intrusion. The patient had shortness of breath on scene and complained of back pain. Due to agitation and mental status changes, the patient was intubated for airway protection. His heart rate was 82 beats per min (BPM), and blood pressure was 68/40 mmHg. The patient had a placement of two 18-gauge IVs and was given 3 liters of crystalloid fluids for hemodynamic instability.

The presentation of this patient is typical for admissions to a level 1 trauma center. As the quality of prehospital treatment of trauma patients improves, the acuity of trauma admissions has increased immensely. This presents a unique challenge to the trauma providers as they need to make potentially lifesaving decisions with incomplete and inaccurate information. For both the trauma surgeon and trauma ICU physician, the best approach is a broad differential diagnosis and preparation for the worse possible scenarios.

Emergency Room Course

Following Advanced Trauma Life Support (ATLS) protocol [1], the patient was first evaluated with the *primary survey*.

Airway:	Intubated with good end tidal CO_2
Breathing:	Bilateral breath sounds; O_2 saturation 100%
Circulation:	HR 87 BPM; BP 72/39 mmHg; Intact distal pulses
Disability:	GCS 3 – intubated; EMS reports that the patient has not moved his lower extremities
Exposure:	No skin lacerations or abrasions

Since he had already received >2 liters of crystalloid fluid, he was given two units of unmatched type O Rh negative packed red blood cells (pRBCs). As his age was suggestive of beta-blocker usage, he was given a dose of glucagon for beta-blocker reversal. This measure did not significantly increase his blood pressure. While the nursing staff was drawing labs and placing monitors, the trauma team completed the *secondary survey*, obtained initial chest and pelvic x-rays, placed femoral arterial and central venous introducer lines, and evaluated the patient with a focused assessment with sonography for trauma (FAST) exam. Throughout the evaluation, the patient was maintained on strict spine precautions per ATLS protocol [1]. The chest x-ray showed good positioning of the endotracheal tube and was negative for injury. The pelvis x-ray was negative for pelvic fractures. The secondary survey was significant for sedated patient with pinpoint pupils and abdominal distention. *Patient's FAST exam was positive for pericardial fluid stripe and intra-abdominal free fluid.* He was taken emergently to the operating room due to concern for both cardiac tamponade and intra-abdominal hemorrhage. The provider had noted that the patient's heart rate remained very low which was inconsistent with cardiac tamponade and hemorrhagic shock.

A comprehensive discussion of the indications for the operating room for trauma patients is beyond the scope of this chapter. While hemorrhage in the most common cause of shock in trauma, the provider must keep in mind other causes of hypotension. For older patients, cardiogenic shock is often a factor. Evaluation by EKG or ultrasound evaluation of ventricular function can help rule out massive myocardial infarction. In our case, the FAST exam was an expedient way to evaluate ventricular squeeze. Massive head trauma and spinal cord injuries are two other common causes of hemodynamic instability. Evaluation by imaging are often not feasible if the patient is unstable, but external signs of injury should prompt neurosurgical consultation and request for intracranial pressure (ICP) monitoring. Lastly, the location of the hemorrhage needs to be determined prior to the OR. Hence, the use of chest x-ray, pelvis x-ray, and FAST exam are essential for the evaluation of the unstable trauma patient and operative planning.

Past Medical/Surgical History

1. BPH (benign prostatic hyperplasia)
2. Depression
3. Hyperlipidemia
4. Hypertension
5. OSA (obstructive sleep apnea) – on CPAP at home

Home Medications

1. Simvastatin (Zocor) 40 mg tablet
2. Fenofibrate micronized (Lofibra) 134 mg capsule
3. Doxycycline hyclate (Oraxyl) 20 mg capsule
4. Losartan-hydrochlorothiazide (Hyzaar) 100–12.5 mg per tablet
5. Fluoxetine (Prozac) 20 mg capsule

Social History

1. Former smoker with 45 pack-year history
2. Occasional ETOH use
3. Works as a pharmacist

The past medical and surgical histories are often unattainable during the initial emergency room evaluation. When possible, trauma providers try to obtain a brief history by the AMPLE acronym: A, allergies; M, medications; P, past medical history; L, last meal; E, event history [1].

Admission Laboratory Results

	Ref. range	
WBC	4.2–9.1 thou/uL	6.4
RBC	4.6–6.1 mil/uL	2.5 (L)
Hemoglobin	13.7–17.5 g/dL	8.0 (L)
Hematocrit	40–51%	25 (L)
Platelets	150–330 thou/uL	115 (L)

	Ref. range	
Sodium, plasma	133–145 mmol/L	141
Potassium, plasma	3.4–4.7 mmol/L	4.3
Chloride, plasma	96–108 mmol/L	107
CO_2, plasma	20–28 mmol/L	16 (L)
Anion gap, PL	7–16	18 (H)
UN, plasma	6–20 mg/dL	28 (H)
Creatinine	0.67–1.17 mg/dL	1.60 (H)
Glucose, plasma	60–99 mg/dL	266 (H)
Lactate	0.5–2.2 mmol/L	5.4 (HH)

	Ref. range	
Protime	9.2–12.3 s	13.8 (H)
INR	1.0–1.2	1.2
aPTT	25.8–37.9 s	22.8 (L)
R Time	4.0–10.0 min	3.8 (L)

	Ref. range	
K Time	1.0–3.0 min	1.7
A Angle	53.0–73.0°	68.0
Maximum amplitude	50.0–72.0 mm	57.8
LY30	−0.1–7.5%	0.0
Coagulation index	−3.0–3.0	1.4

Admission laboratory values are often not useful in the acute trauma setting as they frequently do not reflect acute changes. In this particular case, the lab values were useful and quite clearly indicated blood loss that has been ongoing for some time. The patient's thromboelastogram (TEG) values indicate mild hypercoagulopathy which is often seen as the initial laboratory values.

Operating Room Course

The patient was taken emergently to the operating room for pericardial window and exploratory laparotomy. The anesthesia team was present during the evaluation in the trauma bay and aware of patient's instability. Massive transfusion protocol was initiated, alerting the blood bank to rapidly prepare coolers of blood products. The surgeon proceeded first with a surgical pericardial window. Upon opening the pericardium, relatively small amount of bloody fluid was evacuated. The pericardial sac was irrigated with warm saline and return of fluid was clear. More importantly, there was no major improvement in blood pressure with evacuation pericardial fluid, suggesting that cardiac tamponade was not a factor for patient's hypotension. The surgeon then moved onto exploratory laparotomy. The team evacuated approximately 1 liters of blood upon entrance to the abdomen; the abdomen was packed with laparotomy sponges in four quadrants. At this point, the surgical team alerted the anesthesia team and the intensive care team that this would likely be a damage control operation.

The most active bleeding was observed in the left upper quadrant. The spleen had multiple sites of injury, including at the splenic hilum. A splenectomy was performed with some difficulty due to patient's large body habitus and a distended stomach that could not be decompressed with nasogastric tube. The remaining quadrants were then examined. A large parenchymal laceration was seen on the liver just adjacent to the falciform ligament fossa. The falciform ligament was taken down and used as a buttress, and the laceration was repaired with large chromic sutures. A large capsular disruption was seen over the dome of the liver; this was packed with hemostatic agent and two laparotomy pads. The small bowel was examined in its entirety as was the colon to ensure no enteric injuries.

During the operation, the anesthesia team had been working continuously to keep up with operative bleeding. In total, the patient received 15 units of pRBCs, 12 units of fresh frozen plasma (FFP), 2 units of platelets, 1 unit of cryoprecipitate, and 3 liters of crystalloid. They were able to "catch up" with resuscitation as indicated by the arterial blood gas results below. However, the patient began to have diffuse oozing on all raw surfaces, the team was concerned for trauma-induced coagulopathy. As no active vessel bleeding was observed, the decision was made to pack the abdomen with a temporary vacuum dressing and take the patient to the ICU for correction of coagulopathy and hypothermia.

INITIAL ARTERIAL BLOOD GAS AND FINAL ARTERIAL BLOOD GAS VALUES

	Ref. range	**9PM**	**10.30PM**
pH	7.35–7.43	7.21 (L)	7.42
pCO_2, arterial	36–46 mmHg	48 (H)	38
pO_2, arterial	80–100 mmHg	197 (H)	395 (H)
CO_2, ART (Calc)	21–28 mmol/L	21	25
HCO_3, arterial	19–23 mmol/L	19	24 (H)
Base excess, arterial	−3–1 mmol/L	−9 (L)	0
FO_2 Hb, arterial	90–95%	98 (H)	99 (H)

For modern trauma surgeons, the treatment of severely injured patients (Injury Severity Score > 15) has been guided by the paradigm of damage control surgery (DCS). DCS has been defined as "planned temporary sacrifice of normal anatomy to preserve vital physiology" [2]. *Although DCS was originally described as an approach to patients with acute abdominal injury, the principle has been extended to the treatment of patients with vascular, thoracic, and orthopedic injuries as well. The overarching theory of DCS is that severely injured patients are too sick to survive the time period and physiological challenge needed for definitive repair. By definition, the patient who undergoes DCS is on the verge of physiological exhaustion. The three components of DCS are initial abbreviated laparotomy, ICU resuscitation, and subsequent reoperation for closure and definitive repair* [3].

*The trauma surgeon decides to perform DCS based on a number of factors (*Table 4.1*). Patients with high-energy blunt trauma, multiple torso penetrating trauma, hemodynamic instability, coagulopathy, and/or hypothermia on admission are much more likely to undergo DCS. Patients who are rec-*

Table 4.1 Damage control: key factors in patient selection

Conditions	High-energy blunt torso trauma
	Multiple torso penetrations
	Hemodynamic instability
	Coagulopathy and/or hypothermia
Injury complexes	Major abdominal vascular injury with multiple visceral injuries
	Multicavitary exsanguination with concomitant visceral injuries
	Multiregional injury with competing priorities
Critical factors	Severe metabolic acidosis (pH <7.3)
	Hypothermia (temperature <35 °C or <95 °F)
	Resuscitation and operative time >90 min
	Coagulopathy as evidence of nonmechanical bleeding
	Massive transfusion (>10 units of packed red blood cells)

Adapted from Rotondo and Zonies [6]

ognized to have complex vascular injuries, multicavitary injuries, or multiregional injuries are also best served by an abbreviated operation with an initial aim of controlling hemorrhage. Other indicators for DCS include acidosis, hypothermia, operative time greater than 90 min, ongoing coagulopathy as recognized by nonmechanical bleeding, and transfusion requirements of greater than ten units of packed red blood cells (RBCs) [4]. *Early recognition of the need for DCS is essential for optimal team communication and favorable patient outcomes.*

The operative goals of DCS are control of hemorrhage and gross contamination. The abdomen is opened with a generous midline incision. Hemorrhage control is gained with a variety of techniques depending on the type of injury, including packing, ligation, clamp application, and balloon catheter tamponade. Once bleeding is controlled, attention is turned to control of contamination. The bowel is examined along its entire length; small defects are closed with simple suture closure, and larger defects are quickly resected with staplers. No reconstructive efforts are made. Bowel is left in discontinuity and vessels may be kept patent with temporary shunts. The abdomen is then rapidly "closed" with a vacuum-type abdominal dressing [5]. *The abdominal dressing serves multiple purposes: (1) provides temporary abdominal coverage to allow for second-look surgery, (2) optimizes chances of eventual fascial closure by fully separating the abdominal contents from the abdominal wall and minimizing fascial retraction, (3) allows for means of continuous evacuation of fluid from the abdomen, and (4) allows for the expected expansion of bowel secondary to edema from fluid resuscitation.*

Trauma ICU Course

The ICU provider team was prepared to receive the patient with a pre-warmed room, hemodynamic monitoring tools, rapid infusion device, and additional nursing staff. Patient was transferred on ventilator support. His body temperature measured around 36°C in the operating room. In addition to increasing ambient room temperature, the patient was covered by a Bair Hugger forced-air warming system (3M, Saint Paul, MN). The IVF and blood products were warmed by the Level 1 ® H1200 infusion device (Smith Medical, Minneapolis, MN) prior to administration. He initially had acceptable systolic blood pressure around 110 mmHg. Soon after, the abdominal vacuum dressing volume output began to increase. The drainage appeared sanguineous and averaged 500–1000 mL per hour. He continued to have hypotension requiring blood products and low-dose vasopressors. His TEG results remained relatively normal, ruling out the possibility that hypercoagulability was the cause of rapid bleeding. After 6 h of resuscitation and warming attempts, patient was taken back to the operating room for re-exploration.

*Postoperatively, the patient arrives at the ICU with ongoing resuscitation needs and multiple complicating factors. Damage control resuscitation (DCR) is the subsequent aspect of the damage control paradigm. DCR is a systematic approach to the management of the trauma patient with severe injuries that starts in the emergency room and continues through the operating room and the ICU (*Fig. 4.1*). In the simplest sense, the goal of DCR is to halt the lethal triad of the bleeding trauma patient: hypothermia, acidosis, and coagulopathy. When combined with DCS, DCR has been shown to improve 30-day patient survival* [6]. *The five goals of DCR are (1) body rewarming, (2) correction of acidosis, (3) permissive hypotension, (4) restrictive fluid administration, and (5) hemostatic resuscitation* [7]. *Initial and recurrent communication between the surgeon and the intensivist is paramount for an efficient and successful resuscitation. The ICU team needs to comprehend the extent of injury, the overall stability of the patient, and extent of unresolved shock.*

Hypothermia

While there has been dozens of publications discussing the nuances of treating coagulopathy and acidosis, hypothermia has been a rare topic in the trauma literature. Perlman et al. *recently produced a concise review of hypothermia and its treatment in the trauma setting* [8]. *Hypothermia for trauma patients is defined as mild hypothermia (34–36 °C, 93.2–96.8 °F), moderate hypothermia (32–34 °C, 89.6–93.2 °F), and severe hypothermia (<32 °C, <89.6 °F), where normothermia is 37 ± 0.5 °C (98.6 °F). There are a number of risk factors for hypothermia, including high severity of injury (ISS > 40), extremes of age, wet clothing, general anesthesia in the field or in hospital, intubation, infusion of cold IV fluids, skin and organ exposure, and prolong operations. Hypothermia in the trauma patient contributes to worse coagulopathy, worse metabolic acidosis, and cardiac dysrhythmias and serious electrolyte disorders. Although hypothermia can have deleterious effects on a number of physiological processes, it is most*

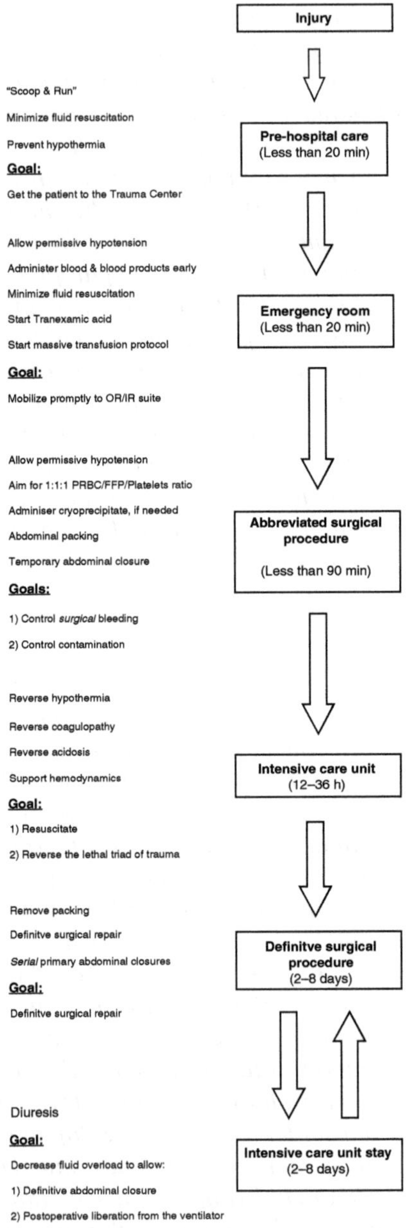

FIGURE 4.1 Damage control resuscitation goals and components. (Used with permission, Kaafarani and Velmahos [7])

prominent as a contributor of trauma-induced coagulopathy. Platelets and clotting factor enzymes are optimally active at 37 °C (98.6 °F). Platelet function is impaired between 33 and 37 °C (91.4–98.6 °F). Temperatures below 33 °C (91.4 °F) also inhibit thrombin, glycoprotein Ib-IX complex, platelet aggregation, and thromboxane B2 production. The prevention of hypothermia should be a priority for the prehospital and emergency room providers, as it becomes more difficult to rewarm the trauma patient once heat is lost. When preparing for patient to arrive from the ED or OR, the ICU room temperature should be elevated with assumption that hypothermia will be present. There are a variety of methods to rewarm a cold patient. Perlman et al. *suggested a temperature-guided protocol to rewarming using warmed IV fluids, warm blankets, and forced-air blankets as part of the ICU treatment.*

Acidosis/Circulatory Support

Although the patient will often arrive with central venous access, these lines are placed in the throes of initial ED resuscitation and in subpar sterile conditions. It is advisable to replace central venous access within 24 h of ICU admission. The initial arterial blood gas values including pH, lactate level, and base deficit are helpful in determining the extent of perfusion/oxygenation deficit. Volume loading is the mainstay of post-trauma circulatory support. Vasopressors should be used with extreme caution as they often compromise microvascular perfusion and mask ongoing hypovolemia and blood loss [9]. *Rather than aiming for normal blood pressure (BP), there has been a growing practice of allowing for permissive hypotension in the approach to an acutely bleeding patient. Permissive hypotension targets for a lower than normal BP, usually a systolic blood pressure of 80–90 mmHg or a mean arterial pressure (MAP) of 50 mmHg. The idea is that by lowering BP goals and decreasing the volume of resuscitative fluid, one can decrease the incidence and severity of dilutional coagulopathy and avoid the theoretical "pop the clot" effect. The case exception to permissive hypotension is in the setting of neurogenic injury. Patients with concomitant spinal cord or brain injuries may require vasopressor support to treat neurogenic shock or to maintain cerebral perfusion pressure; however, efforts need to be made to ensure adequate blood volume.*

The finding of acidosis is a reflection of poor tissue perfusion, and reversal of sodium bicarbonate has not been shown to improve clinical outcomes. Correction of the metabolic acidosis is better achieved through aggressive blood and blood product resuscitation and/or vasopressor support until surgical control of hemorrhage is achieved, shock is reversed, and end-organ perfusion is restored.

Coagulopathy

Trauma-induced coagulopathy (TIC) is attributed to one of the four basic mechanisms including (1) a qualitative platelet defect, (2) diffuse endothelial cell injury, (3) depletion of coagulation factors and platelets through hemorrhage and deposition into injuries, or (4) consumption of platelets and coagulation factors secondary to disseminated intravascular coagulation (DIC) or hyperfibrinolysis [10]. *TIC is worsened by acidosis and hypothermia. Acidemia diminishes coagulation factor enzymatic activity, depletes fibrinogen, and reduces the number of circulating platelets. Hypothermia is an independent risk factor for death during hemorrhagic shock. Complicating matters still further, patients may manifest a clotting issue initially but subsequently convert within hours to a hypercoagulable state and acquire risk for thromboembolic complications.*

Prior to the implementation of damage control resuscitation, severely injured patients received multiple liters of crystalloids and multiple units of pRBCs to maintain hemodynamics. The "unbalanced" fluid administrations in the bleeding trauma patient invariably led to depletion of coagulation factors, exacerbation of dilutional coagulopathy, and more bleeding. With the lessons learned from the military experience in the 1990s, the trauma community has produced multiple studies showing that decreasing use of crystalloid and an increased plasma to

RBC transfusion ratio have improved survival rates [11]. *While the exact ratio of FFP to RBC is still being debated, it is now an accepted practice that large-volume blood transfusion necessitates a balanced product ratio. Once the patient is recognized to having massive hemorrhage (fast rate of bleeding or requirement of more than ten units of blood), most centers now initiate the massive transfusion protocol (MTP). The details of the MTP vary with institutions; the basic tenants are protocol initiation by trauma, anesthesia or ICU team when large-volume hemorrhage is suspected, early and rapid type and cross of patient's blood, initial transfusion of uncrossed O-negative units, and rapid and frequent delivery of cooler packs with set ratio of pRBC and plasma/cryoprecipitate/platelets units* [12].

Once the patient becomes relatively stabilized, massive transfusion protocol can be transitioned to a goal-directed therapy. However, conventional coagulation tests, like prothrombin time and partial thromboplastin time, only describe isolated fragments of the hemostatic process and are poorly associated with bleeding and transfusion requirements. The platelet count itself does not reflect platelet function. Another problem with the conventional coagulation analysis is that the availability of the results is too slow to be of clinical relevance in the massively bleeding patient. Newer assays such as TEG (Haemonetics Corp., Braintree, MA) and ROTEM (Roche, Basel, Switzerland) assess the viscoelastic properties of coagulation in whole blood under low-shear conditions. Viscoelastic assays can identify coagulopathies secondary to impaired thrombin generation. Importantly, these assays can differentiate between low fibrinogen and reduced platelet function as the cause of impaired clot strength, as well as can identify systemic hyperfibrinolysis [13]. *Based on the tracings of clot formation, providers are able to identify component deficiency and use it to guide product replacement during trauma resuscitation.*

This case presents a good demonstration that aggressive warming, blood volume resuscitation, and treatment of acidosis should reverse the effects of the "lethal triad"; ICU intervention would not be effective for ongoing mechanical bleeding.

Frequent communication between the surgical and ICU teams is paramount for making the timely decision to return to the operating room.

Second Operating Room Course

Re-exploration of the abdomen simply required the removal of the vacuum dressing. As expected, a large quantity of clot and blood was encountered once the dressing was removed. After careful examination, the surgical team was able to locate a small vessel bleed along the tail of the pancreas. Once the bleeding vessel was ligated, the abdomen was again examined for additional bleeders. The injured areas of the liver appeared hemostatic, and the liver laparotomy pads were left in place. Three additional laparotomy pads were placed in the left upper quadrant in the splenic fossa and along the tail of the pancreas. The abdominal vacuum dressing was placed. From arrival to the ICU to the completion of the second exploration, the patient required an additional 12 units of pRBCs, 10 units of FFP, and 1 unit each of platelets and FFP.

Despite best clinical practices and diligent care, emergent reoperation is always a possibility. Unplanned return to the operating room usually occurs in three types of clinical scenarios: (1) ongoing bleeding, (2) missed enteric injury resulting in sepsis and shock, and, less frequently, (3) the development of abdominal compartment syndrome (ACS). If continuous mechanical hemorrhage is suspected, the surgeon and the ICU team must establish a transfusion threshold over a period of time as a trigger to return to the operating room. The close communication between ICU and surgical team is key for the immediate post-operative period. The goal of reoperation is to find the mechanical bleed or the source of contamination. Typically, the patient then returns to the ICU with an open abdomen and ongoing resuscitation needs as described above.

Subsequent Trauma ICU Course and Abdominal Closure

The patient returned to the ICU with stable hematocrit but continued to have need for low-dose norepinephrine drip for low BP and bradycardia. His abdominal drainage output slowed down, and the fluid appeared more serous. A formal bedside echocardiogram was performed shortly after surgery. It confirmed that he had good ventricular function.

The patient then completed his trauma evaluation by a *tertiary survey*, which includes a thorough physical exam, CT scans, and x-ray imaging, obtaining further details of the accident. After weaning from sedation, he was responsive and able to follow commands. It was immediately noted that the patient had loss of sensory and motor function in his lower extremities with high suspicion for spinal cord injury. The increased vagal tone from the spinal cord injury accounted for patient's persistent bradycardia and hypotension.

Patient's complete list of injuries:

1. Grade V splenic laceration.
2. Grade II liver laceration.
3. Grade I pancreatic contusion.
4. Complete three-column fracture-dislocation injury through the superior T3 vertebral level, with complete disruption of the facets and spinal canal. There was therefore presumed cord injury.
5. Extensive fractures involving the bilateral ribs and fracture dislocation involving the upper thoracic spine.
6. Left pubic symphysis fracture, left superior and inferior pubic rami fractures.
7. Nondisplaced fracture of the left sacral ala.

Orthopedic surgery was consulted for his spine and pelvis fractures. They recommended non-operative management of his pelvis fractures and surgical fixation for the spine fracture when medically ready. During the first 10 days of hospitalization, the patient returned to the OR multiple times for abdominal washouts and placement of a Wittman patch (Starsurgical, Burlington, WI) before his peritoneal cavity could be closed. The patient had placement of tracheostomy tube and gastrostomy feeding tube due to prolonged weaning from the ventilator and expected need for long-term enteral feeding access. He was initially very sensitive to turns and position changes, with severe bradycardia despite inotropic drugs. Over the course of week, the vasopressor drip was gradually weaned off and patient's heart rate remained normal.

Once the resuscitation phase has been completed, the patient is typically taken back to the operating room with 24–48 h for a second look and definitive repair surgery. The goals of the second-look surgery are to remove any surgical packing, anastomose any portions of resected bowel, repair laceration or install vascular grafts where temporary vascular shunts were placed, possible maturation of ostomy if indicated, and strategic placement of surgical drains. In many instances, surgeons choose to leave the abdominal fascia open after this second-look surgery. In the past, fascia edges were sewn together under tremendous pressure in an effort to close the abdomen as soon as possible. This led to high incidences of acute abdominal syndrome (ACS) after trauma laparotomies. Unrecognized ACS can be fatal, and its treatment requires return trip to the operating room and opening the abdominal cavity to relieve the intra-abdominal hypertension.

The general accepted practice now is to test the tightness of the fascia and abandon efforts to close the abdomen if the edges do not come together easily. In cases where the fascia is closed, the surgical team would ask the anesthesia team to keep close eye on the peak inspiratory pressure (PIP). If a large jump in PIP is noted once the closure is complete, the surgeon may choose to remove some or all of the stitches as elevated PIP is indicative of intra-abdominal hypertension and possible abdominal compartment syndrome. The abdomen is then dressed in a similar fashion to the first surgery. The commercially available negative pressure devices seem to be favored, because they allow fluid collection into a designated canister and can facilitate fluid loss measurements. In addition, many surgeons would install commercially available devices that allow tension to be placed on the fascial edges, such as the Wittmann patch in conjunction with the vacuum dressing. These dressings are changed in the intensive care unit every 2–3 days, and the Wittmann patch can be tightened during these sessions, bringing the fascia edges progressively closer as edema improves. The surgical team then determines the timing to return to the operating room for definitive closure. If fascia closure is no possible, most surgeons would utilize an absorbable mesh to bridge the defect and accept the large ventral hernia that will require eventual repair.

Patients should be monitored closely for fluid balance because patients with an open abdomen have increased fluid loss. These fluid losses may or may not need to be replaced based on the overall fluid status of the patient. An isotonic solution is commonly used for replacement. An open abdomen dressing does not necessitate antibiotic coverage unless there was concern of contamination during the surgery. Similarly, with a secure abdominal dressing, paralytic use is not necessary. Paralytic use is reserved for a very edematous, swollen abdomens where excess abdominal pressure would put the patient at risk for evisceration. As with any critically ill patients, the nutritional status is of great concern. In the past, patients were started on parenteral nutrition with the assumption that the GI tract of an open abdomen would not tolerate tube feeds. Recently, studies have demonstrated that enteral feeds can be commenced within 36 h of completion of acute resuscitation. There were no differences between patients receiving enteral or parenteral nutrition in terms of ventilator days, length of stay, or mortality. There was a lower rate of ventilator-associated pneumonia in the tube feed group [14].

Epilogue

The patient had a long hospital course in the trauma ICU, complicated by many typical ICU patient issues such as volume overload, mucus plugs, large pleural effusions, hospital acquired pneumonia, and clinical depression. After many weeks, the patient was able to maintain on minimal trach collar oxygen support and tolerating bolus gastric tube feeds. He was transferred to physical medicine and rehabilitation unit 3 months after his motor vehicle accident.

Summary

The severely injured trauma patient presents unique resuscitation challenges to the ICU provider. These patients arrive on the units in varying degrees of stability. The intensivist must be prepared to provide massive resuscitative measures to treat severe physiological derangements. The surgeon and the intensivist must have an efficient and communicative relationship to ensure the survival of these critically ill patients. The field of trauma surgery and trauma resuscitation has undergone tremendous change over the past few decades. The ICU provider is challenged to be more flexible and knowledgeable of the treatment paradigms of the trauma patient.

References

1. American College of Surgeons Committee on Trauma. Advanced trauma life support, student course manual, 9th ed. Chicago: American College of Surgeons, 2012. Print.
2. Scalea T. What's new in trauma in the past 10 years. Inter Anesth Clin. 2002;40:1–17.
3. Lee JC, Peitzman AB. Damage-control laparotomy. Curr Opin Crit Care. 2006;12(4):346–50.
4. Rotondo MF, Zonies DH. The damage control sequence and underlying logic. Surg Clin N Am. 1997;77(4):761–77.
5. Sagraves SG, Toschlog EA, Rotondo MF. Damage control surgery--the intensivist's role. J Intensive Care Med. 2006;21(1):5–16.

6. Cotton BA, Reddy N, Hatch QM, et al. Damage control resuscitation is associated with a reduction in resuscitation volumes and improvement in survival in 390 damage control laparotomy patients. Ann Surg. 2011;254(4):598–605.
7. Kaafarani HM, Velmahos GC. Damage control resuscitation in trauma. Scand J Surg. 2014;103(2):81–8.
8. Perlman R, Callum J, Laflamme C, Tien H, Nascimento B, Beckett A, et al. A recommended early goal-directed management guideline for the prevention of hypothermia-related transfusion, morbidity, and mortality in severely injured trauma patients. Crit Care. 2016;20(1):107.
9. Beloncle F, Meziani F, Lerolle N, Radermacher P, Asfar P. Does vasopressor therapy have an indication in hemorrhagic shock? Ann Intensive Care. 2013;3:13.
10. Pohlman TH, Walsh M, Aversa J, Hutchison EM, Olsen KP, Lawrence Reed R. Damage control resuscitation. Blood Rev. 2015;29(4):251–62.
11. Holcomb JB, del Junco DJ, Fox EE, et al. The prospective, observational, multicenter, major trauma transfusion (PROMMTT) study: comparative effectiveness of a time-varying treatment with competing risks. JAMA Surg. 2013;148(2):127–36.
12. Stephens CT, Gumbert S, Holcomb JB. Trauma-associated bleeding: management of massive transfusion. Curr Opin Anaesthesiol. 2016;29(2):250–5.
13. Johansson PI, Stensballe J, Oliveri R, et al. How I treat patients with massive hemorrhage. Blood. 2014;124:3052–8.
14. Dissanaike S, Pham T, Shalhub S, Warner K, Hennessy L, Moore EE, et al. Effect of immediate enteral feeding on trauma patients with an open abdomen: protection from nosocomial infections. J Am Coll Surg. 2008;207(5):690–7.

Chapter 5
Liver Failure in the ICU

Priyanka Rajaram and Ram Subramanian

Case 1

History of Present Illness

The patient is a 40-year-old woman with a history of alcohol abuse who presented to the emergency room with abdominal pain and fatigue progressively worsening over the past 3 days. The patient returned from the Bahamas 5 days prior to presentation where she endorsed drinking four mixed drinks per day along with taking large amount of acetaminophen for daily headaches. She complained of subjective fevers but denied chills, cough, chest pain, emesis, or diarrhea.

P. Rajaram · R. Subramanian (✉)
Emory University School of Medicine, Department of Medicine, Atlanta, GA, USA
e-mail: priyanka.rajaram@emory.edu; rmsubra@emory.edu

J. A. LaRosa (ed.), *Adult Critical Care Medicine*,
https://doi.org/10.1007/978-3-319-94424-1_5

Past Medical History

Alcohol abuse
Methicillin-resistant *Staphylococcus aureus* (MRSA) liver abscess

Physical Exam

On initial presentation, she was alert and answering questions appropriately. She was afebrile with a heart rate of 110 beats per minute (BPM) and blood pressure of 98/60 mmHg. Notable findings on physical exam included mild tenderness to palpation in the epigastric region and right upper quadrant. The remainder of her exam was unremarkable.

Laboratory Parameters and Diagnostic Testing

Her labs on presentation were notable for aspartate aminotransferase (AST) 1450 Unit/L, alanine aminotransferase (ALT) 680 Unit/L, alkaline phosphatase 70 Unit/L, total bilirubin 5.1 mg/dL, international normalized ratio (INR) of 2.1, and acetaminophen level of 65 mcg/ml. The rest of her laboratory testing including a basic metabolic panel (BMP) and complete blood count (CBC) were normal. A computerized tomography (CT) of her head did not show evidence of acute intracranial abnormalities.

Differential Diagnosis

Her labs raise suspicion for acute liver injury. While alcohol abuse and acetaminophen overdose are at the top of our list as causes of direct liver injury, we should also consider acute viral hepatitis and Budd-Chiari syndrome as possible precipitants. At this time, she does not appear to be in fulminant liver failure based on her mental status and synthetic function; however, the key is to closely monitor her over the next several hours for changes in her mentation and liver function tests.

Case Summary

She was admitted to the ICU and initiated on N-acetylcysteine infusion per protocol. Over the next 24 h, she was noted to have a significant decline in her mental status with inability to maintain eye contact and answer questions appropriately. An ultrasound of her liver with Doppler did not show evidence of hepatic or portal vein thrombosis. She was noted to have significant worsening of her liver function tests and synthetic function as shown in Table 5.1. She was electively intubated and placed on mechanical ventilation for grade 3 hepatic encephalopathy. Given the risk for developing intracranial hypertension, the patient was initiated on hypertonic saline to achieve a serum Na level of 145–155 mEq/L. On day 3 of admission, she was noted to be in anuric renal failure with ongoing fulminant liver failure. The patient was initiated on continuous renal replacement therapy and listed for liver transplantation. On hospital day 5, she received a suitable organ offer. A preoperative head CT did not demonstrate any evidence of cerebral edema. She subsequently underwent uneventful liver transplantation, without any intraoperative or postoperative complications. Her postoperative course

Table 5.1 Summary of liver function tests, creatinine, and synthetic function

Parameters	Initial	8 h	24 h	30 h
AST (U/L)	1450	5420	7819	8206
ALT (U/L)	680	2949	4502	5702
INR	2.1	5.6	7.9	9.9
Total bilirubin (mg/dl)	5.1	6.5	7.8	8.1
Creatinine (mg/dl)	0.99	1.64	2.71	3.32
Ammonia (umol/L)	65	299	600	490

Key Points

1. Acute liver failure, previously known as fulminant hepatic failure, is defined as the development of hepatocellular dysfunction manifesting as coagulopathy and encephalopathy in patients without preexisting liver disease over a period of less than 6 months.
2. Early recognition and close monitoring of liver function tests and mental status during the first several hours to days are of utmost importance.
3. All patients should undergo diagnostic imaging with abdominal ultrasound with Doppler or abdominal CT/ MRI to assess patency of hepatic and portal veins, presence of ascites, and liver size.
4. Hepatic encephalopathy (HE) is considered a precursor to the development of cerebral edema and intracranial hypertension (ICH) in these patients. Therapy for advanced HE in ALF (such as hypertonic saline) should be targeted at mitigating the development of ICH.
5. Early transfer to the nearest liver transplant center is recommended, given the potential for rapid deterioration as in this case.

was characterized by the resolution of her multi-organ system dysfunction; of note, her encephalopathy resolved without any neurologic sequelae, and she was extubated on postoperative day 4.

Case 2

History of Present Illness

The patient is a 62-year-old male with a history of cirrhosis secondary to alpha-1 antitrypsin deficiency, who was hospitalized for hematemesis. This was his fourth episode in a period of 2 months. Esophagogastroduodenoscopy (EGD) was performed which showed esophageal varices that were amenable to banding. During this period, he received transfusion of blood products to maintain hemoglobin level > 7 gm/dl, octreotide infusion, and proton pump inhibitor infusion. MELD score was 16.

Past Medical History

1. Alpha-1 antitrypsin deficiency
2. End-stage liver disease
3. Coronary artery disease

Physical Exam

He was afebrile with a HR 110 bpm, BP 111/51. He appeared comfortable with no abdominal tenderness, distention, or fluid wave. The most notable finding on exam was gynecomastia and spider nevi.

Laboratory Parameters

After transfusion of two units of packed red blood cells, his hemoglobin was 6.7 gm/dl. Other notable labs included a serum creatinine of 1.12 mg/dl, total bilirubin of 3.8 mg/dl, and INR 1.39.

Diagnostic Considerations

The patient continued to have recurrent episodes of significant hematemesis along with confusion which required endotracheal intubation and mechanical intubation. Given his recurrent bleeding that was refractory to endoscopic therapy, a transjugular intrahepatic portosystemic shunt (TIPS) was performed by interventional radiology. In addition, an urgent liver transplant evaluation was initiated.

Case Summary

Over the next few days, he continued to remain hypotensive requiring vasopressor support. He was initiated on broad spectrum antibiotic coverage despite no evidence of spontaneous bacterial peritonitis or other infectious etiology. During this time, his MELD continued to rise to 27 and eventually to 40. He was deemed to be a candidate for liver transplantation after a review of his prior recent cardiopulmonary evaluation and was listed urgently for transplant. While awaiting transplant, he developed type 1 hepatorenal syndrome (HRS) and anuric acute kidney injury (AKI) with an increase in his volume status, hyperkalemia, and an anion gap metabolic

Key Points

1. In the setting of variceal bleeding that is refractory to endoscopic therapy, TIPS should be considered to achieve hemostasis.
2. Type 1 hepatorenal syndrome (HRS) is characterized by a rapid and progressive decline in renal function, which can exacerbate preexisting metabolic acidosis and hypervolemia.
3. The management of HRS is multifaceted, with liver transplantation being the ultimate cure. Pharmacologic interventions that can be considered prior to CRRT include octreotide and midodrine, terlipressin, and norepinephrine.
4. Continuous renal replacement therapy (CRRT) continues to remain an important option in patients who fail medical therapy and serves as a bridge to liver transplantation.

acidosis. The patient was started on octreotide and midodrine without significant improvement. Continuous renal replacement therapy (CRRT) was initiated, with a subsequent improvement in his acid base and volume status. Following a suitable organ donor offer, the patient underwent successful liver transplantation without any intraoperative complications. In the postoperative period, CRRT was discontinued after 10 days as the patient regained his intrinsic renal function.

Case 3

History of Present Illness

The patient is a 52-year-old lady with autoimmune cirrhosis and a MELD score of 17, who presents for a liver transplant evaluation. She complains of progressive dyspnea on exertion associated with palpitations, lower extremity edema, and near-syncopal events. No history of chest pain or cardiac events in the past. She is a never smoker.

Past Medical History

1. Autoimmune cirrhosis
2. Gastroesophageal reflux disease

Physical Exam

At her clinic visit, she has a heart rate of 110 bpm and blood pressure of 98/60 mmHg. Pertinent findings on exam include mild abdominal distention with a fluid wave, trace lower extremity pitting edema, and a pronounced P2 component of the second heart sound along with a faint holosystolic murmur in the left upper sternal border.

Laboratory Parameters and Diagnostic Testing

Her labs were notable for a brain natriuretic peptide (BNP) of 200 pg/ml, creatinine 1.20 mg/dl, bilirubin 2.0 mg/dl, INR 1.4, and sodium 135 mEq/L. Her echocardiogram showed evidence of normal left ventricular function, grade 1 diastolic dysfunction, elevated right ventricular systolic pressure of 68 mmHg, moderately dilated right ventricle, and moderately reduced right ventricular systolic function. Her chest radiograph showed cardiomegaly and enlarged pulmonary artery without any evidence of pulmonary edema or pleural effusions.

Differential Diagnosis

Based on her symptoms and echocardiogram, there is a high suspicion for pulmonary hypertension (PH). Two distinct types of PH are seen in cirrhotics – portopulmonary hypertension and pulmonary venous hypertension. The gold standard for diagnosis is a right heart catheterization (RHC) to assess pulmonary hemodynamics, particularly the pulmonary artery wedge pressure (PAWP) to distinguish between the two forms.

Case Summary

The patient underwent a RHC which showed a mean pulmonary artery pressure of 54 mmHg, PAWP 6 mmHg, cardiac output 7 L/min, and pulmonary vascular resistance of 6.8 Wood units. Her central venous saturation during the RHC was 58%. These RHC findings were consistent with a diagnosis of portopulmonary hypertension (POPH). Given her significant symptoms with the near-syncopal episodes and low cardiac output, she was admitted to the ICU after the RHC and initiated on intravenous epoprostenol 2 ng/kg/min. Over the next few days, the epoprostenol was titrated up to a dose of 18 ng/kg/min with improvement in central venous saturation

Key Points

1. Portopulmonary hypertension (POPH), a rare subset of pulmonary arterial hypertension, is defined as the presence of portal hypertension with a mPAP ≥25 mmHg, PAWP ≤15 mmHg, and PVR > 3 Wood units or 240 dyne/s/cm – 5 as measured during RHC.
2. All cirrhotic patients undergoing evaluation for liver transplantation or those with worsening dyspnea on exertion undergo an echocardiogram to screen for pulmonary hypertension.
3. Following a diagnosis of POPH on RHC, treatment includes oral or intravenous medications such as phosphodiesterase 5 inhibitors, endothelin receptor antagonists, and, in severe cases, prostacyclin receptor agonists such as IV epoprostenol.
4. The goal is to improve pulmonary hemodynamics to mPAP <35 mmHg and PVR < 3 Wood units prior to liver transplantation in order to minimize the intraoperative risk of acute right heart failure.

to 69%. The patient was discharged home with a Hickman catheter for continuous epoprostenol infusion and repeat right heart catheterization in 3 months.

Case 4

History of Present Illness

The patient is a 60-year-old male with end-stage liver disease secondary to Budd-Chiari syndrome and hepatocellular carcinoma who is postoperative day 1 from an orthotopic liver transplant (OLT). Patient was successfully extubated in the postoperative setting. He was noted to have mild abdominal tenderness and complained of nausea. No fevers or chills. Review of systems was otherwise unremarkable.

Past Medical History

1. End-stage liver disease secondary to Budd-Chiari syndrome
2. Hepatocellular carcinoma
3. Obstructive sleep apnea
4. Gastroesophageal reflux disease

Physical Exam

He was afebrile with a heart rate of 85 bpm, blood pressure 135/87 mmHg, and breathing comfortably on 2 liters of supplemental oxygen via nasal cannula. His physical exam was notable for mild tenderness to palpation around his incision site without significant drainage or bleeding. He was noted to have diminished bowel sounds, and the abdominal drain had serosanguinous drainage. The remainder of his exam was unremarkable.

Laboratory Parameters

On postoperative day 1, his total bilirubin was 1.6 mg/dL, AST 2233 unit/L, ALT 2981 unit/L, and ALP 230 unit/L. His INR was noted to be 1.7 with elevation in white blood cell count to 16.3 /mcl. His hemoglobin level remained stable at 10.1 g/dL. An echocardiogram was obtained which showed normal left ventricular systolic function, grade 1 diastolic dysfunction, and normal right ventricular size and function.

Differential Diagnosis

Common issues to be aware of in the immediate postoperative period after liver transplantation are hemorrhage, vascular complications, allograft dysfunction, and cardiopulmonary complications. Given no significant changes in his hemoglobin, there is a low concern for life-threatening abdominal hemorrhage. Likewise, cardiopulmonary complications can be ruled out based on his vital signs and echocardiogram. The acute rise in his liver function tests is concerning for vascular complications such as hepatic artery thrombosis, which can be detected on ultrasound of the abdomen with Doppler or CT angiogram of the abdomen.

Case Summary

A right upper quadrant ultrasound with Doppler was performed which showed normal liver parenchyma without intrahepatic dilatation and mild perihepatic fluid. The hepatic and portal veins were patent with appropriate flow; however, the hepatic artery was not visualized, raising suspicion for hepatic artery thrombosis. A CT scan with angiogram of the abdomen was obtained which confirmed the diagnosis. The patient immediately underwent hepatic artery thrombectomy

Key Points

1. Thrombosis of the hepatic artery is one of the most frequent complications seen in the postoperative period, particularly in the pediatric population.
2. Risk factors for the development of hepatic artery thrombosis include poor arterial flow, increased sinusoidal resistance, and stenosis of the anastomosis.
3. Immediate complications include ischemia or necrosis of the allograft. In addition, since the hepatic artery is the sole arterial supply for the biliary system, long-term biliary complications characterized by diffuse non-anastomotic biliary stricturing can be seen several weeks to months after the transplant.
4. Thrombolysis and arterial thrombectomy are options in the acute setting which can be performed by interventional radiology or surgically. However, if this fails, urgent re-transplantation is required.

with infusion of tissue plasminogen activator (tPa) into the hepatic allograft. After the procedure, patient continued to have sustained elevation in his liver function tests which was deemed due to massive hepatocellular injury in the setting of the hepatic artery thrombosis. At this point, he was re-listed as status 1 for liver transplantation and underwent re-transplantation 6 days later.

Suggested Reading

1. Arroyo V, Moreau R, Jalan R, et al. Acute-on-chronic liver failure: a new syndrome that will re-classify cirrhosis. J Hepatol. 2015;62:S131–43.
2. Kandiah P, Olson J, Subramanian RM. Emerging strategies for the treatment of patients with acute hepatic failure. Curr Opin Crit Care. 2016;22:142–51.
3. Bernal W, Wendon J. Acute liver failure. N Engl J Med. 2014;370:1170–1.
4. Larsen FS, Schmidt LE, Bernsmeier C, et al. High-volume plasma exchange in patients with acute liver failure: an open randomized controlled trial. J Hepatol. 2016;64:69–78.
5. Karvellas CJ, Fix OK, Battenhouse H, et al. Outcomes and complications of intracranial pressure monitoring in acute liver failure: a retrospective cohort study. Crit Care Med. 2014;42:1157–67.
6. Shami VM, Caldwell SH, et al. Recombinant activated factor VII for coagulopathy in fulminant hepatic failure compared with conventional therapy. Liver Transpl. 2003;9:138–43.
7. Ede RJ, Gimson AE, Bihari D, et al. Controlled hyperventilation in the prevention of cerebral oedema in fulminant hepatic failure. J Hepatol. 1986;2:43–51.
8. Ford RM, Sakaria SS, Subramanian RM. Critical care management of patients before liver transplantation. Transplant Rev. 2010;24:190–206.
9. Arroyo V, Gines P, Gerbes AL, et al. Definition and diagnostic criteria of refractory ascites and hepatorenal syndrome in cirrhosis. International Ascites Club. Hepatology. 1996;23:164–76.
10. Runyon BA. Management of adult patients with ascites due to cirrhosis: an update. Hepatology. 2009;49:2087–107.

11. Garcia-tsao G, Sanyal AJ, Grace ND, et al. Prevention and management of gastroesophageal varices and variceal hemorrhage in cirrhosis. Hepatology. 2007;46:922–38.
12. Abraldes JG, Villanueva C, Banares R, et al. Hepatic venous pressure gradient and prognosis in patients with acute variceal bleeding treated with pharmacologic and endoscopic therapy. J Hepatol. 2008;48:229–36.
13. Krowka MJ, Wiesner RH, Heimbach JK. Pulmonary contraindication, indications and MELD exceptions for liver transplantation: a contemporary view and look forward. J Hepatol. 2013;59:367–74.

Chapter 6
Harm and Quality in the ICU

Jennifer A. LaRosa

Case Study

History of present illness: FC is a 59-year-old 77-kg African-American male admitted to the intensive care unit (ICU) through the emergency department (ED) 6 days ago after he presented with 2 weeks of worsening shortness of breath, dyspnea on exertion, cough with production of yellow-green sputum, anorexia, and malaise. At the time of admission, he denied sick contacts but does report that he had a similar, self-limited illness about a month ago.

Review of systems on admission was positive for the following findings:

Intermittent palpitations with strenuous exertion
Difficulty sleeping with occasional night sweats and periods of feeling very cold

J. A. LaRosa
Newark, NJ, USA
e-mail: Jennifer.LaRosa@RWJBH.org

J. A. LaRosa (ed.), *Adult Critical Care Medicine*,
https://doi.org/10.1007/978-3-319-94424-1_6

Past medical history:

Essential systemic hypertension ×14 years
Hyperlipidemia ×14 years
Benign prostatic hypertrophy ×3 years

Social history:

Tobacco use – started smoking cigarettes at age 20; smokes ½ pack per day.
EtOH – patient reports 2–4 beers per night on weekend nights only.
The patient denies the use of illicit drugs now or ever.
He works as a driver and delivery representative for UPS.
He is married and has three children.

Family history:

The patient reports that he was adopted as a baby and does not know any genetic family history. His children are 22, 17, and 13 years old and all are in good health.

Medications:

Lisinopril	20 mg PO QD
Atorvastatin	20 mg PO QD
Tamsulosin	0.4 mg PO QD

Hospital course: In the ED, the patient was intubated for both hypoxemia and hypercarbia, and vasopressors were started through a right internal jugular catheter after resuscitation with crystalloid for hypotension and organ hypoperfusion. Strict intake and output measurements were noted, the latter through an intra-urinary catheter.

During the first 3 days in the ICU, he improved clinically. The mechanical ventilator was weaned to the following settings with the associated ABG.

Volume-controlled ventilation:

- FiO2 0.6
- Tidal volume 450 mL

- Respiratory rate 16 breaths per minute (no overdrive breathing triggered by the patient)
- PEEP 5 cmH_2O

ABG: 7.38/45/62/28/96 reported as $pH/PaCO_2/PaO_2/HCO^3/SpO_2$.

Maintenance intravenous fluids with electrolyte repletions were continued, and norepinephrine infusion was weaned down to 4 μg/min on ICU day #3 (from a peak of 24 μg/min). Extremities were warm with 2+ distal pulses, the patient was arousable and followed commands during a brief sedation vacation, and urine output was brisk.

Over the last 24 h, however, going from ICU day #5 into ICU day #6, the patient spiked a temperature of 39.6 °C (103.3 °F), he became restless and agitated with a blood pressure dip to 73/44 (MAP 54) and a prolonged desaturation to an SpO_2 of 78%. In response to these events, respiratory therapy was able to accelerate ventilation with the Ambu-bag and increase his SpO_2 to 92%. Physical exam revealed tachycardia with frequent premature atrial complexes, diffuse rhonchi bilaterally, warm extremities, faint distal pulses, and poor capillary refill. Ventilator support was augmented by increasing FiO2 to 1.00 and PEEP to10 cm H_2O. Two additional liters of crystalloid were administered following which norepinephrine dose was increased to 20 μg/min to achieve a consistent MAP >65 mmHg. Urine output dwindled for a 24-h output of 560 mL and a current rate of 3–5 mL/h.

Physical examination: On ICU day #6, current vital signs are as follows:

T – 39.6 °C (103.3°F)
BP – 93/42 (MAP 59) mmHg
HR – 117
RR – 16/22 (ventilator/patient overdrive)
HEENT: endotracheal tube in place measured at 20 cm at patient's teeth, neck supple, shoddy anterior cervical lymphadenopathy
Cardiovascular: tachycardia, no murmurs or rubs

Pulmonary: diffuse rhonchi throughout both lung fields, normal chest movement and excursion, diffuse percussion dullness
Abdomen: faint bowel sounds, no organomegaly, or tenderness
Extremities: warm to touch, faint distal pulses, sluggish capillary refill, scant but notable mottling on both feet
Neurologic: sedated with little purposeful movement, even with reduced sedation

Pertinent laboratory values and radiographs:

Study	ICU day #1	ICU day #2	ICU day #3	ICU day #4	ICU day #5	ICU day #6
WBC in __× 10^3MCL	16.4	14.4	11.5	15.5	22.1	33.8
Bands	11	6	6	3	22	38
Hemoglobin in G/DL	14.6	12.5	12.0	12.7	11.9	12.2
BUN & Cr in MG/DL	45 & 1.7	30 & 1.2	28 and 1.3	32 and 1.3	40 and 2.2	45 and 3.4
PaO_2/FiO_2	77/0.7	72/0.5	64/0.45	66/0.4	54/0.8	58/1.0
CXR	RML consolidation	RML consolidation	Improvement in RML consolidation	Clearing RML consolidation	Diffusion bilateral air space disease, no lobar consolidation	Dense diffuse, worsening bilateral air space disease

Day #1 sputum culture and 1 out of 2 peripheral blood cultures grew *Klebsiella pneumoniae*. Initial broad-spectrum antimicrobials (maxipime and vancomycin) were de-escalated to piperacillin-tazobactam to which the *Klebsiella* was noted to be sensitive.

Differential Diagnoses

This patient was admitted with a diagnosis of community-acquired pneumonia with acute respiratory failure and septic shock with end-organ dysfunction. He was appropriately resuscitated with intravenous fluids, broad spectrum antimicrobials, mechanical ventilation, and optimization of end-organ perfusion. His improvement was marked by a reduced A-a gradient as well as reduced need for ventilator and vasopressor support. This improvement was abruptly thwarted on days #5 and #6 when the patient became febrile and hemodynamically unstable. Though the differential diagnoses for this deterioration are broad, nearly every potential etiology falls into the category of hospital-acquired condition (HAC) or, more specifically, a HAC subset known as healthcare-acquired infections (HAIs). Potential HACs in this patient include the following:

- CAUTI Catheter-associated urinary tract infection
- CLABSI Central line-associated bloodstream infection
- VAE Ventilator-associated event (ventilator-associated pneumonia)
- VTE Venous thromboembolism

Introduction

To Err is Human was published by the Institute of Medicine (IOM) in 1999 and catalyzed the study of reproducible and sustainable safety and quality and prevention of unintended harm in healthcare arenas [1]. This report estimated that as many as 98,000 US deaths occur annually as a result of preventable medical harm. More recent figures have re-estimated this figure to be almost 4 ½ times higher with an annual death toll as high as 440,000, a figure that may contribute to 1/6 of all hospital deaths [2]. The National Patient Safety Foundation now reports preventable medical harm as the number one cause of death in the United States [3]. As impressive as these figures are, they are likely a mere fraction of the morbidity that occurs as a result of medical errors but is much harder to capture due to variability and inconsistency in reporting and attribution. As many as 33% of patients are estimated to be the victims of some preventable harm during their hospital stay [4]. In addition to the massive human cost, healthcare expenditures have reached an all-time high with estimates at over $36 billion dollars spent on medical errors and adverse events together [5].

Healthcare aims to provide evidence-based safe care that is consistent, predictable, reproducible, and sustainable. It sounds easy but it is not. Successfully translating these principles to the bedside is constantly thwarted by variability, inconsistency, sloppiness, and ego. In 2006, Dr. Peter Pronovost and colleagues demonstrated, through their landmark Michigan Keystone Project, that a simple checklist could reduce their rates of CLABSI by as much as 66% [6].

Critical care units are ideal venues for studying these concepts since they are inherently chaotic and house the most vulnerable patients, undergoing the most invasive diagnostics and therapeutics. A 1995 investigation by Donchin and colleagues found that nearly two errors per day occurred for every patient in the intensive care unit (ICU) [7]. The team introduced a real-time error-reporting system with notation of the following:

- Severity
- Body system
- Type of medical activity
- Date and time of discovery
- Identities of those who committed and discovered the error
- Presumed cause

Investigators concluded that a severe or potentially detrimental error occurred, on average, 1.7 times per day per patient. This study introduced an accurate and precise measurement tool for collecting information about adverse events. Uncovering the reasons why such events occur is critical to developing strategies and processes that reduce their recurrence.

Risk and harm rarely occur as the result of one single error. They occur when each and every barrier of protection has been violated at some level. This is known as the Swiss cheese model, and it has been used to describe the mechanism of harm when each safety layer is breached, allowing harm a pathway directly to the patient [8].

Take the four stages of medication management, by way of example – prescribing, transcribing, dispensing, and administering. Each of the four steps has to be violated for harm to occur [9]. For example:

- The physician prescribes a medication using poor handwriting.
- The pharmacist transcribes it as he believes it is written but does not clarify.
- The pharmacy technician dispenses the medication even though it means splitting pills because he doesn't want to bother the pharmacist with clarification.
- The nurse does not check the patient's identification or the drug and dose before she administers it.
- The wrong patient gets the wrong medication at the wrong dose and dies.

If, at any step along this way, one or more individuals had followed their process precisely, an error would likely not have occurred. The Checklist Manifesto, published in 2009 by Dr. Atul Gawande, was the first earnest attempt to translate the rigorous and wildly successful use of the checklist as a safety tool in aviation to the practice of medicine [10]. Dr. Gawande notes, "the volume and complexity of what we know has exceeded our individual ability to deliver its benefits correctly, safely, or reliably." Healthcare providers are not asked or expected to remember everything all the time. We are, however, expected to follow protocols, to use job aides, and to perform consistently. These fundamental concepts make up the structure of high reliability organizations [11]. The remainder of this chapter will focus on the following two areas as they apply to quality and safety in critical care units.

- Reportable metrics
- Quality and safety basics

Reportable Metrics

Healthcare costs in the US are currently funded via three sources. Out-of-pocket patient expense and insurance company reimbursements make up close to half of this cost. The remaining 50% plus is absorbed by federal, state, and local governments [12]. Needless to say, this financial responsibility strongly incentivizes the government to consolidate services, mitigate risk, and avoid unnecessary cost. Hospital-acquired conditions (as listed in Table 6.1) are the natural starting place for such restrictions, and in 2008, the Centers for Medicare and Medicaid Services (CMS) included ten categories of hospital-acquired conditions (HACs) that were selected for HAC payment penalties [13]. Payment penalties for failure to prevent harm in these areas commenced on October 1, 2008. In addition to payment penalties, private organizations like The Joint Commission and The Leapfrog Group collect, assimilate, and analyze data from CMS [14]. They then publicize a score that reflects aggregated safety outcomes in each healthcare facility.

Hospital-acquired infections (HAIs) are a subset of HACs and are also exceedingly common in critical care settings. The National Quality Forum (NQF) estimates that as many as two million HAIs occur annually in the United States, accounting for an estimated 90,000 deaths [15]. A 2009 CDC study estimated costs associated with HAI at more than $5 billion annually – greater than the cost of either diabetes mellitus with complications ($4.5 billion) or chronic obstructive lung disease ($4.2 billion) [16].

Patient safety indicators (PSIs) are another repository of reportable means of harm with considerable crossover with HACs and HAIs [17]. They are listed in Table 6.2. Like HACs, PSIs are based on documentation and coding data and are entirely retrospective. There are currently 25 PSIs, all of which are related to harm from or related to a surgery, invasive procedures, or childbirth. Like HACs and HAIs, PSIs incur both considerable patient harm and financial penalties with CMS.

A comprehensive summary of all HACs (including HAIs) and PSIs is beyond the scope of this chapter. That said, the case study above represents harm that falls into the categories of HAC, HAI, and PSI. Now that we appreciate the means and gravity of much healthcare-induced harm, it is

TABLE 6.1 CMS hospital-acquired conditions

Foreign object retained after surgery
Air embolism
Blood incompatibility
Stage III and IV pressure ulcers
Falls and trauma
Fractures
Dislocations
Intracranial injuries
Crushing injuries
Burn
Other injuries
Manifestations of poor glycemic control
Diabetic ketoacidosis
Nonketotic hyperosmolar coma
Hypoglycemic coma
Secondary diabetes with ketoacidosis
Secondary diabetes with hyperosmolarity
Catheter-associated urinary tract infection (UTI)
Vascular catheter-associated infection
Surgical site infection, mediastinitis, following coronary artery bypass graft (CABG):
Surgical site infection following bariatric surgery for obesity
Laparoscopic gastric bypass
Gastroenterostomy
Laparoscopic gastric restrictive surgery

(continued)

TABLE 6.1 (continued)

Surgical site infection following certain orthopedic procedures
Spine
Neck
Shoulder
Elbow
Surgical site infection following cardiac implantable electronic device (CIED)
Deep vein thrombosis (DVT)/pulmonary embolism (PE) following certain orthopedic procedures:
Total knee replacement
Hip replacement
Iatrogenic pneumothorax with venous catheterization

TABLE 6.2 AHRQ patient safety indicators

PSI 02 Death rate in low-mortality diagnosis related groups (DRGs)
PSI 03 Pressure ulcer rate
PSI 04 Death rate among surgical inpatients with serious treatable conditions
PSI 05 Retained surgical item or unretrieved device fragment count
PSI 06 Iatrogenic pneumothorax rate
PSI 07 Central venous catheter-related blood stream infection rate
PSI 08 Postoperative hip fracture rate
PSI 09 Perioperative hemorrhage or hematoma rate
PSI 10 Postoperative acute kidney injury requiring dialysis
PSI 11 Postoperative respiratory failure rate
PSI 12 Perioperative pulmonary embolism or deep vein thrombosis rate

TABLE 6.2 (continued)

PSI 13 Postoperative sepsis rate
PSI 14 Postoperative wound dehiscence rate
PSI 15 Accidental puncture or laceration rate
PSI 16 Transfusion reaction count
PSI 17 Birth trauma rate – injury to neonate
PSI 18 Obstetric trauma rate – vaginal delivery with instrument
PSI 19 Obstetric trauma rate – vaginal delivery without instrument
PSI 21 Retained surgical item or unretrieved device fragment rate
PSI 22 Iatrogenic pneumothorax rate
PSI 23 Central venous catheter-related blood stream infection rate
PSI 24 Postoperative wound dehiscence rate
PSI 25 Accidental puncture or laceration rate
PSI 26 Transfusion reaction rate
PSI 27 Postoperative hemorrhage or hematoma rate
PSI 90 Patient safety for selected indicators
PSI Appendices

imperative that we understand how to mitigate risk and provide predictable, comprehensive, and sustainable excellence in the care we provide.

Quality: Six Sigma, CUSP, and Just Culture

"Variety is the spice of life," said William Cowper in his 1785 poem, "The Task." While that may be true for matters of the heart (i.e., nonmedical matters), it is largely not so for the delivery of healthcare [18].

Dr. David Shaywitz said in his 2009 op-ed piece in The Healthcare Blog, "Businesses have long known about the benefits of standardization – lower costs, higher baseline quality — and have aspired to achieve it. The ability to make the same product in the exact same way every single time has contributed materially to the success of companies from McDonalds to Intel. The global adoption of the "Six Sigma" program, an initiative originally developed by Motorola to reduce variability and ensure consistency, is perhaps the most visible example of the value most industries place upon achieving uniformity" [19].

Similarly, Dr. Don Berwick of the Institute for Healthcare Improvement defines quality as encompassing six fundamental principles – safety, effectiveness, patient-centeredness, timeliness, efficiency, and equity. Such delivery requires structure, process, and predictability [20].

Six Sigma

W. Edwards Deming led one of the earliest and most robust efforts to define structure around improved efficiency, effectiveness, and productivity in business venues. Deming was an engineer by trade and a proponent of the Shewhart cycle, a concept he morphed into the PDSA (plan-do-study-act) cycle. It is closely related to DMAIC (define, measure, analyze, improve, control), a similar (and some believe more practical) way to assess barriers and invoke sustainable change. In post-World War II Japan, Deming used these methodologies to guide the automobile manufacturing industry out of utter ruin and into position as one of the world's leaders in this field, a position they continue to hold even to today. Deming originally summarized these processes in 14 key points and 7 deadly diseases, all of which, in aggregate, make up the backbone of the disciplines of Six Sigma and Lean Six Sigma [21]. They have been used in innumerable businesses, healthcare included, as a means to understand process failure and invoke and implement sustainable change.

Dr. John Haughom summarizes the five most applicable and relevant points related to healthcare [22]. They are:

- Quality improvement is the science of process management.
- If you cannot measure it, you cannot improve it.
- Managed care means managing the processes of care, not managing physicians and nurses.
- The right data in the right format at the right time in the right hands.
- Engaging the "smart cogs" of healthcare.

CUSP

Another concise and deliverable means to understand this structure is the Agency for Healthcare Research and Quality's (AHRQ) Comprehensive Unit-based Safety Program (CUSP) [23]. The program was originally developed and endorsed by Dr. Pronovost and the team and has become one of the leading platforms for safety structure worldwide. Initial CUSP efforts were directed at reducing rates of CLABSIs and CAUTIs, an effort that was not only successful but sustainable. One such project, called On the CUSP: Stop BSI, reduced CLABSI in 44 US states by 40% and has saved an estimated 500 lives.

CUSP is one strategy to overcome these barriers and to effectively implement a sustainable safe culture. It is a long, if not, permanently ongoing, effort that focuses on the engagement of both frontline and leadership staff, job prompts and checklists, performance improvement tools, learning from errors, and teamwork and patient/family engagement.

CUSP implementation occurs in three phases. They are pre-CUSP work, CUSP implementation, and post-CUSP work. Pre-CUSP work involves assembling a team, assigning roles and responsibilities, and engaging and including senior executives in promoting the mission. Pre-CUSP work also includes realistically assessing the current safety climate in your organization. This requires honesty and thoughtfulness and must be free from blame. Though the results may be sobering, the purpose of engaging in CUSP is to identify, learn from, and overcome barriers to consistent excellence.

Steps 1–5 as noted in Table 6.3 summarize CUSP implementation. Considerably more detail as well as user-friendly toolkits can be found on the AHRQ website.

Post-CUSP work is the maintenance phase. Though we all want to achieve zero harm and consistent and sustainable quality, this process remains a lifelong journey and not a destination. Ongoing vigilance of risk and a culture of always-asking-why are critical to ongoing success.

Communication and Culture

The merits of Six Sigma, CUSP, and other safety and quality initiatives do not exist without communication and a fair and just culture. In *Being Mortal*, Dr. Atul Gawande writes, "Culture is the sum total of shared habits and expectations." [24] Communities, families, hospitals, and even ICUs have personalities, biases, preconceived notions, and habits – *Cultures*. How many times have you heard "That's not the way we do it here" or "That's just the way it's always been?" Such statements are at the root of unit-based culture and can seem insurmountable.

In 2005, the AHRQ published "Silence Kills," a terrifying missive that described several areas of poor performance in healthcare and the coercive enabling silence that allows them to go unchecked [25]. For example, 84% physicians and 62% nurses observed colleagues taking potentially harmful shortcuts. Fifty-three percent of surveyed nurses felt reluctant to ask for help, and 83% reported peer complaints when asked to assist. Eighty-one percent of physicians and 53% of nurses had concerns about the competency of one of more peers with whom they worked. While these staggering statistics were a wake-up call about clinical competency, they also highlight a national (perhaps even international) culture where deficiencies are covered up, secrets are buried, and speaking up is discouraged. In the "Silence Kills" report, fear

TABLE 6.3 CUSP 5 steps

Step 1 (*Educate Staff on the Science of Safety Training*) The learning objectives include the following: (a) understand that safety is a property of the system; (b) understand the basic principles of safe design that include: standardize work, create independent checks (checklists) for key processes, and learn from mistakes; (c) recognize that the principles of safe design apply to technical as well as team work; and (d) understand that teams make wise decisions when there is diverse and independent input. A video presentation for this training is available at http://safetyresearch.jhu.edu/qsr.
Step 2 (*Staff Identify Defects*) Identify defects from incident reports, liability claims, sentinel events, and most importantly ask staff how the next patient will be harmed through a two-item written survey.
Step 3 (*Executive Partnership*) Partners a senior hospital executive with a unit to open lines of communication, improve frontline providers' attitudes about leadership, educate leaders about the clinical issues and safety hazards, provide staff resources to mitigate hazards, and hold staff accountable for reducing patient risks.
Step 4 (*Begin Learning from Defects*) Staff use a practical yet valid tool to learn from defects by answering (1) what happened, (2) why it happened, (3) what you did to reduce risk, and (4) how do you know risks were actually reduced. Staff are encouraged to learn from at least one defect per month.
Step 5 (*Implement Teamwork Tools*) Provides tools to improve teamwork, communication, and other systems of work in the unit.

of confrontation and/or retaliation was cited as a primary factor for respondents' silence.

In a 2015 online publication of The Joint Commission (TJC), the top three "most frequently identified root causes for Sentinel Events" (in order) were [26]:

Human factors
Leadership
Communication

Prior to this publication, communication was cited as the number one root cause identified for almost every Sentinel Event released by TJC.

After the disastrous events of September 11, 2001, New York City adopted a "see something, say something" campaign [27]. We have used this same slogan to encourage staff to share everything they see and to use this as the foundation for where we need to focus our process change. If staff feel that speaking up will lead to punitive measures, they will be forever silent. In his book "*Safe Patients, Smart Hospitals*," Dr. Pronovost writes, "It has been shown in business meetings that once a person has been given the opportunity to speak, that person is more likely to speak up again during the meeting" [28].

In October of 1999, Dr. Lucian Leape of the Harvard School of Public Health spoke before a subcommittee of the US Congress and reported that "the single greatest impediment to error prevention is that 'we punish people for making mistakes'" [29]. Two years later, David Marx, JD, reacted with a 28-page summary known as Patient Safety and the "Just Culture": A Primer for Health Care Executives [30]. The fundamental tenet of this document is the same as the principle of negative reinforcement. If you shock a lab rat every time he eats a cookie, he will no longer try to eat the cookie. Similarly, if you punish employees for speaking up about potential risk in the workplace, they will fear retribution or retaliation and remain silent. A Just Culture, alternatively, is one in which speaking up is not only encouraged but lauded and harm is largely blameless to the individual with process and structure being the fundamental means of correction. Sadly, this chapter is being written 17 years after the introduction of this concept, and while it has enjoyed some success, it is far from being a ubiquitously accepted element of our healthcare culture.

Summary

Critical care units are ideal for studying preventable harm. The patients they house are exceedingly vulnerable, undergoing the most invasive and unpredictable therapies, and at risk for the greatest unexpected and unintended harm. Fortunately, recent efforts have shed light on means to prevent such harm and to deliver sustainable, predictable, consistent care. Such delivery requires knowledge of process and structure, implementation of every-changing evidence-based practice guidelines, and a relentless commitment to ongoing vigilance with assessment, repair, and improvement of dynamic processes.

References

1. Kohn LT, Corrigan J, Donaldson MS. To err is human: building a safer health system. Washington, DC: National Academy Press; 2000.
2. The National Trial Lawyers. 440,000 deaths annually from preventable hospital mistakes. LawyersandSettlements.com; 2015.
3. Preventable health care harm is a public health crisis and patient safety requires a coordinated. NPSF Call to Action. www.npsf.org; 2013.
4. Szczerba RJ. Six frightening facts you need to know about healthcare. Jersey: Forbes/Tech; 2013.
5. Van Den Bos J, Rustagi K, Gray T, et al. The $17.1 billion problem: the annual cost of measurable medical errors. Health Aff. 2011;30(4):596–603.
6. Pronovost P, Needham D, Berenholtz S, et al. An intervention to decrease catheter-related bloodstream infections in the ICU. NEJM. 2006;355:2725–32.
7. Donchin Y, Gopher D, Olin Y, Badihi Y, Biesky M, Sprung CL, et al. A look into the nature and causes of human errors in the intensive care unit. Qual Saf Health Care. 2003;12(2):143–8.
8. Reason J. Human error: models and management. BMJ. 2000;320(7237):768–70.
9. Hughes RG, Blegen MA. Chapter 37: Medication administration safety. In: Hughes RG, editor. Patient safety and quality: an evidence-based handbook for nurses. Rockville: Agency for Healthcare Research and Quality (US); 2008. Available from: https://www.ncbi.nlm.nih.gov/books/NBK2656.
10. Gawande A. The checklist manifesto: how to get things right. New York: Metropolitan Books; 2010.
11. Baker DP, Day R, Salas E. Teamwork as an essential component of high-reliability organizations. Health Serv Res. 2006;41(4 Pt 2):1576–98. https://doi.org/10.1111/j.1475-6773.2006.00566.

12. Rollins E. Guess who really pays for healthcare? CNN.com; 2010.
13. Hospital-Acquired Conditions [Internet]. Centers for Medicare and Medicaid Services. [revised 2015 Aug 19; cited 2015 Sep 2]. Available from: https://www.cms.gov/Medicare/Medicare-Fee-for-Service-Payment/HospitalAcqCond/Hospital-Acquired_Conditions.html. Accessed 29 Dec 2017.
14. The Leapfrog Group. http://www.leapfroggroup.org. Accessed 29 Dec 2017.
15. Healthcare-Associated Infections. National Quality Forum. http://www.qualityforum.org/Projects/h/Healthcare-Associated_Infections_(HAI)/Healthcare-Associated_Infections_(HAI).aspx. Accessed 29 Dec 2017.
16. Pollock DA, editor. The direct medical costs of healthcare-associated infections in U.S. hospitals and the benefits of prevention. 2009. https://www.cdc.gov/hai/pdfs/hai/scott_costpaper.pdf. Accessed 29 Dec 2017.
17. Patient safety indictors. Agency for Healthcare Research and Quality. https://www.qualityindicators.ahrq.gov/modules/psi_overview.aspx. Accessed 29 Dec 2017.
18. The Project Gutenberg eBook. The task, by William Cowper, Henry Morley, editor. 2015. https://www.gutenberg.org/files/3698/3698-h/3698-h.htm.
19. Shaywitz D. Balancing consistency and innovation in healthcare. Salt Lake: Health Catalyst, John Irvine; 2009.
20. Berwick D. http://www.ihi.org/education/IHIOpenSchool/resources/Pages/Activities/DefiningQualityAimingforaBetterHealthCareSystem.aspx. Accessed 29 Dec 2017.
21. Deming WE. Out of the crisis. Cambridge, MA: Massachusetts Institute of Technology, Center for Advanced Engineering Study; 1986.
22. Haughom J. Five Deming principles that help healthcare process improvement. Salt Lake: Health Catalyst Insights; 2014.
23. Comprehensive Unit-Based Safety Program. AHRQ. https://www.ahrq.gov/professionals/education/curriculum-tools/cusp-toolkit/index.html. Accessed 29 Dec 2017.
24. Gawande A. Being mortal: medicine and what matters in the end. New York: Metropolitan Books, Henry Holt and Company; 2014.
25. Maxfield D, Grenny J, McMillan R, et al. Silence kills: the seven crucial conversations for healthcare. Provo: VitalSmarts; 2005.

26. The Joint Commission online. https://www.jointcommission.org/issues/detail.aspx?Issue=8t1c%2F2QyDr8EUZycx%2F9Jle7jZ8f6u4jhOmsakH3xcO8%3D – April 29th 2015. Accessed 29 Dec 2017.
27. If you see something, say something. Department of Homeland Security. https://www.dhs.gov/see-something-say-something. Accessed 29 Dec 2017.
28. Pronovost PJ, Vohr E. Safe patients, smart hospitals: how one doctor's checklist can help us change health care from the inside out. New York: Hudson Street Press; 2010.
29. Lucian Leape Institute. Through the eyes of the workforce: creating joy, meaning, and safer health care. Boston: National Patient Safety Foundation; 2013.
30. Marx D. Patient safety and the "just culture": a primer for health care executives. New York: Columbia University; 2001.

Chapter 7
Surveillance and Prevention of Hospital-Acquired Infections

Christian A. Engell

Hospital-acquired infections are defined as symptomatic infections that result after hospitalization with no evidence that the infection was present or incubating at the time of admission to the acute care setting [1]. In 1992 it was estimated that approximately two million patients per year develop an HAI, and approximately 90,000 of these patients die [2]. In 2014, an HAI prevalence survey estimated that there were 722,000 HAIs in US acute care hospitals. Additionally, about 75,000 patients with HAIs died during their hospitalizations. Approximately 35% of these infections occurred in the ICU setting [3]. These numbers suggest a recent decrease in the incidence of HAI. Unfortunately, the recent reductions in HAIs do not seem to have led to a proportional reduction in mortality rates.

In the 2014 prevalence survey of HAIs, 49,900 ventilator-associated pneumonias, 35,600 catheter-associated urinary

C. A. Engell
Rutgers University New Jersey School of Medicine, Newark, NJ, USA
e-mail: christian.engell@rwjbh.org

J. A. LaRosa (ed.), *Adult Critical Care Medicine*,
https://doi.org/10.1007/978-3-319-94424-1_7

tract infections, and 15,600 central-catheter-associated primary bloodstream infections can be attributed to US ICUs every year. The survey did not break down which of the 157,500 surgical site infections, 80,400 *Clostridium difficile* infections, and 9700 MRSA bacteremias developed in the ICU, but clearly a sizeable proportion of them were of ICU origin [3].

Given the sheer number of ICU-acquired HAIs, how does an ICU physician identify whether they are dealing with a possible hospital-acquired infection and how are they best be avoided? The aim of the rest of this chapter will be to provide a review of the most recent NHSN criteria for defining the most common hospital-acquired infections. A case will be presented for each of the common infections, and the definitions of a hospital-acquired infection will be reviewed and applied to the case following which a review of prevention bundles including a discussion of recent developments in prevention. Given the amount of focus on these infections in recent years, the goal is not to be comprehensive but rather to give an overview of these HAIs. The following HAIs will be reviewed in this chapter.

1. VAE
2. CAUTI
3. CLABSI
4. *C. difficile*

Case 1

A 65-year-old male with a past medical history of type II diabetes and grade D COPD requiring home O2 presents with a COPD exacerbation. In the emergency room, the patient is intubated after noninvasion methods of ventilation fail. The patient is afebrile and is not producing large amounts of secretions. During her first 3 days intubated in the ICU, her minimum FiO2 is 0.40 and her minimum PEEP is 7. On days 5 and 6 of admission, the patient develops a fever of 102.2 and is maintained on and FiO2 of 0.6 with PEEP of 10.

The patient is started on broad-spectrum antibiotics. Purulent tracheal aspirate culture subsequently grew methicillin sensitive *Staphylococcus aureus*.

Reporting of Ventilator-Associated Events (VAE)

The above patient was diagnosed with a ventilator-associated pneumonia (VAP) by her clinical team. However, since 2013, the surveillance definition of VAP has been supplanted by VAE. The definition of VAE was first developed by a CDC Working Group composed of members of several stakeholder organizations to address the limitations of the current ventilator-associated pneumonia definition [4]. The VAP definition used at the time was neither sensitive nor specific which had implications for surveillance and thereby prevention [5, 6]. The inaccuracy of the surveillance measure made assessment of prevention strategies difficult. One of the difficulties with the VAP definition was the reliance on the chest X-ray interpretation and reporting which has an amount of subjectivity. The VAE surveillance definition algorithm implemented in the NHSN in January 2013 was designed based on objective, streamlined, and potentially automatable criteria that identify a broad range of conditions and complications occurring in mechanically ventilated adult patients [7]. The full classification is shown in Fig. 7.1 [8]. The VAEs are defined progressively from a ventilator-associated condition (VAC) based on changes in PEEP and FiO2 values and progressing through infection-related ventilator-associated condition (iVAC) to possible ventilator-associated pneumonia based on increasing systemic and microbiologic features suggesting infection [8]. In our patient above, the increase from baseline in FiO2 by 0.2 or the increase in minimum PEEP from baseline would both have qualified the patient as a ventilator-associated condition. The fever would qualify the patient for an infection-related ventilator-associated condition. Once purulent secretion cultures resulted, it was possible to report the patient as an episode of possible VAP.

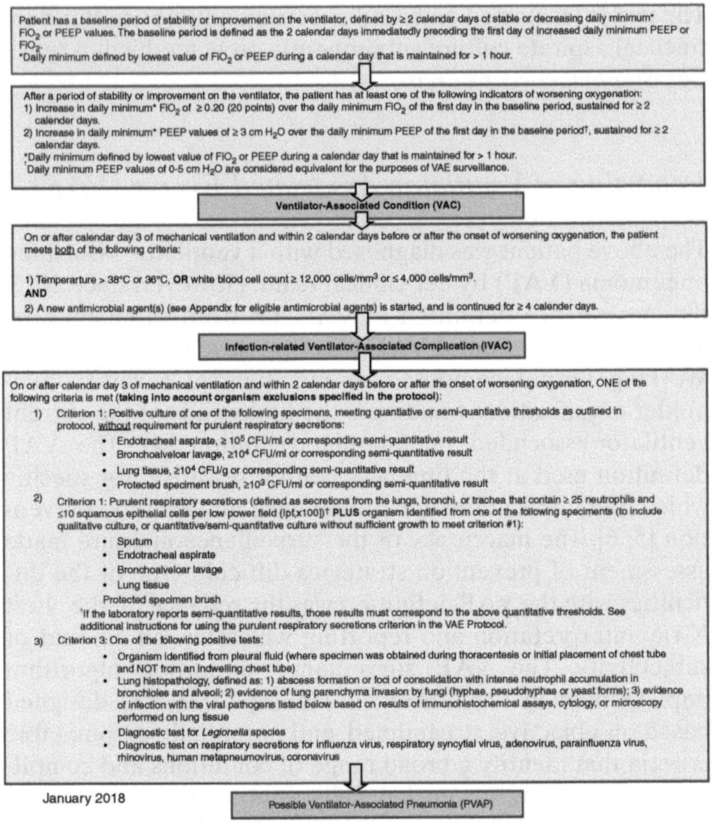

FIGURE 7.1 Ventilator-associated events (VAE) surveillance algorithm. (CDC [8] [cited 2018 Jan 12])

VAE

The incidence of ventilator-associated events has changed as the transition from the VAP definition to VAE definition has occurred. In 2012, VAP rates of 3.3 per 1000 ventilator days were reported in the United States [9]. In 2014, NHSN reported the incidence of VAE to be between 2% and 12% in different types of critical care units with VAEs meeting at least the iVAC definition comprising 30–40% of the VAEs which interestingly approximates the incidence of VAP in 2012 [10].

Although VAE is now the CDC's recommended surveillance metric for ventilated patients in adult critical care units, the existing literature on VAP prevention is primarily based on traditional VAP definitions rather than VAE definitions. A guideline sponsored by the Joint Commission and American Hospital Association was published by the Society for Healthcare Epidemiology of America in 2014 [11]. Six major elements of VAP prevention were outlined in the document and are summarized below:

Avoidance of Intubation If Possible

Use of noninvasive positive-pressure ventilation whenever feasible has been shown to decrease likelihood of intubation and thereby VAE [12]. Caution is recommended when considering NIPPV to manage patients with impaired consciousness, acute lung injury, acute respiratory distress syndrome, severe hypoxemia, and severe acidemia [13].

Minimize Sedation

Managing ventilated patients without sedatives whenever possible is recommended. Managing agitation by addressing its source and avoiding benzodiazepines can reduce duration of intubation [14]. Daily spontaneous awakening trials for patients without contraindications have been studied in two randomized controlled trials that showed a decreased net use of sedatives and a 2–4-day reduction in duration of mechanical ventilation [15, 16]. Finally, spontaneous breathing trials have been associated with shorter intubation times especially when combined with awakening trials [17].

Maintain and Improve Physical Conditioning

Providing early exercise and mobilization has been associated with quicker extubation, decreased length of stay, and increased the rate of return to independent function in multiple studies [11]. Furthermore, early mobility programs may be cost-saving [18].

Minimize Pooling of Secretions Above the Endotracheal Tube Cuff

Provide endotracheal tubes with subglottic secretion drainage ports for patients likely to require greater than 48 h or 72 h of intubation. A meta-analysis suggested that the use of endotracheal tubes with subglottic drainage reduced VAP rates by 55% while decreasing the mean ICU stay by 1.5 days [19]. However, reductions in duration of mechanical ventilation with subglottic secretion drainage appear to be limited to patients on a ventilator for more than 48–72 h [20]. Identifying the subset of patients requiring subglottic secretion drainage tubes can be tricky especially since extubating patients to place a subglottic secretion drainage tube is not recommended [11].

Elevate the Head of the Bed

Elevating the head of the bed to 30–45° has been evaluated in three randomized controlled trials with only 387 patients in all [21–23]. Only one trial reported a significant 76% decrease in VAP rates [21]. However, a meta-analysis pooling the three studies did find a significant impact on VAP [24]. Furthermore, enteral feeding in the supine position substantially increases the risk of developing VAP [21]. The guidelines note that there was insufficient data to determine the impact of head-of-bed elevation on duration of mechanical ventilation or mortality, but given the simplicity, ubiquity, minimal risk, lack of cost, and potential benefit of this intervention, it should be classified as a basic practice while awaiting further data [11].

Maintain Ventilator Circuits

Changing the ventilator circuit as needed rather than on a fixed schedule has no impact on VAP rates or patient outcomes but decreases costs. The ventilator circuit should only be changed if visibly soiled or malfunctioning [11].

Summary of VAE

Like all new surveillance definitions, the ability of the VAE surveillance definition to help reduce the incidence of VAE remains to be seen. It does appear that the new definition has succeeded in reducing the time need to collect data while at the same time increasing the objectivity of data collection [25]. As can be suspected from the guidelines which focus on interventions to reduce days of mechanical ventilation, it has been suggested that there should be direct focus on reducing days of mechanical ventilation instead of VAE [26].

Case 2

A 53-year-old male with a past medical history of diabetes presents to the CCU after experiencing sudden retrosternal chest pain. After experiencing urinary retention, a urinary catheter is placed. The patient is diagnosed with NSTEMI. On hospital day 2, a cardiac catheterization suggests that the patient is a candidate for coronary artery bypass grafting which is completed on hospital day 4. On hospital day 5, the urinary catheter is removed and the patient voids successfully. On hospital day 5, the patient starts to complain of dysuria and suprapubic tenderness. A urine analysis is positive and reflex urine cultures show 100,000 colony forming units of *E. coli*.

Reporting of Catheter-Associated Urinary Tract Infections

The above patient was diagnosed with symptomatic catheter-associated urinary tract infection. This case was a hospital-acquired infection. The CMS reporting requirements include two distinct types of hospital-acquired CAUTI to be reported, symptomatic CAUTI and asymptomatic CAUTI. For the definitions below, all elements must be satisfied within a 7-day infective window period comprising the diagnostic event day and 3 calendar days before and after the event [27].

Symptomatic Catheter-Associated UTI [27]

All three criteria must be met:

1. Patient had an indwelling urinary catheter that had been in place for >2 days on the date of event (day of device placement = day 1) *AND* was either still present for any portion of the calendar day on the date of event or removed the day before the date of event.
2. Patient has at least one of the following signs or symptoms: (a) fever (>38.0 °C), (b) suprapubic tenderness, (c) costovertebral angle pain or tenderness, (d) urinary urgency, (e) urinary frequency, and (f) dysuria.
3. Patient has a urine culture with no more than two species of organisms, at least one of which is a bacterium of ≥100,000 CFU/ml.

Asymptomatic Catheter-Associated UTI [27]

All three criteria must be met:

1. Patient with or without an indwelling urinary catheter has no signs or symptoms of symptomatic UTI.
2. Patient has a urine culture with no more than two species of organisms, at least one of which is a bacterium of ≥100,000 CFU/ml.

3. Patient has a positive blood culture with at least one matching bacterium to the urine culture. All elements of the ABUTI criterion must occur during the Infection Window Period.

CAUTI

Approximately 12–16% of adult hospital inpatients will have an indwelling urinary catheter at some time during hospitalization [3]. For each day an indwelling urinary catheter remains, a patient has a 3–7% increased risk of acquiring a catheter-associated urinary tract infection (CAUTI) [28]. It is estimated that there are annually approximately 35,000 episodes of catheter-associated urinary tract infection in US ICUs [3]. The overall mortality rate associated with CAUTI has been calculated at around 3% [29].

In April 2013, the Centers for Disease Control and Prevention (CDC) released the National Healthcare Safety Network (NHSN) data summary report for 2011. The CAUTI pooled means for intensive care units (ICUs) ranged from 1.2 per 1000 urinary catheter days in medical surgical ICUs to 4.1 in burn ICUs. Non-ICU rates ranged from 1.3 to 1.5 per 1000 urinary catheter days in medical, surgical, or medical surgical units [29]. Although there has been modest improvement in CAUTI rates, progress has been much slower than other device-associated infections, such as central line-associated bloodstream infections (CLABSIs), where significant improvement has been made. An estimated 17–69% of CAUTI may be preventable with implementation of evidence-based practices. This means that 380,000 infections and 9000 deaths related to CAUTI per year could be prevented [27].

Prevention of CAUTI

CAUTI prevention is the cornerstone of reducing its associated cost, morbidity, and mortality. Considerable work has been done to clearly pinpoint which factors are most critical for CAUTI reduction, and the findings are not yet entirely clear. What is well known is that minimization of urinary catheter use and early removal is the most effective tools for reducing CAUTI rates.

Although there are clear indications for the use of indwelling urinary catheters, adherence to these guidelines are often lower than they should be [30]. There are a number of reasons for this discrepancy. Physician and nursing culture is foremost among these. A 2012 Scandinavian study revealed that early removal of urinary catheters after thoracic surgery did not result in a need for increased catheterization [31]. A 2011 study revealed not only that urinary catheters were unnecessary for patients undergoing Caesarean section but also that there was no increased risk of urinary retention or intraoperative difficulties without their use [32]. As could be expected, the investigators did cite higher rates of urinary tract infections when catheters were used [32]. Despite these studies, a 2013 study still revealed that 26.1% of patients did not have an appropriate indication for their catheter [33]. In summary, urinary catheters are simply overused and are used many times for nonindicated reasons.

CAUTI prevention strategies must focus on clear indications for the insertion of a urine catheter, proper maintenance while in use, and early catheter removal. However, adherence to these strategies appears to be variable. A 2009 survey of 25 hospitals revealed that there does not seem to be one particular strategy that is being used by all hospitals. Of the hospitals surveyed, 9% used stop orders or discontinuation reminders, 14% attempted the use of condom catheters, and 30% used bladder scanners to avoid reinsertion [34]. In 2012, another study showed similar findings—9.5–12.4% of ICUs used nurse-driven removal protocols or reminders for discontinuation, 20% used condom catheters, and 25.9% had a policy related to the use of a bladder scanner [35]. Numerous guidelines have attempted to standardize strategies for CAUTI prevention. A 2014 update of strategies for preventing CAUTI was published by the Society for Healthcare Epidemiology of America with sponsorship from the Joint Commission and the American Hospital Association. It recommendations are summarized below [36]:

Provide appropriate infrastructure for preventing CAUTI

This broad recommendation is a reminder that appropriate resources need to be dedicated to preventing CAUTI. The necessary infrastructure includes but is not limited to providing hospital guidelines on placement, indication, and removal of catheters [37], availability of frontline staff trained in the aforementioned guidelines, adequate supplies for catheter placement, and a medical record documentation system that is capable of documenting compliance with guidelines [38].

Perform surveillance for cauti

Utilization of the NHSN reporting mechanism for CAUTI is the most commonly used approach for surveillance of CAUTI. Hospitals can easily calculate their standardized infection ratio for different target populations to evaluate which areas need improvement.

Provide education and training

Educate healthcare personnel involved in the management of urinary catheters and assess their competency in an ongoing manner. A 2012 study reported that through education and heightened surveillance, urinary catheter insertion could be reduced significantly from 18.5% to 9.2% [39].

Use appropriate technique for catheter insertion

The following basic techniques should be employed: (1) Insert urinary catheters only when necessary. (2) Consider alternative methods for bladder management, such as intermittent catheterization or external collection devices. (3) Practice hand hygiene while managing urinary catheter. (4) Use aseptic insertion technique with catheter insertion. (5) Use sterile gloves, drape, sponges, antiseptic solution, and single-use packet of lubricant for insertion. (6) Use the smallest catheter as possible [36].

Ensure appropriate management for maintenance of indwelling catheters

The following basic maintenance techniques should be employed: (1) Properly secure catheters to prevent urethral trauma. (2) Maintain a sterile, closed drainage system. (3) Replace the catheter and collecting system when breaks in aseptic technique, disconnection, or leakage occur. (4) Collect necessary urine samples from sampling port with a sterile adaptor after cleansing port with disinfectant. (5) Obtain larger volumes of urine for special analyses aseptically from the drainage bag. (6) Maintain unobstructed urine flow. (7) Employ routine hygiene [36].

Championing a team and using hospital-specific pilots to implement recommendations are critical in the reduction of CAUTI rates. A 2013 study reported a 50% reduction in the use of urinary catheters and a 70% reduction in CAUTI rates by implementation of a nurse-driven protocol [40]. Similarly, another study reported that the use of a daily interdisciplinary team to implement recommendations in a combined medical and surgical ICU could significantly reduce both catheter days (5304 vs 4541) and CAUTI rates (4.71 vs 1.98 infections per 1000 ICU days) [41].

Summary of CAUTI

CAUTI remains a challenging hospital-acquired infection. The surveillance definitions take into account that some patients may have clinically asymptomatic infection as well as symptomatic infection. There are no single factors responsible for CAUTIs, but they certainly do not occur in the absence of catheters. Though streamlining utilization, insertion, and management of catheters through guideline-based practice may reduce CAUTI rates, reducing catheter use is probably the single most effective means of preventing CAUTI.

Case 3

A 63-year-old female is admitted to CCU on July 4 after having a heart attack. A femoral central line was placed in the catheterization lab on the day of admission. On July 7, the patient's central line was removed. On July 8, a blood culture was collected because she became confused and was having chills and a fever of 101. Blood cultures resulted *E. faecalis*. No other source of infection was identified.

Reporting of a Hospital-Acquired Central-Line Bloodstream Infection (CLABSI)

The above patient was diagnosed with a hospital-acquired CLABSI. An NHSN defined CLABSI requires two main elements: (1) A laboratory confirmed bloodstream infection with a qualifying central line in place for over two calendar days before the positive culture *AND* (2) the qualifying central line must be in place on the date of culture or the day before the culture was drawn. In our patient above, the central line was present for 3 days. Though the culture was collected on the day after removal of the line, it still qualifies as a potential CLABSI. Since the infection cannot be attributed to another source, this infection was reported as a CLABSI [42].

CLABSI

CLABSIs are a major source of morbidity and cost in modern hospitals. In US ICUs, the majority of patients have at least one central venous catheter (CVC), for a total of 15 million CVC days per year. It is thought that 80,000 CRBSIs occur in US ICUs each year. These episodes are independently associated with increased hospital cost and length of stay, but they have generally not been shown to independently increase mortality [43].

Prevention of CLABSI

Prevention of CLABSIs requires an interdisciplinary endeavor. Education, training, and staffing is paramount. Factors that have been associated with increased CLABSI rates include understaffing and lack of an effective educational program on insertion and maintenance of catheters [44]. Personnel with competency in CVC placement and maintenance should place and maintain CVCs. One study from 2014 revealed that electronic medical systems, standardization of insertion kits, and simulation training, all reduced the rate of CRBSI [45].

Selection of catheters and sites are important in reducing the rate of CLABSIs. The decreased rate of infections from placement of short-term subclavian catheters should be weighed against the risk of pneumothorax, subclavian artery puncture, subclavian vein laceration, subclavian vein stenosis, hemothorax, thrombosis, and air embolism [46]. Although a meta-analysis from 2012 suggested that there was no difference in CLABSI rates between access sites in ICU patients, femoral vein access should be avoided in adult patients [47]. Subclavian vein access should be avoided in patients with advanced kidney disease and patients undergoing dialysis in order to avoid subclavian stenosis. When catheters are placed, ultrasound guidance should be used but only by those fully trained in its technique [48]. If a catheter is placed in an emergency without strict adherence to aseptic technique, the catheter should be replaced as soon as possible, at the most within 48 h. Choice of catheter type is important. Since the infection risk increases with the number of ports or lumens, the clinician should use the catheter type with the minimum necessary number of lumens. When a catheter is no longer essential, it should be removed. The best way to avoid CLABSIs is to avoid unnecessary CVCs, which may include early fistula or graft placement in patients with chronic renal failure. Routine replacement of catheters is not recommended by the IDSA guidelines for prevention of catheter infections [46].

Hand hygiene and aseptic technique are vital in both insertion and maintenance of catheters. Use of maximal sterile barrier precautions, including a cap, mask, sterile gown, sterile gloves, and a sterile full-body drape, for the insertion of catheters is recommended [49]. The insertion site should be prepared with a 0.5% chlorhexidine preparation with alcohol before catheter insertion and during dressing changes [46].

Maintenance of catheter sites is part of the ongoing effort to prevent CLABSIs. After oozing has been controlled with gauze dressing, transparent dressing can used. The transparent dressings should be changed every 7 days. If the dressing becomes damp, loosened, or visibly soiled, it should be replaced. Catheter sites should be monitored daily for evidence of infection which is made easier by transparent dressings [46].

In setting where the CLABSI rates remain a problem, chlorhexidine-impregnated sponge dressings can be used for temporary short-term catheters. Likewise, there may be a role for antimicrobial- or antiseptic-impregnated catheters and cuffs if standard prevention measures have been unsuccessful. Antibiotic or antiseptic ointments, locks, and hub caps may play a role in select situations [46].

Summary of CLABSI

The best way to avoid CLABSI is to avoid unnecessary use of catheters. Extensive IDSA guidelines for prevention of catheter infections provide recommendations as summarized above to reduce the overall burden of infections. Since the introduction of CMS non-payment rules in 2008 led to the widespread adoption of the aforementioned recommendations, the incidence of CLABSI has been reduced by approximately half [50].

Case 4

A 27-year-old woman with a past medical history of severe asthma is admitted to the ICU on December 24th after being intubated in the emergency room. She is febrile to 102.7 and is suspected of having pneumonia. Antibiotics are started on admission. However, her chest X-ray shows no evidence of infiltrates, her influenza A antigen is positive, and her procalcitonin is within normal limits. The patient is diagnosed with an asthma exacerbation and influenza. Antibiotics are discontinued and the patient is extubated on the second day of admission. On December 26th, she has three watery bowel movements. A stool *C. difficile* pcr is ordered. However, a specimen is not sent until December 27 in the morning. The specimen is positive for *C. difficile.*

Reporting of Hospital-Acquired Clostridium difficile Infection

The above patient was diagnosed with *Clostridium difficile*, and the episode was reported as hospital acquired. Hospital-acquired *Clostridium difficile* infections are reported to NHSN as LabID events. LabID event reporting is based strictly on laboratory testing data without clinical information allowing for much less labor-intensive tracking for *C. difficile*. (MRSA bacteremia is also reported as a LabID event.) The definition for hospital-acquired *Clostridium difficile* infection termed healthcare facility-onset is simply a specimen collected >3 days after admission to the facility (i.e., on or after hospital day 4) [51]. Whether or not the patient had diarrhea or other clinical signs of infection may be clinically significant, but it is not significant when LabID events are used for reporting purposes. In our case above, the patient was diagnosed with suspected *C. difficile* on the third calendar day of admission which was likely the first clinical day of *C. difficile* infection. However, the *C. difficile* pcr test was not sent until the fourth calendar day. The above case was classified as a hospital-acquired *C. difficile* infection. If the specimen had been sent on the third day, the infection would have been classified as a community-onset infection.

CDI

Clostridium difficile is an anaerobic, spore-forming bacillus that causes pseudomembranous colitis, presenting with diarrhea that often recurs and can progress to toxic megacolon, sepsis, and death [52]. It is estimated that there are upward toward 80,000 cases in acute care hospitals per year [3]. The average total cost for a single inpatient *C. difficile* infection (CDI) has been estimated at more than $35,000 and the estimated annual cost burden for the healthcare system exceeding $3 billion [53].

Prevention of Hospital-Acquired Clostridium difficile Infections

Development of CDI can be thought of as a two-step process: (1) the patient needs to be susceptible to *C. difficile*, and (2) the patient needs to be exposed to the infectious spores of *C. difficile*. Prevention of CDI is aimed at mitigating the risk of these two steps occurring. In a 2014 update of practice strategies to prevent *Clostridium difficile* infections [54], the Society for Healthcare Epidemiology of America reviewed the recommendations for prevention of CDI as shown below:

Encourage appropriate use of antimicrobials

Exposure to antibiotics has not been a risk factor linked to increased susceptibility to CDI. A major risk factor for hospitalized patients to acquire *C. difficile* is previous antimicrobial exposure [55]. Furthermore, multiple studies have demonstrated that outbreaks often abate with focus on, among other areas, antimicrobial utilization [54]. Appropriate utilization includes both using antimicrobials for the appropriate indications as well as selecting the antibiotic with the least risk of increasing susceptibility to CDI [56]. Choosing the appropriate treatment for CDI as well as discontinuing other antibiotics has been associated with decreased risk of recurrence [57].

Use contact precautions for infected patients and ideally single-patient rooms

To reduce the environmental burden of *C. difficile* spores and thereby risking infection of susceptible patients, contact precautions are recommended. Place patients with CDI under contact precautions to help reduce patient-to-patient spread of the organism. Contact precautions for CDI include gown and gloves in addition to CDC compliant hand hygiene upon exiting the room. It is important to maintain adequate supplies for contract precautions on each ward. Though this may sound like a simple task, it can in reality be a quite challenging task, and leaders, nurses, and physicians need to be engaged [54]. Continuing contact precautions for at least 48 h after diarrhea resolves has been recommended; however, the ideal length of isolation is not known [58].

Ensure cleaning and disinfection of equipment and the environment

Directly reducing the environmental burden *C. difficile* spores by disinfection and cleaning prevents contamination and potential exposure of susceptible patients. Almost all aspects of the patient environment have been documented to allow for colonization including patient rooms and the equipment used to provide care [59]. For disinfection of this environment, facilities should consider using household bleach or other products with sporicidal activity. The solution needs to have a contact time that meets manufacturers' recommendations, and routine monitoring of adherence to cleaning protocols should be assessed regularly [54].

Implement a laboratory-based alert system

A patient with diagnosed but unrecognized CDI has the potential to contaminate the environment until isolated.

A laboratory alert system can ensure that this scenario does not occur. Once a diagnosis of *C. difficile* is made, alert system relying on telephone, pager, or electronic alerts should be sent to the provider and to the patient care area so that the patient can be placed on isolation. Clear protocols for the process should be available [54].

Monitor CDI rates

As the burden of CDI in a hospital increases, there is the potential risk for further increased transmission. Calculating CDI rates regularly at the unit and organizational level can provide vital information for key stakeholders. This data will be necessary as outcome measures for the performance improvement necessary to bring down rates [54].

Education

Hospital leadership, healthcare providers, environmental services, patients, and families all should have educations on CDI. This education should include risk factors, routes of transmission, local CDI epidemiology, patient outcomes and treatment, and prevention measures. Proper education may help to alleviate patient and family fears regarding being placed in isolation [60, 61]. Information should be included about frequently asked questions such as the risk of transmission to family while in the hospital and at home.

Measure compliance with CDC or WHO hand hygiene and contact precaution recommendations

Finally, patient-to-patient transmission of *C. difficile* is thought to occur primarily through contamination of the hands of healthcare providers. Unfortunately, baseline hand hygiene adherence rates have been found to be approximately 40–60% in multiple studies [61]. Evidence-based recommendations for implementation of hand hygiene programs in healthcare settings have been published. Glove use upon entering rooms has been shown to be effective at preventing the transmission of *C. difficile* [61]. Given the lack of sporicidal effect of alcohol-based hand hygiene products compared with the relatively inefficient spore removal of handwashing, the proper way to perform hand hygiene is an area of controversy [54].

Summary of CDI

Hospital-acquired CDI is diagnosed as a lab event. Any positive test for CDI after calendar day 3 of admission is defined as hospital acquired. In order to develop CDI, patients have to be susceptible to infection often due to antibiotic exposure, and they have to be infected by *C. difficile* spores either before or during hospitalization. The preventive measures aimed at reducing CDI rates are aimed at reducing the number of susceptible patients by reducing inappropriate antibiotic use or by reducing environmental spread of *C. difficile* spores.

References

1. Horan TC, Andrus M, Dudeck MA. CDC/NHSN surveillance definition of health care-associated infection and criteria for specific types of infections in the acute care setting. Am J Infect Control. 2008;36:309–32.
2. CDC. Public health focus: surveillance, prevention and control of nosocomial infections. MMWR Morb Mortal Wkly Rep. 1992;41(42):783–7.
3. Magill SS, Edwards JR, Bamberg W, Zintars GB, Ghinwa D, Kainer MA, et al. Multistate point-prevalence survey of health care-associated infections. N Engl J Med. 2014;370:1198–208.
4. Magill SS, Klompas M, Balk R, et al. Developing a new, national approach to surveillance for ventilator associated events. Crit Care Med. 2013;41:2467–75.
5. Klompas M. Interobserver variability in ventilator-associated pneumonia surveillance. Am J Infect Control. 2010;38:237–9.
6. Klompas M, Kulldorff M, Platt R. Risk of misleading ventilator-associated pneumonia rates with use of standard clinical and microbiological criteria. Clin Infect Dis. 2008;46:1443–6.
7. Klompas M, Khan Y, Kleinman K, et al. Multicenter evaluation of a novel surveillance paradigm for complications of mechanical ventilation. PLoS One. 2011;6:e18062.

8. CDC. Device associated module, ventilator associated events. January 2018 [Cited 2018 Jan 8] Available from: https://www.cdc.gov/nhsn/pdfs/pscmanual/10-vae_final.pdf.
9. Rosenthal VD, Bijie H, Maki DG, et al. International Nosocomial Infection Control Consortium (INICC) report, data summary of 36 countries, for 2005–2009. Am J Infect Control. 2012;40:296–407.
10. Magill SS, Qunna L, Gross C, Dudeck M, Alle-Bridson K, Edwards J. Incidence and characteristics of ventilator-associated events reported to the National Healthcare Safety Network in 2014. Crit Care Med. 2016;44(12):2154–62.
11. Klompas M, Branson R, Eichenwald EC, Greene LR, Howell MD, Lee G, et al. Strategies to prevent ventilator-associated pneumonia in acute care hospitals: 2014 update. Infect Control Hosp Epidemiol. 2016;35(8):915–36.
12. Hess DR. Noninvasive positive-pressure ventilation and ventilator-associated pneumonia. Respir Care. 2005;50(7):924–9.
13. Carron M, Freo U, BaHammam AS, et al. Complications of non-invasive ventilation techniques: a comprehensive qualitative review of randomized trials. Br J Anaesth. 2013;110(6):896–914.
14. Barr J, Fraser GL, Puntillo K, et al. Clinical practice guidelines for the management of pain, agitation, and delirium in adult patients in the intensive care unit. Crit Care Med. 2013;41(1):263–306.
15. Kress JP, Pohlman AS, O'Connor MF, Hall JB. Daily interruption of sedative infusions in critically ill patients undergoing mechanical ventilation. N Engl J Med. 2000;342(20):1471–7.
16. Schweickert WD, Gehlbach BK, Pohlman AS, Hall JB, Kress JP. Daily interruption of sedative infusions and complications of critical illness in mechanically ventilated patients. Crit Care Med. 2004;32(6):1272–6.
17. Girard TD, Kress JP, Fuchs BD, et al. Efficacy and safety of a paired sedation and ventilator weaning protocol for mechanically ventilated patients in intensive care (awakening and breathing controlled trial): a randomized controlled trial. Lancet. 2008;371(9607):126–34.
18. Lord RK, Mayhew CR, Korupolu R, et al. ICU early physical rehabilitation programs: financial modeling of cost savings. Crit Care Med. 2013;41(3):717–24.
19. Muscedere J, Rewa O, McKechnie K, Jiang X, Laporta D, Heyland DK. Subglottic secretion drainage for the prevention of ventilator-associated pneumonia: a systematic review and meta-analysis. Crit Care Med. 2011;39(8):1985–91.

20. Frost SA, Azeem A, Alexandrou E, et al. Subglottic secretion drainage for preventing ventilator associated pneumonia: a meta-analysis. Aust Crit Care. 2013;26(4):180–8.
21. Drakulovic MB, Torres A, Bauer TT, Nicolas JM, Nogue S, Ferrer M. Supine body position as a risk factor for nosocomial pneumonia in mechanically ventilated patients: a randomized trial. Lancet. 1999;354(9193):1851–8.
22. van Nieuwenhoven CA, Vandenbroucke-Grauls C, vanTiel FH, et al. Feasibility and effects of the semi-recumbent position to prevent ventilator-associated pneumonia: a randomized study. Crit Care Med. 2006;34(2):396–402.
23. Keeley L. Reducing the risk of ventilator-acquired pneumonia through head of bed elevation. Nurs Crit Care. 2007;12(6):287–94.
24. Alexiou VG, Ierodiakonou V, Dimopoulos G, Falagas ME. Impact of patient position on the incidence of ventilator-associated pneumonia: a meta-analysis of randomized controlled trials. J Crit Care. 2009;24(4):515–22.
25. Boyer AF, Schoenberg N, Babcock H, et al. A prospective evaluation of ventilator-associated conditions and infection-related ventilator-associated conditions. Chest. 2015;147:68–81.
26. Trevino SE, Kollef MH. Ventilator-associated events: are we missing the forest for the trees? Crit Care Med. 2015;43(9):2017–8.
27. CDC. NHSN. CAUTI definition and case studies. March 2017 [cited 2017 Dec 26]. Available from: https://www.cdc.gov/nhsn/pdfs/training/2017/Scalise_March22.pdf.
28. McGuckin M. The patient survival guide: 8 simple solutions to prevent hospital and healthcare-associated infections. New York: Demos Medical Publishing; 2012.
29. Klevens RM, Edward JR, et al. Estimating healthcare-associated infections and deaths in U.S. hospitals. Public Health Rep. 2007;122:160–6.
30. Toughill E. Indwelling urinary catheters: common mechanical and pathogenic problems. AJN Am J Nurs. 2005;105:35.
31. Zaouter C, Wuethrich P, Miccoli M, et al. Early removal of urinary catheter leads to greater post-void residuals in patients with thoracic epidural. Acta Anaesthesiol Scand. 2012;56:1020–5.
32. Li L, Wen J, Wang L, et al. I routine indwelling catheterization of the bladder for caesarean section necessary? A systemic review. BJOG. 2011;118:400–9.
33. Fernandez-Ruiz M, Calvo B, Vara R, et al. Inappropriate use of urinary catheters in patients admitted to medical wards in a university hospital. Enferm Infecc Microbiol Clin. 2013;31:523–5.

34. Saint S, Olmsted RN, Krein SL. Translating health care–associated urinary tract infection prevention research into practice via the bladder bundle. Jt Comm J Qual Patient Saf. 2009;35:449–55.
35. Conway LJ, Pogorzelska M, Larson E, et al. Adoption of policies to prevent catheter-associated urinary tract infections in United States intensive care units. Am J Infect Control. 2012;40:705–10.
36. Lo E, Nicolle L, Coffin SE, et al. Strategies to prevent catheter associated urinary tract infections in acute care hospitals: 2014 update. Infect Control Hosp Epidemiol. 2014;35:464–79.
37. Gould CV, Umscheid CA, Agarwal RK, Kuntz G, Pegues DA. Healthcare infection control practices advisory committee (HICPAC): guideline for prevention of catheter-associated urinary tract infections. 2009. http://www.cdc.gov/hicpac/cauti/001_cauti.html.
38. Hooton TM, Bradley SF, Cardenas DD, et al. Diagnosis, prevention and treatment of catheter-associated urinary tract infection in adults: 2009 international clinical practice guidelines from the Infectious Diseases Society of America. Clin Infect Dis. 2010;50:625–63.
39. Marigliano A, Barbadoro P, Pennacchietti L, et al. Active training and surveillance: 2 good friends to reduce urinary catheterization rate. Am J Infect Control. 2012;40:692–5.
40. Parry MF, Grant B, Sestovic M. Successful reduction in catheter-associated urinary tract infections: focus on nurse directed catheter removal. Am J Infect Control. 2013;41:1178–81.
41. Arora N, Patel K, Engell CA, et al. The effect of interdisciplinary team rounds on urinary catheter and central venous catheter days and rates of infection. Am J Med Qual. 2013;29:329–34.
42. CDC. NHSN. CLABSI definition and case studies. March 2017 [cited 2017 Jan 12]. Available from: https://www.cdc.gov/nhsn/pdfs/training/2017/Puckett_March22.pdf.
43. O'Grady NP, Alexander M, Burns LA. Et al; healthcare infection control practices advisory committee. Guidelines for the prevention of intravascular catheter-related infections. Am J Infect Control. 2011;39(4 suppl 1):S1–S34.
44. El-Kholy A, Saied T, Gaber M, Younan MA, Haleim A, ElSayed H, et al. Device-associated nosocomial infection rates in intensive care units at Cairo University hospitals: first step toward initiating surveillance programs in a resource-limited country. Am J Infect Control. 2012;40(6):e216–20.
45. Allen GB, Miller V, Nicholas C, Hess S, Cordes MK, Fortune JB, et al. A multitiered strategy of simulation training, kit

consolidation, and electronic documentation is associated with a reduction in central line associated bloodstream infections. Am J Infect Control. 2014;42(6):643–8.
46. Mermel LA, Allon M, Bouza E, et al. Clinical practice guidelines for the diagnosis and management of intravascular catheter-related infection: 2009 update by the Infectious Diseases Society of America. Clin Infect Dis. 2009;49:1–45.
47. Marik PE, Flemmer M, Harrison W. The risk of catheter-related bloodstream infection with femoral venous catheters as compared to subclavian and internal jugular venous catheters: a systematic review of the literature and meta-analysis. Crit Care Med. 2012;40(8):24–79.
48. Miller AH, Roth BA, Mills TJ, Woody JR, Longmoor CE, Foster B. Ultrasound guidance versus the landmark technique for the placement of central venous catheters in the emergency department. Acad Emerg Med. 2002;9(8):800–5.
49. Pronovost P, Needham D, Berenholtz S, et al. An intervention to decrease catheter-related bloodstream infections in the ICU. N Engl J Med. 2006;355:2725–32.
50. Waters TM, Daniels MJ, Bazzoli GJ, Perencevich E, Dunton N, Staggs VS, et al. Effect of Medicare's nonpayment for hospital-acquired conditions: lessons for future policy. JAMA Intern Med. 2015;175(3):347–54.
51. CDC. NHSN. MRSA bacteremia and CDI LabID event reporting. 2017 [cited 2017 Dec 27]. Available from: https://www.cdc.gov/nhsn/acute-care-hospital/cdiff-mrsa/index.html.
52. CDC. Vital signs: preventing Clostridium difficile infections. MMWR Morb Mortal Wkly Rep. 2012;60(09):157–62.
53. Walsh N. *C. difficile* inpatient stays long, costly. MedPage Today. 2012, December 8.
54. Dubberke ER, Carling P, Carrico R, Donskey CJ, Loo VG, McDonald LC, et al. Strategies to prevent Clostridium difficile infections in acute care hospitals: 2014 update. Infect Control Hosp Epidemiol. 2014;35(s2):s48–65.
55. Loo VG, Bourgault AM, Poirier L, et al. Host and pathogen factors for Clostridium difficile infection and colonization. N Engl J Med. 2011;365(18):1693–703.
56. Doernberg SB, Winston LG, Deck DH, Chambers HE. Does doxycycline protect against development of Clostridium difficile infection? Clin Infect Dis. 2012;55(5):615–20.
57. Le F, Arora V, Shah DN, Salazar M, Palmer HR, Garey KW. A real-world evaluation of oral vancomycin for severe Clostridium

difficile infection: implications for antibiotic stewardship programs. Pharmacotherapy. 2012;32(2):129–34.
58. Sethi AK, Al Nassir WN, Nerandzic MM, Bobulsky GS, Donskey CJ. Persistence of skin contamination and environmental shedding of Clostridium difficile during and after treatment of C. difficile infection. Infect Control Hosp Epidemiol. 2010;31(1):21–7.
59. Cohen SH, Gerding DN, Johnson S, et al. Clinical practice guidelines for Clostridium difficile infection in adults: 2010 update by the Society for Healthcare Epidemiology of America (SHEA) and the Infectious Diseases Society of America (IDSA). Infect Control Hosp Epidemiol. 2010;31(5):431–55.
60. Lewis AM, Gammon J, Hosein I. The pros and cons of isolation and containment. Hosp Infect. 1999;43(1):19–23.
61. Johnson S, Gerding DN, Olson MM, et al. Prospective, controlled study of vinyl glove use to interrupt Clostridium difficile nosocomial transmission. Am J Med. 1990;88:137–40.

Chapter 8
Sepsis and Septic Shock

Anand Kumar and Victor Tremblay

Case Study

A 67-year-old man is brought to the emergency department by his wife for fever and flank pain for 24 h. He has a previous medical history of type 2 diabetes, gout, and recurrent nephrolithiasis. His medications include glyburide and allopurinol. He has no known allergy. On physical examination, the patient is confused and cannot answer questions appropriately. His blood pressure is 85/40 mmHg and his heart rate is 128 beats per minutes. His respiratory rate is 26/min with an oxygen saturation of 97% on 2 L/min nasal prongs. He is febrile at 38.8 °C. He has costovertebral tenderness on the right. His extremities are warm with bounding pulses.

Laboratory studies show a white blood cell count of 23,000/mm^3, platelets of 98,000/mm^3, creatinine of 256 micromol/L, and lactate of 6.2 mmol/L. Urinalysis is positive for nitrite and numerous white blood cells. Chest x-ray is normal.

A. Kumar (✉)
Section of Critical Care Medicine, Section of Infectious Diseases, University of Manitoba, Winnipeg, MB, Canada

V. Tremblay
Section of Critical Care Medicine, University of Manitoba, Winnipeg, MB, Canada

J. A. LaRosa (ed.), *Adult Critical Care Medicine*,
https://doi.org/10.1007/978-3-319-94424-1_8

Diagnosis

The patient presents with hypotension and signs and symptoms compatible with an infection. The patient most likely has sepsis, and possibly septic shock, from a urinary tract infection.

Sepsis is a very common diagnosis. As many as 800,000 cases of sepsis are admitted every year to American hospitals. This is comparable to the incidence of first myocardial infarctions. The overall mortality is around 200,000 cases per year [1]. The incidence of septic shock seems to be increasing recently [2].

Sepsis is defined as life-threatening organ dysfunction caused by a dysregulated host response to infection according to the 2016 Sepsis-3 consensus definition [3]. For clinical purposes, organ dysfunction is defined by an acute increase in SOFA score by 2 or more points. The baseline score can be assumed to be zero for patients with no known organ dysfunction.

Septic shock is a subcategory of sepsis with higher mortality and organ dysfunction. It can be defined as patient with sepsis with ongoing hypotension requiring vasopressors to maintain MAP greater than or equal to 65 mmHg *and* having a serum lactate equal or greater to 2 mmol/L *despite* adequate volume resuscitation. Mortality for patients with sepsis without septic shock is around 10%, while the mortality for patients with septic shock is around 40%. The term "severe sepsis" which was in the old definition has disappeared in the new Sepsis-3 definition.

The previous definition of sepsis as the presence of a suspected infection and two out of four systemic inflammatory response syndrome (SIRS) criteria has been abandoned.

The SIRS criteria were:

1. Temperature >38 °C or <36 °C.
2. Heart rate >90/min.
3. Respiratory rate >20/min or $PaCO_2$ < 32 mmHg.
4. White blood cell count >12,000/mm^3 or <4000/mm^3 or >10% immature bands).

The SIRS criteria were thought to reflect an inflammatory reaction to an insult, but not necessarily a sign of a dysregulated response. It was found to be poorly sensitive. About 12% of patients admitted to ICU in Australia and New Zealand with sepsis and organ dysfunction did not have at least two out of four SIRS criteria [4]. The old definition of sepsis using SIRS criteria was also found to poorly predict mortality compared to the Sepsis-3 definition.

Diagnosing sepsis and septic shock in a timely fashion is important so that treatment can be initiated early. A score that can be used outside of the intensive care unit is the quick SOFA (qSOFA) score. It has three components that are each allocated 1 point, and a score of 2 or more is considered positive:

- Respiratory rate ≥ 22/min.
- Altered mentation.
- Systolic blood pressure ≤ 100 mmHg.

Clinical presentation and investigation: The differential diagnosis of shock includes cardiogenic shock, obstructive shock, hypovolemic shock, and distributive shock (see Table 8.1). Septic shock is a form of distributive shock which is characterized by a loss of venous tone and peripheral resistance. Clinically, the patient with fluid-resuscitated septic shock will present with tachycardia, tachypnea, and hypotension with a high or normal pulse pressure (systolic blood pressure at least double the diastolic blood pressure). The skin is usually warm and extremities well perfused as opposed to the nondistributive types of shock. The pulse pressure can be low, and skin can be poorly perfused in case of very severe or unresuscitated septic shock or a mixed shock like a patient with superimposed hypovolemic elements (due to venous pooling) along with septic shock.

The presentation of septic shock frequently involves elements of other forms of shock. Hypovolemia is common given that patient often have diarrhea or decreased their fluid intake prior to coming to hospital. Sepsis-induced cardiac dysfunction is also very common. Other forms of distributive shock, including adrenal insufficiency and anaphylaxis, are not uncommon.

Table 8.1 Classification of shock

1. Hypovolemic
Hemorrhagic
Fluid depletion (nonhemorrhagic)
Interstitial fluid redistribution
Thermal injury
Trauma
Anaphylaxis
Increased vascular capacitance (venodilatation)
Sepsis
Anaphylaxis
Toxins/drugs
2. Cardiogenic
Myopathic
Myocardial infarction
Myocardial contusion (trauma)
Myocarditis
Cardiomyopathy
Septic myocardial depression
Pharmacologic
Mechanical
Valvular failure
Hypertrophic cardiomyopathy
Ventricular septal defect
Arrhythmic
3. Extracardiac obstructive
Tension pneumothorax
Pulmonary embolus
Cardiac tamponade

(continued)

TABLE 8.1 (continued)

Status asthmaticus/auto-PEEP
Constrictive pericarditis
Intrathoracic obstructive tumors (direct vena cava obstruction)
4. Distributive
Septic
Toxic shock syndrome
Anaphylactic
Neurogenic
Endocrinologic
Adrenal crisis
Thyroid storm

Adapted with permission from Parrillo and Dellinger [21]

Post-fluid resuscitation, septic shock is hemodynamically characterized by a hyperdynamic circulatory profile, decreased systemic vascular resistance (<900 dynes per second/cm^5), normal or increased cardiac index (>4.2 L/min/m^2), normal or decreased pulmonary capillary wedge pressure (<15 mmHg), and normal or high SvO2 or ScvO2 (>65 or 70%). Before fluid resuscitation, however, severe septic shock may exhibit a hypodynamic profile similar to hypovolemic shock with narrow pulse pressures and low central filling pressures, cardiac output, and SvO2 with reduced cardiac output.

Given that right heart catheterizations are used less often given their invasive nature and multiple studies showing absence of clinical benefit for their use, bedside ultrasonography has emerged as a useful way of assessing shock in a noninvasive way. Many clinicians now use it as part of their physical examination in critically ill patients. There have been several protocols (RUSH, ACES) on bedside ultrasonography in undifferentiated shock [5, 6].

On bedside ultrasonography, septic shock will classically present with normal heart function (although both increased and decreased contractility can be seen in some circumstances), small to normal inferior vena cava with normal inspiratory variation, and absence of bilateral B-lines in lungs (localized B-lines could point out to a diagnosis of pneumonia). Cardiac output as measured by left ventricular outflow tract velocity time integral (LVOT VTI) method should be preserved or high in the majority of cases.

Laboratory results are useful to identify organ dysfunction. White blood cells can be either elevated or decreased. Elevation in creatinine, bilirubin, and INR and decrease in PaO_2/FiO_2 ratio and platelets are associated with organ dysfunction and worse outcomes and are included in SOFA score. Glucose is often elevated even in patients without diabetes. C-reactive protein is often elevated more than two standard deviations. Procalcitonin is elevated in bacterial sepsis, but its ability to differentiate between sepsis and other causes of SIRS is questioned [7].

Lactate is a very important laboratory test. An elevated serum lactate (>2 mmol/L) is associated with poor outcome. The pathophysiology of lactate elevation in septic shock is complex. While local or global tissue hypoxia can be responsible, often, the rise in lactate can be due factors other than anaerobic metabolism. Impaired microcirculation, increased glycolytic flux through beta2-adrenergic receptor activation due to the activation of endogenous catecholamine systems, and decreased lactate clearance are other causes of increased lactate [8].

Nevertheless, failure to clear lactate despite fluid resuscitation is part of the diagnostic criteria for septic shock and portends a high mortality. Its use is therefore important in the initial evaluation of patients with potential sepsis or septic shock. Even in the setting of normal blood pressure, an elevated lactate (>4 mmol/L) is associated with a poor prognosis [9].

Collection of cultures from all potential sites of infection is important. If possible these cultures should be obtained prior to antimicrobials. Every patient with suspected sepsis or septic shock should get blood cultures from at least two sites (including at least one peripheral site). Site cultures, including sputum, urine, cerebrospinal fluid, abscess, or pleural effusion, should be obtained depending on the clinical picture and clinical suspicion.

Approximately one-third to one-half of sepsis patients do not have any positive culture. It is thus not absolutely necessary for the diagnosis, but it can help guide management and treatment.

Management

The most important part of management of sepsis and septic shock is early recognition. Delayed recognition is frequent and leads to delay in treatment. The diagnosis of sepsis is primarily based on clinical criteria. The qSOFA score can be used to identify patients with infection at greater risk of poor outcome and does not require any laboratory test. The full SOFA score is more accurate at predicting mortality but requires laboratory tests. An elevated lactate is also useful in recognizing sepsis and potential septic shock.

Once the empiric diagnosis of sepsis is made, treatment should be rapidly instituted. It is useful to separate management of sepsis in five different categories:

1. Early antimicrobials.
2. Hemodynamic management (fluid and vasopressors).
3. Source control.
4. Adjunctive therapies.
5. De-escalation.

While they are discussed separated here, it is important to remember that in real life clinical environment, these things should be happening rapidly and simultaneously.

Early Antimicrobials

Early administration of appropriate antimicrobials is a keystone of sepsis care. Several studies have shown that delays in administrating antimicrobials in septic shock are associated with worse outcome. Each hour delay in antimicrobials in septic patient with hypotension was associated with a 7.6% decrease in survival [10]. These results have been validated in numerous newer studies [11].

When considering the delay in antimicrobials, it is important to realize that there can also be a substantial delay between the time of the order to give the antimicrobials and the actual time it is administered. At least one study has shown that delay to be in the order of hours for various reasons [12]. Every effort should be made to ensure that the antimicrobials are given as soon as possible. This requires that the doctors, nurses, and pharmacists are aware of the importance of giving antimicrobials early and good communication between different health-care professionals.

While it is critical to give antimicrobials early, the physician should ensure that the appropriate antimicrobials are given. This choice has to take into account the suspected anatomic site of infection, past medical history of the patient (including receipt of antimicrobials within the preceding 3 months), and previous documented infection of the patient. Studies have shown that if inadequate antimicrobials are given initially, mortality increases in critically ill patients [13]. It is better to give broad-spectrum antimicrobials initially and narrow it down once the patient is more stable and/or an organism has been identified in culture.

Consequently, most patients with sepsis and septic shock are treated with a broad-spectrum beta-lactam such as piperacillin-tazobactam, ceftriaxone, ceftazidime, cefepime, or meropenem. Coverage for MRSA should be strongly considered if the patient has risk factors or if the local flora mandates. If the patient has pneumonia, atypical coverage particularly for Legionella should be initially considered. If the patient is immunocompromised in any way or has a health-care-associated infection, pseudomonas coverage should be included. During influenza season, patient presenting with respiratory symptoms and flu-like illness should generally also be covered with oseltamivir empirically until tests are negative.

Antifungal treatment should not be routinely used if risk factors are absent. If the patient has risk factors for invasive

Candida infection such as neutropenia, abdominal perforation, long-standing central venous access, chemotherapy, transplant, or total parenteral nutrition, it may be appropriate to consider the addition of an echinocandin (particularly for septic shock) pending culture results. If aspergillus is suspected, such as a profoundly neutropenic patient with new lung opacities, empiric voriconazole or amphotericin B can be considered.

Another factor to consider when choosing empiric coverage of antimicrobials is whether one should double cover the most likely bacterial pathogens. While studies have failed to show benefit in sepsis of double coverage of the most likely organism, meta-analysis seems to show benefit for the sickest patients: the ones with septic shock [14]. The Surviving Sepsis Campaign Guidelines of 2016 thus permits the use of two different antibiotics of different mechanistic classes (e.g., a β-lactam with an aminoglycoside or a fluoroquinolone) to cover the most likely organism only in patients with septic shock [15].

Often multiple antimicrobials have to be given to cover multiple potential organisms. In this situation, it is preferable to start with the antimicrobial with the highest likelihood of covering the offending organism. This will often be a broad-spectrum β-lactam which also has the advantage that they can be administered fairly rapidly.

When the frontline clinician is confronted with complex case and unsure of the correct empiric treatment, he should get an infectious disease or intensivist consultation as soon as possible as timely administration of the correct antimicrobials is one of the most important things that need to be done in the care of septic patients.

Hemodynamic Management

Shock and hypotension is often found in patient with sepsis. It is important to ensure that patients with sepsis and septic shock are adequately monitored. Peripheral venous access should be established. Arterial cannulation for accurate blood pressure monitoring should be done in unstable patients. A urinary catheter should be inserted for adequate urine output monitoring. Vital signs should be taken frequently, and the patient should be monitored in a resuscitation room or the intensive care unit if they have septic shock. Intubation might be required for hypoxemia, increased work of breathing, or decreased level of consciousness.

Central venous cannulation should be performed for most patients who require vasopressor medications. While it is possible to give vasopressors peripherally for a short period of time, there is a risk of extravasation and soft tissue necrosis. Additionally, the central venous line can give useful information such as the central venous pressure (CVP) and central venous oxygen saturation (ScvO2). Right heart catheterization should be reserved only for cases where the diagnosis of distributive shock is in doubt or in mixed shock (for example septic and cardiogenic shock). It should not be a routine part of management of sepsis or septic shock.

Initial management of hypotension should almost always begin with fluid resuscitation. While there is no consensus on the amount of fluid needed, 30 mL/kg of crystalloid is a good starting point and is recommended by Surviving Sepsis Guidelines.

In 2001 a study showed that early management (<6 h post-presentation) with a protocol targeting a mean arterial pressure ≥65 mmHg, CVP 8–12 mmHg, ScvO2 > 70%, and a hemoglobin of ≥90 g/L using fluids, vasopressors, blood transfusion, and dobutamine had been shown to improve outcome in severe sepsis and septic shock. However, three more recent randomized controlled trials have shown that this protocol is not superior to standard treatment [16–19].

If the patient is still hypotensive after initial fluid resuscitation, the patient should be reassessed. Crystalloid infusion until a CVP of 8–12 mmHg is reached or based on dynamic assessment of fluid responsiveness is appropriate. Fluid responsiveness is defined as an increase in cardiac output by 10–15% following a bolus of 500 mL of crystalloid. There are multiple ways of assessing fluid responsiveness, but a detailed discussion is beyond the scope of this chapter.

Crystalloids, either balanced solutions such as ringers lactate or normal saline, are the fluid of choice initially. Colloids have not been shown to improve outcome in sepsis, and starch solution seems to be associated with increase in renal failure and possibly mortality. Albumin has been shown to be safe with no increase in mortality. Its use might be indicated if several liters of crystalloid have already been given and the physician wants to minimize the amount of fluids given. But given the much higher cost of albumin, the risks of giving a blood products and lack of benefit, crystalloid remains the fluid of choice.

Once the physician has optimized preload and the patient is still hypotensive, the next step is to add vasopressors to maintain a MAP above 65 mmHg. Norepinephrine is the usual first-line vasopressor. It is an endogenous catecholamine with both powerful inotropic (cardiac alpha- and beta-1 receptors) and peripheral vasoconstriction effects (alpha-receptors). In a randomized controlled trial of shock, norepinephrine was found to have less side effects as compared to dopamine (mostly tachyarrhythmia). Dopamine has thus generally fallen out of favor. Phenylephrine (alpha-receptors agonist) can be used if trying to avoid tachycardia.

Vasopressin has been used in sepsis usually as an add-on to norepinephrine at a low dose (2.4 unit/h). It acts to increase systemic vascular resistance through peripheral V1 receptors with no increase in heart rate. Use of vasopressin decreases the amount of norepinephrine given but does not seem to affect mortality.

Some international regions utilize epinephrine more frequently. The main difference with norepinephrine is stronger activation of beta-1 and beta-2 receptors resulting in a stronger inotropic and chronotropic effects. It is worth noting that epinephrine tends to increase lactate, glucose, and lower potassium through its beta-2 activity. A modest lactate rise might be due to epinephrine and not an inadequate resuscitation.

In cases where bedside ultrasonography, low ScvO2, or physical examination show that there is an element of low cardiac output or sepsis-induced myocardial dysfunction, pure inotropes such as dobutamine or milrinone might be needed. There is no utility in increasing cardiac output to supraphysiologic level as studies have failed to show any benefit of this strategy. The goal of inotropes should be to increase cardiac output to normal to normalize tissue perfusion.

Dobutamine is a beta-1 agonist with powerful inotropic and chronotropic but also peripheral vasodilatory effects. Milrinone is a phosphodiesterase inhibitor that acts by blocking the degradation of cyclic AMP. It also has inotropic and chronotropic with peripheral and pulmonary vasodilatory effects. Their effect on blood pressure is variable; sometimes the increase in cardiac output will offset the peripheral vasodilatation, and the blood pressure will increase. Reduced blood pressure may result if the peripheral vasodilatation is more important and central venous pressures are low. The physician should be ready to increase other vasopressors when starting either dobutamine or milrinone in septic shock.

The usual MAP target of 65 mmHg can also be individualized. A randomized controlled trial of MAP target in septic shock failed to show a benefit of MAP target higher than 65 mmHg. A subset of patients with chronic hypertension showed a decreased acute kidney injury with the higher target. Similarly, a patient with signs of good perfusion (good mentation, capillary refill, urine output ≥0.5 mL/kg/h, and decreasing lactate) at lower MAP might benefit from a lower blood pressure target.

Source Control

Several infections only need antimicrobials and hemodynamic support, but there are also many who will not get better unless the infectious burden is decreased with source control. Empyema, abscesses, cholangitis, ruptured intra-abdominal infections, obstructed urinary tract infections, or necrotizing fasciitis are examples of infections requiring source control. Antimicrobials penetration is often poor leading to bad outcome with antimicrobials alone. Depending on the type and anatomical location of infection, source control can be done using surgery, chest tube, endoscopic retrograde cholangiopancreatography, or interventional radiology-guided drainage.

Studies have also shown that survival decrease with delay in achieving source control [20]. It is therefore important to aggressively look for source of infection that might need source control right away when the diagnosis of sepsis or septic shock is made. This will often require additional imaging, such as ultrasound or CT scan. A target of 6–12 h to obtain definitive source control is reasonable.

All intravascular devices should be considered potential source of infection in a septic patients and, if feasible, should be removed as soon as possible.

Adjunctive Therapies

Since sepsis is thought to be a dysfunctional host response to infection, there have been numerous pharmacological attempts to treat this dysfunctional host response. Unfortunately, the vast majority of these attempts have been unsuccessful. The most well-known is activated protein C. While an early study showed improved 28 days survival in the subgroup of patients with severe sepsis and septic shock, this result could not be replicated in a larger randomized controlled trial.

There is no evidence of benefit using early blood purification techniques such as high-volume hemofiltration or hemoperfusion, plasma exchange, or coupled plasma filtration adsorption. The indication for renal replacement therapy is the same as for every other critically ill patient.

There is no role for targeting higher hemoglobin level in septic patients. The target is the same as for general ICU patients: ≥70 g/L although a higher hemoglobin target of 90 g/L is appropriate for patients with septic shock (or those with concurrent acute coronary syndromes).

The only adjunctive therapy still being recommended is corticosteroids. They are recommended only in situation of septic shock with hypotension despite fluids and vasopressors for more than an hour. However, they only reduce pressor requirements but do not appear to improve outcome. They should not be used in other less sick patients.

There are multiple potential adjunctive therapies being studied at this time, including esmolol, anticoagulants, and the combination of vitamin C, hydrocortisone, and thiamine. But the clinical utility of these therapies remains to be proven.

De-escalation

Initial treatment of sepsis and septic patients include broad-spectrum antimicrobials and aggressive fluid resuscitation and vasopressors. Once patients have stabilized and start to improve, it is important to de-escalate to minimize harms. Antimicrobials should be narrowed based on culture or the most likely organism if culture negative. Antimicrobials may also be de-escalated on the basis of clinical improvement despite negative cultures. Duration of antimicrobial therapy should be no more than 7–10 days except for certain circumstances.

Vasopressors should be decreased as the blood pressure tolerates.

Fluid administration should slow down as soon as the patient is deemed euvolemic. Once the sepsis resolves, patients often end up in fluid overload, and diuresis may be required.

Every line or catheter should be reassessed daily and removed as soon as safe. They are sources of infection and discomfort. If the patient is intubated, sedation should be minimized and spontaneous breathing trial done daily as soon as it is safe to do so.

Case Conclusion

The patient was diagnosed with sepsis and possible septic shock. Piperacillin-tazobactam and vancomycin were administrated within 1 h of the clinical diagnosis. A bedside ultrasonography showed normal LV and RV function, no B-lines in the lungs, and a normal sized inferior vena cava but with greater than 50% inspiratory collapse.

30 mL/kg of crystalloid was given initially, but blood pressure remained low and norepinephrine was started. Lactate was still elevated at 5.9 mmol/L after the fluid bolus thus confirming the diagnosis of septic shock. A radial arterial cannula, a central venous line, and a urinary catheter were installed. Further fluid was administrated based on a low CVP. The patient had to be intubated for progressive increase work of breathing and hypoxemia. Vasopressin was added when norepinephrine had to be increased to 0.3 mcg/kg/min. Hydrocortisone was also administered for ongoing hypotension. The patient maintained warm extremities, ScvO2 was 76%, and bedside ultrasonography showed normal left ventricular function so inotropes were not given.

Given the history of renal stone and the hemodynamic instability, the diagnosis of obstructed urinary tract infection was entertained. A CT scan showed an obstructed stone in the distal right ureter and signs of right-sided pyelonephritis. Urology was consulted, and the stone was removed with ureteroscopy 5 h after ED admission. Pus was seen coming out of the ureter following stone removal.

The patient improved once the obstruction was lifted. Culture showed pan sensitive *Klebsiella* pneumonia in the urine and blood. Antimicrobials were narrowed down to ciprofloxacin for 7 days. Vasopressor requirements decreased, lactate decreased to normal, and renal function eventually returned to normal after several weeks although the patient needed renal replacement therapy for 1 week due to oliguria and fluid overload. He was extubated on day 5 and discharged home after 2 weeks.

Future Aims

- The optimal hemodynamic and fluid management strategy is still elusive. Early goal-directed therapy has been shown to not be better than usual management.

The decision to stop giving fluids is not yet defined. There are several studies showing harm of excess fluid administration. The patient should receive as much fluids as needed but not more; there is little agreement on what the amount is and how to individualize these decisions.

- The use of bedside ultrasound is growing as a tool to diagnose shock, assess fluid responsiveness, and monitor treatment response. Whether this will lead to better patient's outcome remains to be seen.
- Studies of adjunctive therapies in sepsis: esmolol, anticoagulations, or the combination of vitamin C, hydrocortisone, and thiamine.

Key Points

- Sepsis is defined as life-threatening organ dysfunction caused by a dysregulated host response to infection. Organ dysfunction is defined as an increase of SOFA score by 2 or more (assume baseline SOFA = 0 if no known organ dysfunction).
- Quick SOFA (qSOFA) is a quick screen to detect patients with potential sepsis. It is positive if two or more of the following are positive: (1) respiratory rate ≥22/min, (2) altered mental status, and (3) systolic blood pressure ≤100 mmHg.
- Septic shock is defined by hypotension requiring vasopressors *and* lactate greater than 2 mmol/L *after* adequate fluid resuscitation.
- Early adequate antimicrobials are extremely important. Delays in antimicrobials administration have been shown to increase death.

- Early source control in infections where it is required has also been shown to improve outcomes.
- Crystalloid administration, vasopressor administration, and sometimes inotropes are part of the hemodynamic management. Resuscitation targets are usually MAP greater than 65 mmHg and normalization of lactate.
- Corticosteroids can be added for vasopressors-dependent septic shock.

References

1. Angus DC, Linde-Zwirble WT, Lidicker J, Clermont G, Carcillo J, Pinsky MR. Epidemiology of severe sepsis in the United States: analysis of incidence, outcome, and associated costs of care. Crit Care Med. 2001;29:1303–10.
2. Kadri SS, Rhee C, Strich JR, Morales MK, Hohmann S, Menchaca J, et al. Estimating ten-year trends in septic shock incidence and mortality in United States academic medical centers using clinical data. Chest. 2017;151(2):278.
3. Singer M, Deutschman CS, Seymour CW, Shankar-Hari M, Annane D, Bauer M, et al. The third international consensus definitions for sepsis and septic shock (sepsis-3). JAMA. 2016;315(8):801–10.
4. Kaukonen KM, Bailey M, Pilcher D, Cooper DJ, Bellomo R. Systemic inflammatory response syndrome criteria in defining severe sepsis. N Engl J Med. 2015;372(17):1629–38.
5. Atkinson PR, McAuley DJ, Kendall RJ, et al. Abdominal and cardiac evaluation with sonography in shock (ACES): an approach by emergency physicians for the use of ultrasound in patients with undifferentiated hypotension. Emerg Med J. 2009;26:87–91.
6. Perera P, Mailhot T, Riley D, Mandavia D. The RUSH exam: rapid ultrasound in SHock in the evaluation of the critically lll. Emerg Med Clin North Am. 2010;28:29–56, vii.

7. Tang BM, Eslick GD, Craig JC, McLean AS. Accuracy of procalcitonin for sepsis diagnosis in critically ill patients: systematic review and meta-analysis. Lancet Infect Dis. 2007;7(3):210.
8. Suetrong B, Walley KR. Lactic acidosis in Sepsis : it's not all anaerobic: implications for diagnosis and management. Chest. 2016;149(1):252–61.
9. Casserly B, Phillips GS, Schorr C, Dellinger RP, Townsend SR, Osborn TM, et al. Lactate measurements in sepsis-induced tissue hypoperfusion: results from the surviving sepsis campaign database. Crit Care Med. 2015;43(3):567.
10. Kumar A, Roberts D, Wood KE, Light B, Parillo JE, Sharma S, et al. Duration of hypotension before initiation of effective antimicrobial therapy is the critical determinant of survival in human septic shock. Crit Care Med. 2006;34(6):1589–96.
11. Seymour CW, Gesten F, Prescott HC, Friedrich ME, Iwashyna TJ, Phillips GS, et al. Time to treatment and mortality during mandated emergency care for sepsis. N Engl J Med. 2017;376:2235–44.
12. Kanji Z, Dumaresque C. Time to effective antibiotic administration in adult patients with septic shock: a descriptive analysis. Intensive Crit Care Nurs. 2012;28(5):288–93.
13. Paul M, Shani V, Muchtar E, et al. Systematic review and meta-analysis of the efficacy of appropriate empiric antibiotic therapy for sepsis. Antimicrob Agents Chemother. 2010;54:4851–63.
14. Kumar A, Zarychanski R, Light B, Parrillo J, Maki D, Simon D, et al. Early combination antibiotic therapy yields improved survival compared with monotherapy in septic shock: a propensity-matched analysis. Crit Care Med. 2010;38(9):1773–85.
15. Rhodes A, Evans LE, Alhazzani W, et al. Surviving sepsis campaign: international guidelines for management of sepsis and septic shock: 2016. Intensive Care Med. 2017;43:304.
16. Rivers E, Nguyen B, Havstad S, et al. Early goal-directed therapy in the treatment of severe sepsis and septic shock. N Engl J Med. 2001;345:1368–77.
17. The Arise Investigators and Anzics Clinical Trials Grou. Goal-directed resuscitation for patients with early septic shock. N Engl J Med. 2014;371:1496. https://doi.org/10.1056/NEJMoa1404380.
18. ProCESS Investigators. A randomized trial of protocol-based care for early septic shock. N Engl J Med. 2014;371:1683–93.
19. Mouncey PR, Osborn TM, Power GS, et al. Trial of early, goal-directed resuscitation for septic shock. N Engl J Med. 2015;372:1301–11.

20. Bloos F, Thomas-Rüddel D, Rüddel H, et al. Impact of compliance with infection management guidelines on outcome in patients with severe sepsis: a prospective observational multicenter study. Crit Care. 2014;18:1.
21. Parrillo JE, Dellinger RP. Critical care medicine: principles of diagnosis and management in the adult. 4th ed. Philadelphia: Elsevier; 2014.

Chapter 9
Advanced Practice Providers in the ICU: Models for a Successful Multiprofessional Team

Heather Meissen and Aimee Abide

Case Presentation

A 65-year-old male is admitted to the intensive care unit (ICU) from the catheterization laboratory (cath lab). Earlier in the day, he presented to the emergency department (ED) with crushing chest pain. His past medical history included hypertension (HTN), hyperlipidemia (HLD), and tobacco use. In the ED, his electrocardiogram (EKG) was positive for ST-elevation myocardial infarction (STEMI). He was taken to the cath lab for emergent percutaneous coronary intervention (PCI). In the cath lab, the cardiologist successfully placed a stent to the culprit coronary lesion and restored blood flow. After completion, the patient was admitted to the ICU for

H. Meissen (✉)
Emory Critical Care Center, Emory Healthcare, Nell Hodgson Woodruff School of Nursing, Emory University, Atlanta, GA, USA
e-mail: heather.meissen@emoryhealthcare.org

A. Abide
Emory Critical Care Center, Emory Healthcare, Atlanta, GA, USA
e-mail: Aimee.Abide@emoryhealthcare.org

J. A. LaRosa (ed.), *Adult Critical Care Medicine*,
https://doi.org/10.1007/978-3-319-94424-1_9

recovery. Upon arrival to the ICU, the patient was drowsy but oriented and chest pain free. The ICU team, consisting of a critical care registered nurse, respiratory therapist, and advanced practice provider (APP), assembled to receive sign out from the cath lab team. As the patient was being transferred from the transport bed into the ICU bed, he groaned loudly, clutched his chest, and became unresponsive. The hospital emergency response team "code blue" was activated, and the APP notified the critical care medicine (CCM) intensivist of the situation. The CCM physician, not immediately available, directed the APP and ICU team to respond.

The ICU APP, recognizing a rhythm change to ventricular fibrillation, acted as the code team leader and initiated advanced cardiac life support (ACLS). As the critical care nurse determined no pulse and began cardiopulmonary resuscitation (CPR), the APP ran the ACLS algorithm, organizing the steps of CPR and defibrillation and directing the respiratory therapist to secure an advanced airway. The EKG technician was immediately called, and EKG confirmed an acute STEMI. As the team suspected, the newly placed stent to the left anterior descending coronary (LAD) was occluded. The swift action of the ICU team maintained successful rounds of CPR to ensure adequate blood flow to vital organs while notifying the cath lab team of an acute STEMI. With the assistance from the nursing staff, respiratory therapy, and APP, the acute signs of stent occlusion were immediately recognized, and rapid, high-quality ACLS enabled the patient to be resuscitated and transported back to the cath lab for repeat intervention.

Discussion

Demand placed on our healthcare system due to an aging American population combined with an increase in patients seeking care is having a significant impact on how care is delivered to some of our sickest patients [1]. Additionally, a shortage of intensivist-trained physicians and physician in-training work hour restrictions has influenced intensive care staffing models as physician groups struggle to stretch limited resources [2–5]. New and innovative changes in the care delivery model are necessary to maintain high-quality, cost-effective care. Specialty prepared nurse practitioners and physician assistants have become integral components to the care delivery model filling the provider shortage. Proper training and utilization are imperative in creating care teams who will perform to the top of their abilities. A well-trained APP working in an efficient staffing model can save health-care systems and federal beneficiaries a significant amount each year [6]. Appropriate staff to patient ratios, specialty-trained personnel, specialized monitoring, and resources for continual care can provide an efficient care delivery model conducive to high-quality cost-effective care [7].

The term advanced practice provider (APPs) collectively refers to nurse practitioners (NPs) and physician assistants (PAs) both of whom have advanced training at the master's or doctoral level. Relieving provider shortage in the ICU can be a challenge; however, most healthcare institutions have filled this gap with APPs. According to surveys from the American Academy of Physician Assistants (AAPA) and the American Association of Nurse Practitioners (AANP), more than 10,000 APPs practice in ICU settings [8, 9]. Additionally, APPs can provide high-quality care similar to care provided by physician residents [10]. The rising cost of healthcare, healthcare reform, and workforce demands have changed the healthcare landscape.

Critical care delivery models have evolved, and innovative, value-based models are emerging to fit the needs of critically ill patients. Current models include open or closed ICUs and 24x7 intensivist staffing. Emerging innovative models include nightly coverage with telemedicine and utilizing APPs to fill intensivist shortages [11]. In an open ICU, the patient's primary care physician, a hospitalist or another specialty physician, who is not critical care trained, assumes the role of managing physician. Closed ICUs employ a critical care specialist or intensivist as the managing physician. The Society of

Critical Care Medicine and the Leapfrog Group recommend a 24-h intensivist staffing model, but the ongoing shortage of trained intensivists limits the ability of hospitals to provide coverage [12–14]. Telemedicine can supply an intensivist-trained physician virtually to the bedside of many more patients compared to traditional staffing models. Benefits of electronic-ICU (e-ICU) or telemedicine include rapid intervention on alarms and abnormal laboratory values resulting in faster initiation of lifesaving treatment [11]. Staffing APPs in-house, who are able to reach ICU patients within minutes and are able to discuss patient care issues virtually with an intensivist via the telephone or telemedicine, can provide a high-quality, value-based alternative care delivery model [15].

Evidence indicates that critically ill patients are better served in an ICU with high-intensity staffing [16]. A recent survey conducted by the Society of Critical Care Medicine Taskforce on ICU staffing investigated provider to patient ratios for APPs in the ICU. Mean provider to patient ratios in the ICU were 1:5 (range, 1:3 or 1:8) for both NPs and PAs. In units which utilized fellows and medical residents, the mean APP to patient ratio was 1:4 (range, 1:3 or 1:8) with additional provider to patient ratio increasing to 1:9 on the night shift in the ICU [17]. Appropriate staffing in the ICU is an area of investigation for maximizing ICU coverage. Several factors influence APP provider to patient ratios, including the number of ICU beds, ICU occupancy rate, provider shifts per day and per week, patients' severity of illness, the level of care, and the clinical, research and teaching workload of the physician [18]. In other cases, some staffing models utilize APPs for procedural tasks only to relieve burden on physician workload.

Some examples of efficient staffing models can be seen in the figures below. Figure 9.1 represents a 20-bed intensive care unit in an academic institution. This unit staffs two APPs per day shift and two per night shift. During the day 4–6 medical residents care for 12 patients. The 2-day shift APPs cover 4 patients each. At night, the APPs cover 10 patients each with in-house support from the medical resident. The

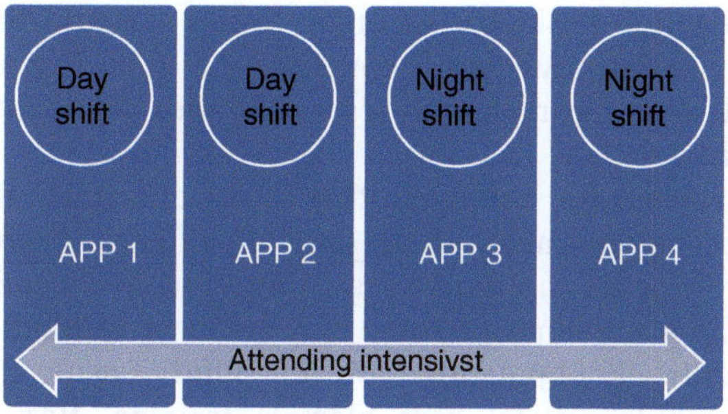

FIGURE 9.1 Staffing models. Academic hospital with a 20-bed ICU. Two APP staff during both day- and nighttime shifts. Day APP ratio is 1:4, and night ratio is 1:10. Teaching team covers the other 12 patients during the day with the attending. Attending intensivist covers 24 h of the day with home night call. Attending covers 7 day blocks, on average 7 weeks of the year. Fellows, if available, take first call at night. One resident is in-house at night

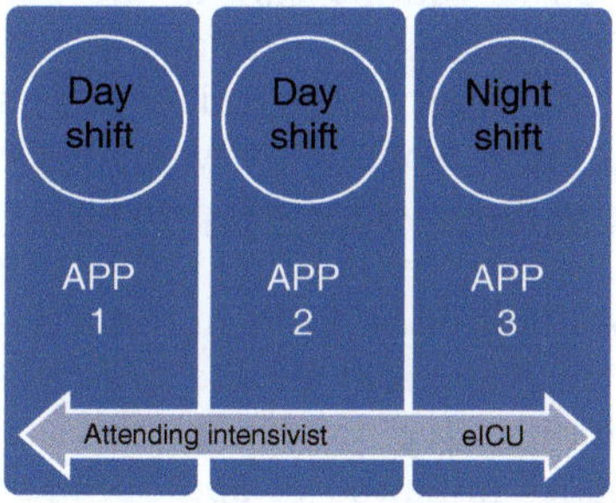

FIGURE 9.2 Staffing models. Community hospital with a 12-bed ICU. Day APPs cover all 12 patients with a staffing ratio of 1:6. Night shift APP covers 1:12. Attending intensivist covers in-house during the day. The e-ICU serves as physician support during the night hours

critical care intensivist rounds in-house during the day and takes call from home. Figure 9.2 represents a 12-bed ICU in a community hospital. This unit staffs 2 APPs per day who cover 6 patients each and 1 APP at night who covers 12 patients. The critical care intensivist is in-house during the day and will not take call at night. In this scenario the night shift intensivist physician is covered by e-ICU. The addition of e-ICU frees up night call responsibilities of the attending on record.

For critical care staffing models to run efficiently, the APP should be highly trained in the specialty of critical care medicine. While acute care nurse practitioners have education and training in acute illnesses, some may graduate with little exposure to critically ill patients. Only a handful of acute care programs include critical care elective training. PAs receive general training in primary medicine with training for advanced responsibilities traditionally provided by the sponsoring physician. Both nurse practitioners (NPs) and physician assistants (PAs) graduate from an accredited program of study and must pass national certifying exams to obtain state licensure.

The general medical areas that comprise the scope of practice for APPs include primary roles in both admissions and discharges, as well as routine care at the bedside, including daily assessment, ordering medications, initiating treatments, and reviewing and interpreting, diagnostic and laboratory tests [19]. Additional work activity involves assessing and implementing nutritional support, providing family updates and counseling, and communicating with consultants [20]. The roles and responsibilities of APPs in the ICU setting include comprehensive management of the critically ill patient in group collaboration with physician intensivists [19]. Their role in the ICU includes initiation of appropriate treatments and medications using established protocols and practices as well as interaction with the multidisciplinary ICU team on rounds, consultation with other providers to optimize care, communication with patients and families, and coordination of multidisciplinary care among admitting services, consultants, and the other members of the ICU team [21]. APPs can also be credentialed to perform a myriad of procedures. Some common procedures in which APPs can perform include arterial lines, central lines, thoracentesis, paracentesis, medical and surgical chest tube placement, and lumbar punctures. In many settings, APPs can manage the airway either by providing bag mask ventilation or inserting endotracheal tubes.

After obtaining licensure and certification, additional training in specialty areas occurs during orientation or structured postgraduate residency and fellowship programs. APPs can provide high-quality, cost-effective care if given time to develop appropriate skillsets relevant to their specialty areas. However, during the practice transition year, many mistakes in patient care can occur due to lack of training and support for the new graduate provider. New graduates can face unorganized orientation periods and experienced mentors lack the time to train due to growing clinical demands. Employers have also recognized the liability new graduates bring, understanding that they need significant mentoring prior to autonomous practice. Orientation quality and structure can differ significantly within ones' own institution as well as across the country. Harris reported inadequate and unorganized orientation leads to job dissatisfaction [22], while Bush reported increased job satisfaction with completion of a postgraduate residency or fellowship program [23]. Evidence is emerging showing deficits in confidence and competence during the first year after graduation for the student transitioning to the provider role [24]. To accommodate this void during the transitional year, many healthcare institutions have created postgraduate residency or fellowship programs [25]. New graduates are seeking out programs which offer specialty training in a structured and safe environment [26]. The first PA residency program originated at Montefiore Medical Center in 1971 [27]. In 2007, Community Health Center in Connecticut created the first nurse practitioner residency [28]. New graduates who complete residency or fellowship programs are provided a robust training structure and a safe place to learn as well as a leadership curriculum in which to grow their skills. Over the last 10 years, postgraduate training for APPs has expanded at an exponential growth. In 2011, the Emory Critical Care Center created a joint NPPA critical care program which received the nation's first accreditation for nurse practitioners from the American Nurses Credentialing Center as a practice transition program [29]. APP residency and fellowship programs fill the workforce void with highly qualified providers while also developing the next generation of provider leaders.

Today, more than 100 APP residency or fellowship training programs successfully train the next generation of providers. Although more healthcare systems are implementing residency and fellowship programs, little evidence exists which supports these programs. Healthcare institutions appreciate a need for structured transition to practice and formal verification of specialty-specific competency despite the deficit in evidence [26]. The cause of the deficit is multifaceted and can mostly be attributed to the low numbers of individuals completing these programs. Currently only a few studies exist to support postgraduate training for APRNs. The obvious gap in robust evidence supporting fellowship programs limits growth and validity. While we may see and feel the benefits at the bedside, healthcare institutions, academic programs of study, and government bodies struggle to financially support these programs. In 2010, the Institute of Medicine published guidelines in the Future of Nursing Report which supported residency and fellowship training for APRNs. These recommendations were upheld in the 2015 update [29, 30]. Despite recommendations, more research is needed to support this initiative.

APPs now work in a variety of ICU settings providing critical care services. Several studies support utilization of APPs within staffing models producing positive impacts on patient care management. APPs enhance patient care flow without altering patient outcomes or direct hospital costs. Implementing APP staffing models produces similar outcomes to resident physician models, while other studies have shown improved clinical and financial outcomes for specific patient populations. Patient satisfaction, enhanced collaboration, and communication in the ICU along with increased compliance with clinical practice guidelines are other positive outcomes associated with the APP workforce [20]. APPs are a viable alternative to traditional staffing models, providing safe and effective care in the critical care environment [20, 31–33].

References

1. Grabenkort R, Meissen H, Gregg S, et al. Acute care nurse practitioners and physician assistants in critical care: transforming education and practice. Crit Care Med. 2017;45(7):1111–4.
2. Singh H, Thomas EJ, Peterson LA, et al. Medical errors involving trainees: a study of closed malpractice claims from 5 insurers. Arch Intern Med. 2007;167:2030–6.
3. Freed GL, Dunham KM, Moran LM, et al. Resident work hour changes in children's hospitals: impact on staffing patterns and workforce needs. Pediatrics. 2012;130:700–4.
4. Cook RI, Render M, Woods DD. Gaps in the continuity of care and progress on patient safety. BMJ. 2000;320:791–4.
5. Pastores SM, O'Connor MF, Kleinpell RM, et al. The accreditation Council for Graduate Medical Education resident duty hour new standards: history, changes and impact on staffing of intensive care units. Crit Care Med. 2011;39:2540–9.
6. Evaluation of hospital-setting HCIA awards: third annual report. 2016. https://downloads.cms.gov/files/cmmi/hcia-hospitalsetting-thirdannualrpt.pdf. Accessed 31 Jan 2018.
7. Gutsche JT, Raiten JM. Staffing models for the ICU: open, closed, MD, NP, or telemedicine? Curr Anesthesiol Rep. 2013;3:65–72.
8. National Survey 2013. AAPA https://www.aapa.org/wpcontent/uploads/2016/12/Annual_Server_Data_Tables-S.pdf. Accessed 31st Jan 2018.
9. National Survey 2015. AANP https://www.aanp.org/research/reports. Accessed 31 Jan 2018.
10. Gershengorn HB, et al. Impact of non-physician staffing on outcomes in a medical ICU. Chest. 139(6):1347–53.
11. Buchman T, Coopersmith C, Meissen H, et al. Innovative interdisciplinary strategies to address the intensivist shortage. Crit Care Med. 2017;45(2):298–304.
12. Haupt MT, Bekes CE, Brilli RJ, et al. Guidelines on critical care services and personnel: recommendations based on a system of categorization of three levels of care. Crit Care Med. 2003;31(11):2677–83.
13. Leapfrog Group. Leapfrog hospital survey. Factsheet: ICU physician staffing. http://www.leapfroggroup.org/sites/default/files/Files/IPS%20Fact%20Sheet.pdf. Last revised April 1, 2016. Accessed 26 July 2016.

14. Krell K. Critical care workforce. Crit Care Med. 2008;36(4):1350–3.
15. Pronovost PJ, Needham DM, Waters H, et al. Intensive care unit physician staffing: financial modeling of the leapfrog standard. Crit Care Med. 2004;32(6):1247–53.
16. Pronovost PJ, Angus DC, Dorman T, et al. Physician staffing patterns and clinical outcomes in critically ill patients: a systematic review. JAMA. 2002;288(17):2151–62.
17. Kleinpell RM, Ward NS, Kelso LA, et al. Provider to patient ratios for nurse practitioners and physician assistants in critical care units. AJCC. 2015;24(3):e16–21.
18. Valentin A, Ferdinande P. ESICM working group on quality improvement. Recommendations on basic requirements for intensive care units: structural and organizational aspects. Intensive Care Med. 2011;37(10):1575–87.
19. Kleinpell, RM, Buchman, TG, Boyle, WA. Meeting 21st-century challenges in critical care delivery and beyond: nurse practitioner and physician assistant providers in the ICU. In: Integrating nurse practitioners and physician assistants in the ICU: strategies for optimizing contributions to care. Mount Prospect: Society of Critical Care Medicine. Chicago Illinois. 2012. p. 1–8.
20. Kirton OC, Folcik MA, Me I, et al. Midlevel practitioner workforce analysis at a university-affiliated teaching hospital. Arch Surg. 2007;142:336–41.
21. Kleinpell RM, Ely EW, Grabenkort R. Nurse practitioners and physician assistants in the intensive care unit: an evidence-based review. Crit Care Med. 2008;36:2888–97.
22. Harris C. Bridging the gap between acute care nurse practitioner education practice: the need for postgraduate residency programs. J Nurse Pract. 2014;10:331–6.
23. Bush CT. Postgraduate nurse practitioner education: impact on job satisfaction. J Nurse Pract. 2016;12:226–34.
24. Hart AM, Bowen A. New nurse practitioners' perceptions of preparedness for and transition into practice. J Nurse Pract. 2016;12:545–52.
25. Development MH. Evaluation, and verification of competencies: what advanced practice providers and physician leaders can learn from each other. In: LaRosa J, Kaufman K, editors. Current concepts in adult critical care, vol. 8. Mt Prospect: Society of Critical Care Medicine; 2017. p. 65–74.
26. Association of Post Graduate APRN Programs. http://www.apgap.org/. Accessed 28 July 2016.

27. Montefiore. Postgraduate residency for physician assistants in surgery. http://www.montefiore.org/postgraduate-residency-physician-assistants-surgery. Accessed 27 July 2016.
28. Flinter M. From new nurse practitioner to primary care provider: bridging the transition through FQHC-based residency training. Online J Issues Nurs. 2011;17:6.
29. Institute of Medicine. The future of nursing: leading change, advancing health. Washington, DC: The National Academies Press; 2010.
30. Institute of Medicine. Assessing progress on the Institute of Medicine the Future of nursing report. Washington, DC: The National Academies Press; 2015.
31. Garland A, Gershengorn HB. Staffin in ICUs: physicians and alternative staffing models. Chest. 2013;143:214–21.
32. Fry M. Literature review of the impact of nurse practitioners in critical care services. Nurs Crit Care. 2011;16:58–66.
33. Gershengorn HB, Johsnson MP, Factor P. The use of nonphysician providers in adult intensive care units. Am J Respir Crit Care Med. 2012;185:600–5.

[illegible]

Chapter 10
Critical Care Billing, Coding, and Documentation

Michael J. Apostolakos

Case Presentation

Day 1

A 75-year-old male presents to the emergency department (ED) of an academic medical center with cough, fever, and shortness of breath. He became sick over the previous week. Symptoms markedly worsened over the past 2 days. He has a 40 pack-year smoking history and moderate chronic obstructive pulmonary disease (COPD). He has hypertension and mild renal insufficiency. His medications include fluticasone/salmeterol inhaler, albuterol inhaler, lisinopril, and metoprolol. His vital signs on arrival to the ED are blood pressure (BP) 85/60 mmHg, respiratory rate (RR) 26 breaths/min, heart rate (HR) 120 beats/min, and regular and temperature of 102 degrees F.

Initial labs reveal a white blood cell count (WBC) of 20,000/microL with 20% bands, creatinine 1.8 mg/dL (baseline 1.3 mg/dL), lactate 3.7 mmol/dL and chest x-ray (CXR) with right

M. J. Apostolakos
University of Rochester Medical Center, Rochester, NY, USA
e-mail: Michael_apostolakos@urmc.rochester.edu

J. A. LaRosa (ed.), *Adult Critical Care Medicine*,
https://doi.org/10.1007/978-3-319-94424-1_10

middle lobe (RML) infiltrate. Oxygen (O_2) saturation is 70%. Arterial blood gas (ABG) on 100% non-rebreather (NRB) mask is pH 7.45/PCO_2 30 mmHg/PO_2 65 mmHg/O_2 sat 93%.

The ED attending spends 45 min assessing and treating this patient. He directs the intravenous fluid (IVF) and antibiotics. He calls the critical care medicine (CCM) attending to discuss the case and to request CCM admission.

A nurse practitioner (NP) who is part of the critical care provider group assesses and continues the treatment of the patient in the ED. The patient's BP remains 85/60 mmHg, HR is 115 beats/min, and RR is 28 breaths/min and mildly labored. Two additional liters of IVF are administered. Repeat lactate is 3.5 mg/dL. Urine output is 15 mL/h. Vancomycin and piperacillin/tazobactam have been administered. The NP places a central line in anticipation of the need for pressors. Total time spent by NP assessing and treating the patient exclusive of time spent for the central line placement was 55 min. The patient is discussed with the CCM attending and admitted to the intensive care unit (ICU).

On arrival to the ICU, the patient is immediately evaluated by the critical care medicine (CCM) attending. The attending assesses the patient, reviews labs, and begins norepinephrine at 1 mcg/min intravenously (IV) and titrates this to a mean arterial pressure (MAP) of 65 mmHg. He boluses two more liters of IVF and assesses intravascular volume by bedside ultrasound (US). The patient becomes progressively tachypneic using accessory muscles, and the patient is semi-electively intubated. Total time spent with the patient exclusive of the intubation was 45 min. The attending spends 20 min updating the family in the waiting room prior to the family seeing the patient.

Day 2

Overnight, the patient stabilizes, and the norepinephrine is slowly titrated down from a peak of 25 mcg/min to off. The patient appears euvolemic on exam. He is on mechanical ventilation settings of volume control (VC) with RR set at 14 breaths/min, tidal volume (TV) 550 mL, positive end expiratory pressure (PEEP) of 10 cm H_2O, and 60% fraction of inspired O_2 (FiO_2). Chest x-ray (CXR) reveals mild pulmonary edema on top of RML infiltrate. The patient's ABG is pH 7.37, PCO_2 40 mmHg, and PaO_2 60 mmHg with O_2 saturation of 91%. The patient's lactate has decreased to 1.9 mmol/L from a peak of 5.5 mmol/L the previous night. The CCM attending rounds on the patient with the ICU team. The CCM attending reviews the labs/data with the team and performs an independent physical exam. The attending reviews the note written by a second year medical resident he is supervising which accurately summarizes the patient's medical problems, how the patient is responding to therapy, and the plans for the day. The CCM attending reviews and cosigns the note stating that he has assessed and discussed the patient with the resident and that he agrees with the note written by the resident. He goes on to say that the patients BP is stabilizing and that the decreasing lactate suggests improving perfusion of tissue and that the patient appears to be responding to the antibiotics.

Early in the afternoon, the patient develops tachycardia and hypotension with systolic blood pressure (SBP) in the 80s mmHg. IVF boluses of lactated ringers 30 mL/Kg x 2 are given with transient improvement in blood pressure. Electrocardiogram (EKG) reveals nonspecific ST-T wave changes. Repeat hematocrit (HCT) reveals a drop to 15%. A nasogastric (NG) tube is placed with return of 500 cc of bright red blood. The patient is started on IV Protonix drip and transfused with two units of packed red blood cells (PRBCs). The attending was at the bedside or on the floor reviewing tests on this patient for 35 min. The advanced practice provider (APP) was there for 30 min caring for the patient as well during the same time period. A gastrointestinal service consult is called, and they perform upper endoscopy on the patient. Severe gastritis with bleeding gastric ulcer with visible vessel is coagulated, and the bleeding stops. The patient stabilizes.

Day 3

The next day, the patient's vital signs remain stable with HR 90 beats/min, BP 120/80 mmHg, RR 18 breaths/min on 50% FiO_2, and 8 cm H_2O PEEP. The patient's HCT is 22%. Troponin T returns and is increased to 1.0 ng/mL. Bedside echocardiogram (ECHO) reveals global mild-moderate hypokinesis with ejection fraction of 40%. A cardiology consult is called. EKG remains with nonspecific ST-T wave changes. Cardiology makes the diagnosis of demand mediated non-ST myocardial infarction (NSTMI). They recommend to continue the patient's ASA, low-dose beta-blocker, and statin.

Days 4–13

Over the next 10 days, the patient's condition changes minimally each day. The patient meets oxygenation criteria to extubate but fails daily pressure support (PS) trials with rapid shallow breathing index above 100 each day.

The patient's failure to wean to date is felt to be due to underlying COPD with recent pneumonia and sepsis complicated by upper gastrointestinal bleed and NSTMI. A family meeting is held with wife and children at the patient's bedside so that the patient can participate. Previously the patient had stated he didn't want prolonged mechanical ventilation. After discussing for 90 min the risks and benefits of tracheostomy and prolonged wean with the patient and family, they decide to proceed with tracheostomy.

Days 14–28

The patient makes slow progress with weaning after tracheostomy and is transferred to a weaning unit.

Overview

This case illustrates the broad array of services that a critical care specialist provides. It describes scenarios in which billing codes for critical care, procedures, and evaluation and management should be used. Furthermore, the case involves critical care services provided by advanced practice providers (APPs) such as nurse practitioners (NPs) or physicians assistants (PAs) as well as care provided by attendings while supervising residents or fellows. One must understand the billing of services under these situations as in order to document, code, and bill accurately and appropriately.

In order to understand the billing, coding, and documentation, one must understand Current Procedural Terminology (CPT) and International Statistical Classification of Diseases and Related Health Problems (ICD) codes as well as relative value units (RVUs).

CPT codes are owned by the American Medical Association [1]. They are a series of numbers generally five numbers long that usually start with 99. They are used to identify services, procedures, and other diagnostic and treatment services performed by physicians. CPT codes are used to communicate with third-party insurance payers.

ICD is a medical classification list by the World Health Organization [2, 3]. As the name implies, ICD assigns a number to describe each of the thousands of possible diseases. Currently, the United States uses a modification of ICD referred to as ICD-10-Clinical Modification or simply ICD-10-CM.

RVUs assign the value to the work required for different medical procedures and services [4]. RVUs are one part of the complicated reimbursement process, which also takes into account geographic differences in costs to provide services that are used to determine an appropriate level of payment to the provider. RVUs are used by insurers to reimburse medical care fairly among different specialties. While private payers vary in their reimbursement rates and policies, most are tied in some form to the Medicare system.

In order to follow the case discussion, one must understand the basics of billing. Evaluation and management (referred to as E/M) describes a series of CPT codes that do not involve a procedure but rather account for physician time, intensity of service, and complexity of the evaluation and treatment. Providers are paid by insurance companies based on which CPT code is submitted. An ICD-10-CM code is attached to the CPT code to reveal the medical complaints and conditions addressed in the visit. This system is complex. The Centers for Medicare and Medicaid Services (CMS) promulgates documentation requirements for use with CPT codes [5]. Most insurers use these documentation requirements as well. The components of medical record documentation for E/M services include the reason for the encounter (history, physical examination, and prior diagnostic studies), assessment, clinical impression or diagnosis, and medical plan. However, documentation also entails time-based E/M codes for which the requirements for documentation and billing are different. Critical care codes are one example of time-based codes. It is the provider's responsibility to ensure that the medical record supports the level of service reported to the payer. More information regarding requirements to meet E/M billing may be found here [6–8].

As stated above, critical care codes are time-based E/M codes. Critical care is defined as the direct delivery by a physician(s) of medical care for a critically ill or critically injured patient. A critical illness or injury acutely impairs one or more vital organ systems such that there is a high probability of imminent or life-threatening deterioration in the patient's condition. The use of critical care codes (CPT 99291-99292) requires a minimum of 30 min of care treating a critical illness using "using high complexity decision-making to assess, manipulate, and support vital systems to treat single or multiple vital organ system failure and/or prevent further life-threatening deterioration of the patient's condition," per CMS. Documentation for each date and encounter must accurately state the appropriateness of care and include the total time spent providing critical care. The critical and unstable nature of the patient's condition should be accurately documented to support the medical necessity of the extended 1:1 care. The complexity of the medical decision-making should be clear as well as the aggregate of the total time spent with the patient. Details of the requirements to bill critical care codes may be found here [5].

Critical Care Billing, Coding, and Documentation: Case Discussion

Day 1

This patient presents with signs and symptoms of pneumonia on top of having significant comorbidities of COPD, renal insufficiency, and hypertension. His vital signs (soft BP, elevated HR and RR) as well as an elevated lactate and creatinine as well as hypoxia all support critical illness. Critical care codes are not site-specific. Critical care may be provided on the hospital floor, in the emergency department, in the post-anesthesia recovery room, or in other areas of the hospital. The ED physician spent 45 min evaluating and stabilizing this patient with IVF, oxygen, and antibiotics for pneumonia. One needs to spend at least 30 min doing so to bill the first hour of critical care (CPT 99291). Once a provider spends 75 min or more, subsequent half hours of critical care (CPT 99292) may be billed per the table (Table 10.1). If less than 30 min is spent caring for the patient, the appropriate E/M code must be billed.

The APP from the critical care medicine team is consulted and subsequently manages the patient in the ED. The patient remains critically ill and requires constant attention. The patient's vital signs (HR, BP, and RR) and persistently elevated lactate and low urine output all support the critical nature of this patient's condition. This provider's evaluation and management of this patient's critical conditions requires

Table 10.1 Critical Care billing code requirements by time

Total Duration	Codes
Less than 30 min	99232 or 99233 or other E/M code
30–74 min	99291 x 1
75–104 min	99291 x 1 and 99292 x 1
105–134 min	99291 x 1 and 99292 x 2
135–164 min	99291 x 1 and 99292 x 3
165–194 min	99291 x 1 and 99292 x 4
194 min or longer	99291 x 1 and 99292 as appropriate (per the above illustration)

55 min of time. This qualifies for the first hour of critical care which will be reimbursed at 85% of the rate for physicians. This time will only be reimbursed if it is not concurrent with the ED physician's critical care. That is, only one provider may bill critical care at a time even if two are at the bedside at the same time. Therefore, it is a good practice to not only document the total time but the exact time during the day that the critical care was provided to clearly demonstrate that critical care was provided at different times and was not "double billed." The APP may also bill for the central line placed in addition to the critical care time spent caring for the patient. Critical care time is exclusive of procedures that may be billed separately (Table 10.2). Certain procedures are billed as part of critical care time and should not be billed separately (Table 10.3).

The patient is transferred to the ICU where the critical care attending evaluates and continues the stabilization process for the patient. He starts a pressor to increase BP and perfusion. He continues volume boluses based on bedside US of the heart and inferior vena cava. Total time spent providing critical care services is 45 min. Routine updates of families (20 min in this case) are not counted as critical care time. Discussions with patients and/or families of critically ill patients leading to important goals of care or treatment decisions may be included in critical care time [5].

TABLE 10.2 Common procedures that may be billed separately from critical care codes (99291–99292)

Procedures	CPT® codes
CPR (while being performed)	92950
Endotracheal intubation	31500
Central line placement	36555, 36556
Intraosseous placement	36680
Tube thoracostomy	32551
Temporary transvenous pacemaker	33210
Electrocardiogram interpretation and report only	93010
Elective electrical cardioversion	92960

TABLE 10.3 Services that are included in critical care codes (99291–99292) and should not be billed separately

Procedures	CPT® codes
Interpretation of cardiac output measurements	93561, 93562
Chest x-rays, professional component	71010, 71015, 71020
Blood draw for specimen	36415
Blood gases, data stored in computers	99090
Gastric intubation	43752, 91105
Pulse oximetry	94760, 94761, 94762
Temporary transcutaneous pacing	92953
Ventilator management	94002-94004, 94660, 94662
Vascular access procedures	36000, 36410, 36415, 36591, 36600

As the APP who billed earlier is in the same billing group as the attending, only one of them may bill the first hour of critical care. There is no split/shared billing for critical care.

One of them alone must meet criteria to bill the first hour of critical care. After that, the times may be added to bill the subsequent half hours of critical care. In this case, 55 min plus 45 min is 110 min of critical care. Therefore the first hour of critical care (APP) and two subsequent ½ hours (CCM attending) may be billed (Table 10.1). In this case, the intubation may be billed separately from total critical care time. Critical care procedures may not be split/shared between APPs and attending physicians. Whoever performs the procedures bills for the procedure.

Day 2

The patient stabilizes overnight, and the overall condition has improved. Pressors have been weaned off, and oxygenation is improved. A medical resident is working with the team and sees the patient prior to rounding with the attending. During rounds, the patient is evaluated by the attending including physical examination, review of data, and discussion with the team. The attending reviews the residents note which accurately summarizes the patient condition and plan. He states such and cosigns the note. He has spent a total of 23 min caring for the patient. The totality of the note (resident and attending) may be used for billing. Based on the complexity of the care, if a detailed history or physical examination is performed, a high-level follow-up visit (CPT 99233) may be billed [7, 8]. As less than 30 min was spent caring for the patient, critical care may not be billed.

If an attending physician is working with a resident(s) and wishes to bill critical care, the teaching physician must meet the criteria for billing on their own. Time spent teaching must not be counted. Only time spent providing critical care together (or the attending alone) may be counted. A combination of the teaching attending and resident documentation may be utilized to support the critical care billing. However, the teaching physician's medical record documentation must provide substantive information, including the following:

(1) the time the teaching physician spent providing critical care, (2) confirmation that the patient was critically ill during the time the teaching physician saw the patient, (3) what made the patient critically ill, and (4) the nature of the treatment and management provided by the teaching physician.

Later in the day, the patient becomes critically unstable with what appears to be a gastrointestinal bleed. The patient's drop in BP and HCT supports this. The patient's attending and NP were at the bedside resuscitating the patient. The attending is there for 35 min, and the NP is there for 30 min. As they were there concurrently, only one may bill. As the APP is only reimbursed at 85% of the physician rate, the physician should be the one to bill for the time. This time may be billed in addition to the E/M code earlier in the day, as two separate services were performed. The patient stabilizes after being seen by the GI specialist, and the gastritis is actively treated.

Day 3

The next day the patient remains stable. The CCM attending evaluated the patient with the APP who is in the same billing group. As opposed to critical care which cannot be split/shared as far as billing goes, E/M codes may be split/shared by a physician and APP in the same group practice so long as the physician provides any "face-to-face" portion of the encounter. Their combined documentation must support the level of billing [7, 8].

Day 4–13

From day 4 through 13, the patient is not critically ill. The appropriate E/M code should be chosen to bill each day. It should be noted for the family meeting that there are time-based E/M codes other than critical care codes. The E/M guidelines have a specific provision to allow physicians to use time as the controlling factor to determine the level of care in certain circumstances. In these instances, the physician must spend the entire allotted time face-to-face with the patient, and at least half of that time must be used for “counseling and coordination of care.” If you choose to code based on time, you must record the duration of the encounter and also state that more than half the time was spent on counseling and coordination of care. In addition, the nature of the counseling and coordination of care must be documented [6–8]. If you code based on time, there are no specific documentation requirements for history, physical examination, and medical decision-making. It is recommended, however, that you record pertinent information about these items in the chart. It is essential to record the time spent. The 90 min spent discussing the tracheostomy with the patient and family should be billed using this method.

Day 14–28

This patient remains stable with slow clinical improvement and weaning. Generally, E/M codes will be billed. One could consider ventilator management codes if the physician is only managing the ventilator. Two codes are used for ventilator management for inpatient services: 94002 and 94003. One code is for the day when the physician initiates ventilator management, and the second code is for a subsequent day. These codes have total RVUs of 2.43 and 1.76, respectively. These codes should be used when ventilator management is the only service provided by the physician. If the patient is not critically ill, this code or another E/M code should be utilized. If the physician is also providing other critical care services, he or she should bill only for the critical care [5]. The ventilator management codes are bundled into the critical care code 99291 and may not be reported (and will not be paid) separately. Ventilator management is also bundled into the other hospital E/M codes. The physician may not report and will not be paid for ventilator management and initial or subsequent hospital (E/M) visits on the same day. The relative

TABLE 10.4 Medicare reimbursement for medical care

Billing code	RVUs	Medicare reimbursement
99291 (1st hour critical care)	6.26	$226
99292 (subsequent critical care)	3.16	$113
99231 (level 1 subsequent hospital care)	1.10	$40
99232 (level 2 subsequent hospital care)	2.03	$73
99233 (level 3 subsequent hospital care)	2.92	$105
99221 (level 1 admission history and physical)	2.87	$102
99222 (level 2 admission history and physical)	3.88	$138
99223 (level 3 admission history and physical)	5.71	$204
94002 (ventilator management, initial)	2.43	$87
94003 (ventilator management, subsequent)	1.76	$63

RVUs and reimbursements for critical care, E/M, and ventilator management codes are listed here (Table 10.4).

Summary

Critical care physicians are drawn to their field to help patients and their families during life-threatening illness. Most critical care physicians are not formally trained on how to bill for services, and to some this may seem an unimportant issue. Billing for services to critically ill patients is complex but necessary for the successful practice of critical care. Knowing how to bill appropriately assures appropriate reimbursement for the important work critical care providers perform. In order to do so, one must understand the environment they work in and thus the requirements for documentation, coding, and billing while working alone or with residents, APPs, and other consultants/physicians. Hopefully, this case study helps critical care providers do just that.

References

1. American Medical Association. CPT (Current Procedural Terminology). https://www.ama-assn.org/practice-management/cpt-current-procedural-terminology. Accessed 12/28/2017.
2. Centers for Medicare and Medicaid Services. ICD-10 (CMS). https://www.cms.gov/Medicare/Coding/ICD10/. Accessed 12/28/2017.
3. Centers for Disease Control and Prevention. International Classification of Diseases, Tenth Revision, Clinical Modification (ICD-10-CM) https://www.cdc.gov/nchs/icd/icd10cm.htm. Accessed 12/28/2017.
4. Beck DE, Margolin DA. Physician coding and reimbursement. Ochsner J. 2007;7:8–15.
5. Centers for Medicare and Medicaid Services. Medicare Claims Processing Manual Chapter 12 – Physicians/Nonphysician Practitioners https://www.cms.gov/Regulations-and-Guidance/Guidance/Manuals/downloads/clm104c12.pdf. Accessed 12/28/2017.
6. Centers for Medicare and Medicaid Services. Evaluation and Management services guide, August 2015. Centers for Medicare & Medicaid Services. https://www.cms.gov/Outreach-and-Education/Medicare-Learning-Network-MLN/MLNProducts/MLN-Publications-Items/CMS1243514.html. Accessed 12/28/2017.
7. Centers for Medicare and Medicaid Services. 1997 Documentation Guidelines for Evaluation and Management Services (Centers for Medicare & Medicaid Services). https://www.cms.gov/Outreach-and-Education/Medicare-Learning-Network-MLN/MLNEdWebGuide/Downloads/97Docguidelines.pdf. Accessed 12/28/2017.
8. Centers for Medicare and Medicaid Services. 1995 Documentation Guidelines for Evaluation and Management Services (Centers for Medicare & Medicaid Services). https://www.cms.gov/Outreach-and-Education/Medicare-Learning-Network-MLN/MLNEdWebGuide/Downloads/95Docguidelines.pdf. Accessed 12/28/2017.

Chapter 11
Shock and Vasopressors: State-of-the-Art Update

Michael Kouch and R. Phillip Dellinger

Introduction

Shock is present when the cardiovascular system is unable to maintain appropriate blood flow to vital organs. Inadequate tissue perfusion (tissue hypoperfusion) is defined by some combination of hypotension, oliguria, and elevated lactate and results in impaired delivery of nutrients to tissues, most notably, oxygen. Based on the type of shock, some combination of intravenous fluids (or blood), inotropic agents, and vasopressors are used to improve perfusion in such pathophysiologic states. With the exception of hypovolemic shock, vasopressors are a key component of shock therapy. Even in hypovolemic shock, vasopressors may be initially required to maintain blood pressure during fluid and/or blood resuscitation. Below, we present a case of shock and a practical

M. Kouch · R. P. Dellinger (✉)
Critical Care Medicine, Cooper University Health Care,
Cooper Medical School of Rowan University, Camden, NJ, USA
e-mail: Kouch-Michael@CooperHealth.edu;
Dellinger-Phil@CooperHealth.edu

J. A. LaRosa (ed.), *Adult Critical Care Medicine*,
https://doi.org/10.1007/978-3-319-94424-1_11

approach to management. At each stage of management in the case, we will pause to describe the reasoning and literature behind each clinical decision. We encourage the reader to answer each clinical question before moving forward.

Case Presentation

A 67-year-old male presents to the emergency department via emergency medical services with the chief complaint of near syncope. His triage vital signs are as follows:

Heart rate (HR) 122 beats per minute (bpm), respiratory rate (RR) 32 breaths per minute, blood pressure (BP) 72/44 mmHg, pulse oximetry 93% on room air, and temperature 101.7 F. He has a past medical history of poorly controlled hypertension, hyperlipidemia, and benign prostatic hypertrophy (urgency, frequency). Upon discussion with the family at bedside, the patient had been complaining of lightheadedness for 2 days.

On exam, the patient is slow to respond but oriented to person, place, and time. He has dry mucous membrane without lesions. He is tachycardic with clear and equal breath sounds bilaterally. His extremities are warm with capillary refill >3 s. His abdomen is moderately tender in the suprapubic region without rebound. No skin lesions are noted. He has 5/5 strength bilaterally with no dysmetria. He has no nuchal rigidity.

The patient is currently retired with no recent travel history. He has no recent hospitalizations and lives at home with his wife. He has taken no new medications recently.

Point-of-care testing reveals a normal glucose and a lactate of 5.1 mmol/L. Intravenous (IV) access is obtained, and laboratory studies are sent.

You perform a focused bedside ultrasound assessment which shows a collapsible inferior vena cava (IVC) with respirations, no free fluid at Morrison's pouch, and an abdominal aorta measuring 2.7 cm at maximum diameter. You note the right ventricle is not well visualized. The left ventricle has moderate depression in contractility. His records show a recent echocardiogram with normal left ventricular function.

What is your differential diagnosis for his current condition?

The differential diagnosis for this patient should initially include all shock etiologies. The history is not consistent with anaphylactic, neurogenic, or hemorrhagic shock. This patient's left ventricular function is depressed with a previous echocardiogram that was normal and could be seen with cardiogenic, septic, or anaphylactic shock. The hallmarks of distributive or vasodilatory shock include relative hypovolemia (venodilation), absolute hypovolemia (capillary leak), arterial vasodilation, and in some patients depression of cardiac contractility. Sepsis-induced cardiomyopathy complicates over half of all sepsis cases [3].

A diagnosis of presumed septic shock is made. Blood cultures are drawn, and broad-spectrum antibiotics are begun. Crystalloid in the form of lactated Ringers is ordered to be administered stat with a dose of 30 ml/kg over 30 min.

Complete blood count shows a leukocytosis of 22 K, with platelets of 110 10^3 /μL.

Basic metabolic panel is notable for a creatinine of 2.2 mEq/L with a BUN of 43 mg/dL, bicarbonate of 15 mEq/L, and an anion gap of 20.

A chest radiograph is obtained and shows no acute pathology. Urinalysis is positive for ketones, leukocyte esterase, and nitrites. There are too numerous to count white blood cells present on microscopic exam. Urosepsis is now the presumed diagnosis.

A formal ultrasound is performed showing no hydronephrosis or perinephric fluid collection.

Following the 30 ml/kg fluid bolus, the patient remains hypotensive with a mean arterial pressure (MAP) of 55 mmHg with continued delayed capillary refill.

You make the decision to start vasopressors to maintain end-organ perfusion.

Consider the following questions:

Within what time frame would you initiate vasopressors in a patient with persistent hypotension?

What is your MAP goal in general and specifically in a patient with a history of poorly controlled hypertension?

Which is your initial choice of vasopressor, and why?

Will you delay vasopressor initiation for central venous catheter placement?
Does this patient require arterial line placement?

The Surviving Sepsis Campaign (SSC) has issued recommendations regarding vasopressors in septic shock [1]. The choice of norepinephrine versus dopamine as the first-line vasopressor had once been an area of staunch debate. However, it has become standard practice to use norepinephrine as the first-line vasopressor to treat septic shock. When compared to dopamine, norepinephrine has demonstrated increased potency in achieving a MAP goal [4]. The superiority of norepinephrine is due primarily to its relatively limited side effect profile without sacrificing efficacy when compared to alternative vasopressors. Norepinephrine typically does not produce significant tachycardia as its venoconstriction effect and associated stimulation of right atrial baroreceptors neutralize the beta-1 chronotropic stimulation. When compared to dopamine, norepinephrine has a lower incidence of arrhythmic events [5, 6]. In a single meta-analysis, dopamine may have an increased relative risk of death when compared to norepinephrine [7]. This information has pushed norepinephrine to the forefront as the preferred vasopressor. Dopamine has been relegated to a niche role as a vasopressor which will be discussed later.

Despite no head-to-head trials showing that norepinephrine is superior to epinephrine for the treatment of septic shock, norepinephrine is, in general, considered to have a more preferable side effect profile. Epinephrine has been associated with tachycardia, transient increase in insulin requirements, and elevated lactic acid levels as displayed in Fig. 11.1 [8]. Epinephrine, along with low-dose vasopressin, is considered the next drug of choice in septic shock patients that do not respond to norepinephrine.

Studies in septic shock have revealed low levels of circulating vasopressin, an unexpected finding as increased levels would be expected with hypotension, a stimulus for vasopressin release [9, 24]. This argument for a relative vasopressin

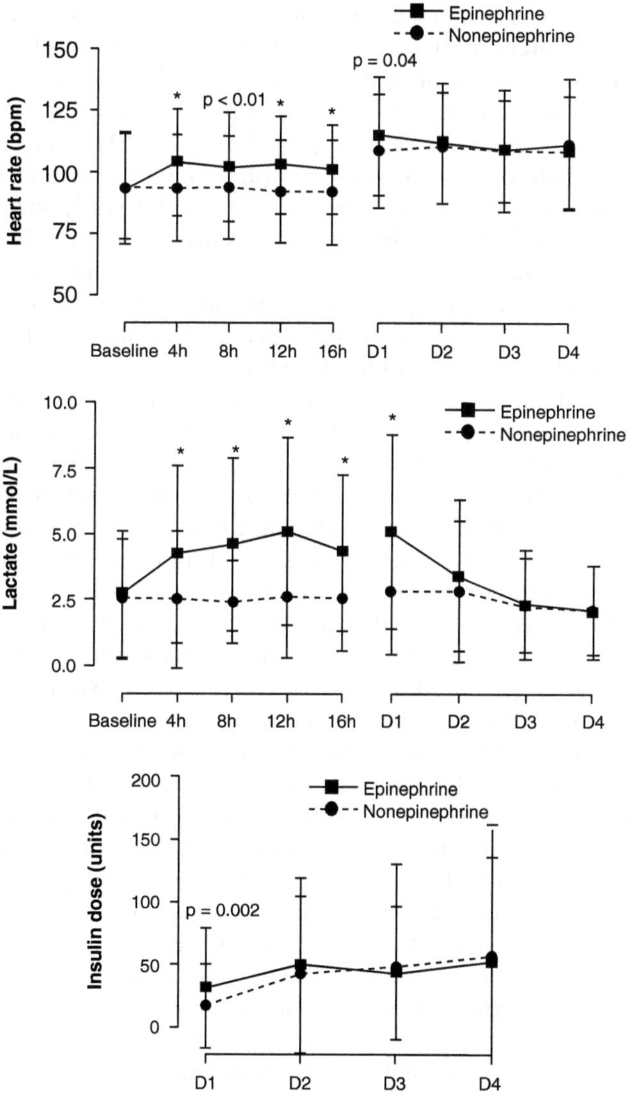

FIGURE 11.1 Comparisons between epinephrine and norepinephrine on heart rate (*top*), arterial lactate (*middle*), and mean daily insulin dose (*bottom*). (Reprinted/adapted with permission from Springer; Myburgh et al. [8])

deficiency has been made by some to support the use of low-dose vasopressin (up to 0.03–0.04 units per minute) as a physiologic replacement therapy in septic shock. The use of higher doses of vasopressin increases the risk of cardiac, digital, and splanchnic ischemia [10]. The VANISH trial used intermediate doses of vasopressin (up to 0.06 U/min) for the treatment of septic shock. The endpoint of this study was the incidence of kidney failure in septic shock. While no difference in kidney failure was demonstrated with the use of higher doses of vasopressin, the vasopressin group had a 2.5% increased risk of adverse events (see more detailed discussion of vasopressin to follow) [11].

The timing of initiation of vasopressors is not addressed in the SSC guidelines. The Centers for Medicare and Medicaid Services (CMS) sepsis quality measures give positive credit for achieving a MAP of 65 mmHg or greater within the first 6 h of diagnosis of septic shock and following 30 ml/kg crystalloid bolus. The classic teaching of "filling the tank" with fluid resuscitation prior to starting vasopressors is often the clinical approach. But this leaves the question: how long should a patient remain hypotensive prior to initiating vasopressors? Recent studies have looked at early versus delayed vasopressor initiation without a clear answer to this question. In a retrospective review, Bai et al. displayed an increase in survival with early administration of norepinephrine. This study noted a 5.3% increase in mortality with each hour delay in starting a vasopressor [12]. Beck et al. was able to show only a weak correlation between vasopressor delay and in-hospital mortality. The authors of this study note the effect to be driven by those patients with delays greater than 1 h [13]. Lastly a third retrospective review by Waechter et al. found the lowest mortality when vasopressors were initiated 1–6 h after the onset of shock and greater than 1 liters of IV fluids were completed [14]. Without clear randomized trials, it is not possible to give a definitive recommendation for timing of vasopressors. However, the severity and duration of hypotension are assumed to drive end-organ injury. It is, therefore, a reasonable approach to begin vasopressors within the first 1–6 h of resuscitation to achieve an adequate MAP and perfusion. In patients with profound hypotension or profound symptoms of hypotension, the decision to begin earlier and in parallel with initial fluid resuscitation would seem appropriate.

The next decision after initiation of a vasoactive medication is what MAP target to choose. Persistent hypotension (MAP <60–65 mmHg) has been associated with worse outcomes including increased risk of death [15]. In 2014, Asfar et al. performed an open-label randomized controlled trial comparing a low-target MAP group (65–70 mmHg) to a high-target group (80–85 mmHg). There was no difference in 30- or 90-day mortality. The low-target group exhibited fewer arrhythmias (primarily atrial fibrillation). In patients with a history of chronic hypertension, targeting a higher MAP did decrease the incidence of increasing creatinine and the rate of renal replacement therapy from days 1 to 7. Overall, there was no difference in major adverse events between the two groups [16]. This literature can be interpreted in different ways. A higher MAP goal may be considered to be safe and useful in patients with chronic hypertension in the hope of decreasing renal compromise (subgroup analysis). Another view would consider the higher MAP goal to be equal to lower MAP goal with a higher risk of arrhythmia (primary analysis). The most recent SSC guidelines recommend a MAP goal of 65 mmHg [1]. A MAP goal of 65 mmHg should be considered in the majority of patients but customized to the individual based on end-organ perfusion and observed side effects.

After choosing initial vasopressor and MAP goals, we move to the decision of how to deliver the vasoactive medication. Is a central venous catheter (CVC) required to initiate therapy? How safe is a peripheral IV (PIV)? Classic teaching has included the need for a CVC for delivery of vasopressors. This general practice has been driven by numerous case reports of vasopressor extravasation and tissue injury. However, recent studies have called this classic teaching into question. In 2013 Ricard et al. randomized patients to receive CVC or peripheral venous catheters at the beginning of fluid resuscitation and concomitantly used for vasopressor administration. The authors of this study concluded CVC to be superior to peripheral venous access, citing less major complications, including a 14% rate of extravasation in those patient receiving vasopressor through a peripheral IV. However, the majority of complications listed were erythema and difficulty with insertion or maintenance of the IV site. Location of peripheral access and clinical outcomes regarding tissue injury were not reported. Of note, approximately half of the peripheral venous access group from this study was transitioned to a CVC [17]. In 2015, Cardenas-Garcia et al. published data on a 20-month period in which vasopressors were delivered via peripheral access. In this single site study, the authors noted extravasation in only 2% of patients and no tissue injury after a protocolized treatment including site checks every 2 h and phentolamine and nitroglycerine treatment if extravasation was discovered. 13% of patients required transition to CVC placement. This study did not have a control group randomized to CVC only [18].

Extravasation of vasopressors is a real risk. But the severity and frequency of that risk are not fully clear. A systematic review by Loubani et al. in 2015 found 83.5% of all extravasation to have occurred in peripheral IV placement distal to the antecubital or popliteal fossae. The median time of administration of peripheral vasopressors before local tissue injury was 24 h [19]. Therefore, it appears to be a reasonable approach to initiate vasopressors via peripheral access as to not delay treatment. Based on the above literature, a well-placed IV proximal to the antecubital fossa is preferred. This site should be checked at a minimum of every 2 h and used for less than 24 h. This may limit the need for CVC if vasopressors can be weaned quickly with further resuscitation. We do not recommend extended use of peripheral IVs for vasopressor infusion.

In a patient requiring vasopressors for shock, an arterial line should be placed when available. Large randomized trials comparing noninvasive versus invasive blood pressure monitoring are not available. However, smaller studies have shown the unreliability of noninvasive blood pressure monitoring in shock [20, 21]. The insertion and maintenance of arterial lines have been shown to have a complication rate of less than 1% [22]. This limited complication risk and the unreliability of noninvasive monitoring lead to the recommendation for arterial line use. An underestimation of MAP would lead to overuse or excessive dosing of vasopressors.

We now return to our case.

Antibiotics and intravenous fluid resuscitation have been completed. Norepinephrine was initiated, but the patient continues to decline. He remains in shock with a norepinephrine dose of 50 ug/min and a MAP of 55 mmHg.

What is the maximum dose of first-line vasopressor before adding a second agent to either join or potentially replace norepinephrine based on response?

Which is your second agent of choice in this patient? What dose will you use?

As discussed previously, norepinephrine is recommended as the first-line vasopressor in septic shock primarily based on its relatively benign side effect profile. There is not a clear maximum dosage recommended prior to initiating a second vasopressor. The threshold for adding a second vasopressor varies by continent (higher doses used in some European countries when compared to the United States) and by individual preference. Case reports note a risk of extremity ischemia when the dose exceeds 1.2 ug/kg/min [23]. However the logic behind association of a dose threshold for extremity ischemia when higher doses of norepinephrine are being used to treat refractory "vasodilatory" shock seems flawed. The likely reason for the use of higher doses is the vasodilatory refractoriness and, in the presence of more intense vasodilation driving the higher doses, poorly linked to tissue ischemia from vasopressor dosing. In fact, we prefer the use of the term "poorly responsive" to norepinephrine when higher and higher doses are not achieving target MAP. We believe this is preferred over the frequently expressed "maxed out" on norepinephrine. One randomized controlled trial used a norepinephrine dose of 0.5 ug/kg/min as cutoff for "catecholamine-resistant" vasodilatory shock [10]. There does not appear to be a clear limit to norepinephrine. Authors of the SSC guidelines users' guide have chosen a titration to 35–90 ug/min as the cutoff [1]. Dosage limits should take into account an individual's tolerance and response to further titration of norepinephrine. Maximum dosages should be lowered with the appearance of side effects such as arrhythmia.

When adding a second agent, it is most often a decision between low-dose vasopressin and epinephrine. With regard to septic shock, both are within the recommendations provided by the SSC to maintain an appropriate MAP.

Although low-dose vasopressin is not recommended as the initial agent in the treatment of septic shock, it can be added to norepinephrine when norepinephrine fails to achieve MAP target or as a norepinephrine-sparing agent once MAP target is achieved with norepinephrine alone (physiologic replacement logic).

While norepinephrine is the recommended first-line vasopressor, both epinephrine and vasopressin have unique characteristics making them useful as second-line agents.

Vasopressin is an endogenous vasopressor hormone which causes vasoconstriction by acting on V1 receptors on smooth muscle. It is a pure vasopressor with no cardiac effects except indirect stimulation of right atrial baroreceptors. At normal physiologic states, vasopressin levels are low. The VASST trial in 2008 compared norepinephrine to norepinephrine and vasopressin (0.01–0.03 U/min). This study showed no difference in mortality. It did demonstrate a "catecholamine-sparing" effect of vasopressin in which lower doses of norepinephrine were required. An a priori subgroup with less severe shock in this study did have a lower mortality (28-day mortality relative risk, 0.74 (95% CI, 0.55–1.01) $P = 0.05$). This group was defined by requiring <15 ug/min norepinephrine at randomization [25]. Several earlier studies have shown decreased norepinephrine requirements and improved cardiac output with the initiation of vasopressin in catecholamine-resistant shock [26, 27]. These studies included doses higher than recommended by the SSC. At higher doses there appears to be higher risk for cardiac, digital, and splanchnic ischemia [10]. Therefore a lower dose of up to 0.03 U/min (some would say 0.04 U/min) is recommended with higher doses used only in salvage therapy (alternative agents have failed to achieve MAP target).

Epinephrine is a catecholamine vasopressor which acts on both alpha- and beta-receptors. This results in a higher MAP due to increased vascular tone and increased cardiac output. As noted previously, the main side effects of epinephrine include an increase in serum lactate and tachycardia making it a second-line agent behind norepinephrine [8]. However, these effects have not been shown to alter a patient's clinical outcome. In 2008, Myburgh et al. performed a prospective, double-blind, randomized controlled trial comparing the use of epinephrine to norepinephrine for patients in shock [8]. There was no difference in mortality between the two groups at 28 and 90 days. Specifically within a subgroup of patients diagnosed with sepsis, there was no difference in time to achieve goal MAP (>70 mmHg) or mortality. While no difference in primary or secondary endpoints was found, this study has been used to advocate for norepinephrine as the first-line agent due to its comparable efficacy and decreased side effects (Fig. 11.1).

The theoretical benefit of epinephrine over other vasopressors in shock is based on the beta-receptor activity. Although norepinephrine is expected to raise cardiac output in septic shock, epinephrine is a more potent inotrope and should produce a greater increase in cardiac output in patients with sepsis-induced cardiomyopathy. In 2007, Annane et al. published a prospective, multicenter, randomized, double-blind study in 330 patients with septic shock. This study compared epinephrine to norepinephrine plus dobutamine. There was no significant difference in mortality at 28 days between the two groups. The epinephrine group did display lower arterial pH on days 1–4 and an increased arterial lactate on day 1. These findings were hypothesized to be due to beta-2 stimulation of the NA + K ATPase pump in skeletal muscles rather than tissue dysoxia [28]. These transient laboratory values did not have a clear impact on clinical outcomes. Within 4 days, there was no difference in mortality, end-organ dysfunction, or hemodynamic stability. The SSC does recommend the consideration of dobutamine in patients who are believed to have been resuscitated to an adequate intravascular volume, have achieved target MAP, and yet have continued tissue hypoperfusion with clinical signs of low cardiac output (see discussion to follow).

The decision for which vasopressor to add to norepinephrine must be based on the efficacy and tolerance in the individual patient. At this time there have been no randomized trials comparing vasopressin to epinephrine in patients currently on norepinephrine. Therefore both options remain a viable choice. Vasopressin appears to lower the norepinephrine requirement and may be especially useful in patients who do not tolerate a high dose of a catecholamine. Epinephrine may be most useful in those patients who require some inotropic and chronotropic support. This is especially helpful in those patients who display decreased cardiac output and would not tolerate the vasodilatory effects of an inotrope such as dobutamine.

We will return to our case.

Vasopressin is started at a dose of 0.03 units/minute. The patient has an initial improvement in blood pressure but again continues to decompensate with a MAP persistently below 65 mmHg. Epinephrine is added as the third vasopressor agent. The patient's blood pressure improves.

The nurse calls you to evaluate the patient. The monitor displays a narrow complex, irregularly irregular rhythm with a ventricular rate of 132. When the abnormal rhythm is present, MAP decreases from 70 to 50 mmHg.

Would you make changes to your vasopressor regimen?

Phenylephrine, although not recommended for empiric therapy, has been used in the setting of serious physiology altering vasopressor-induced tachyarrhythmias. Phenylephrine is a selective alpha-1 agonist with no effect on beta-receptors. It is a pure vasoconstrictor with no cardiac stimulation. Therefore, it should not produce tachyarrhythmias. As a pure vasoconstrictor, it would be expected to decrease stroke volume and cardiac output, a less desirable effect. There has been limited data comparing phenylephrine to other vasopressors. Morelli et al. performed a prospective, randomized controlled trial comparing phenylephrine to norepinephrine as a first-line vasopressor in septic shock. In this study, phenylephrine had similar effects on cardiopulmonary parameters. However, phenylephrine was less effective in treating hypotension as higher doses were required to maintain a goal MAP [29]. This study was limited in that it only enrolled 32 patients and measurements of cardiopulmonary parameters were only measured at 12 h via right heart catheterization. The SSC has recommended a limited use of phenylephrine in septic shock (not as empiric therapy but consideration in high cardiac output septic shock or when tachyarrhythmias are induced with norepinephrine or epinephrine) [1]. Based on the pharmacology of this medication, there may be a role for phenylephrine in this patient population, but there is no confirmatory data.

Not as it pertains to our patient but to the general population of patients with septic shock, what role does dopamine play in a patient with shock? What about a pure inotrope such as dobutamine?

Dopamine has a limited role in the treatment of septic shock. It has effect on both alpha- and beta-receptors similar to norepinephrine and epinephrine. It has the added activity on dopamine receptors which may alter renal and splanchnic perfusion. As discussed earlier, it has been replaced by norepinephrine as the first-line vasopressor for the majority of this patient population. It has subsequently become a potential niche vasopressor for patients with septic shock, sinus bradycardia, and low risk for arrhythmia. There has been no randomized controlled trial using dopamine in this patient population. This thought is based on known pharmacology rather than study results. Low-dose dopamine does not benefit patients at risk for renal failure. In a multicenter, randomized, double-blind, placebo-controlled study, Bellomo et al. showed no significant difference in survival, peak creatinine, or need for renal replacement therapy in patients receiving low-dose dopamine versus placebo [30].

Therefore, the use of dopamine should be held for a specific patient population or a part of salvage therapy.

In patients with continued hypoperfusion despite improvement of preload and MAP, inotrope support may be considered. This recommendation is based on limited data. As discussed prior, the randomized controlled trials comparing dobutamine plus norepinephrine to epinephrine alone did not show a difference in mortality [28]. Previous recommendations for the use of dobutamine in the early resuscitation of septic shock were based on the Rivers et al. early goal-directed therapy trial [31]. Dobutamine was added when there was persistently low ScV02 < 70% despite treatment with vasopressors, IV fluids, and in the presence of appropriate hematocrit. Current recommendations favor considering adding dobutamine later in resuscitation as discussed above.

The patient is continued on norepinephrine and low-dose vasopressin. Given the development of a tachyarrhythmia, he is transitioned off epinephrine and started on phenylephrine with elimination of his episodic tachycardic arrhythmia. Repeat laboratory data returns showing a lactate of 2.4 mmol/L and improving creatinine with adequate urine output of 0.75 cc/kg/h (target 0.5–1.0 cc kg). With continued antibiotic therapy, vasopressor support is titrated down over several days with improving hemodynamics. Although not evidence based, we withdraw phenylephrine first, then vasopressin, and then norepinephrine. Some would reverse the order for the latter two vasopressors.

Future Aims

The future of shock management involves earlier detection of end-organ dysfunction, monitoring of cardiovascular performance, and pharmacologic and mechanical support. As newer noninvasive devices are developed, the reliability of these tools will need to be evaluated. While drug therapy most often includes norepinephrine as the vasopressor of choice, literature comparing combination therapy of vasopressors is limited. Individualized treatment regimens and choices in drug and fluid delivery will likely be tailored to each patient based on physiologic makeup and response to therapy.

Angiotensin II (ATII) has been recently added to the list of FDA-approved vasopressors available in the treatment of distributive shock. ATII is a naturally occurring hormone which interacts with the renin-angiotensin-aldosterone system (RAAS) causing both venous and arterial vasoconstriction. It is a pure vasopressor. Recently, the ATHOS-3 trial randomized 321 patients with distributive shock to receive ATII vs placebo [32]. Prior to enrollment, patients were required to be receiving 0.2 μg/kg/min of norepinephrine or equivalent dose of another vasopressor. The primary outcome was MAP response defined as a MAP increase of 10 mmHg or at least 75 mmHg at 3 h. 69.9% of the ATII group versus 23.4% of the control group reached this primary endpoint (Fig. 11.2). While secondary outcomes did show decreased all-cause mortality at days 7 and 28, these did not reach statistical significance [31]. Although the authors reported an improvement in the cardiovascular sequential organ failure assessment (SOFA) scores at 48 h without a difference in the total SOFA, this is somewhat misleading since this improvement is achieved simply by giving a vasopressor to the active treatment group and a placebo to the control arm.

Criticisms of this study include a MAP goal higher than recommended for the general population, unclear fluid status of the studied patient population, limited information regarding markers of end-organ perfusion such as lactate and urine output, and omission of cardiac output measures. As to the latter, it is likely important to avoid the use of this pure vasopressor in patients with low cardiac output since the only randomized controlled trial studying a pure vasopressor in septic shock was associated with worse outcome with particular concern in the low cardiac output subgroup

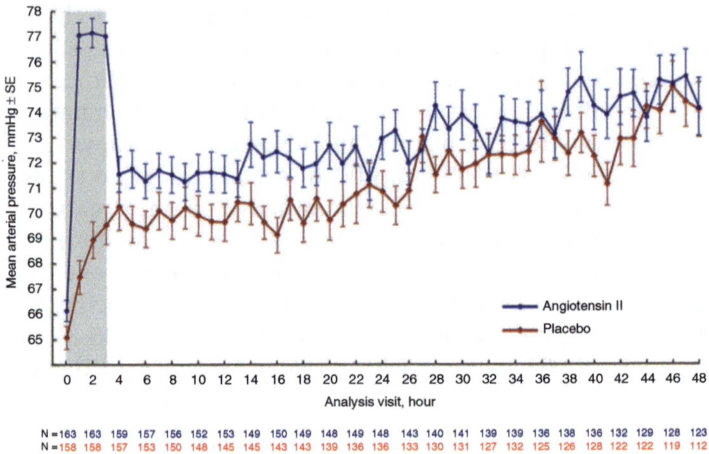

FIGURE 11.2 Comparison of ATII versus placebo on mean arterial pressure (MAP) in patients in distributive shock on vasopressors. (Reprinted/adapted with permission from New England Journal of Medicine Khanna et al. [32])

(directly measured in this study) [33]. The primary composite endpoint of the ATHOS-3 trial focused on the achievement of MAP goal rather than patient-centered mortality. The small population also limits the safety data provided. In particular, the thrombotic risk reported by the FDA is not clearly displayed in this trial but is clearly enunciated on the FDA labeling which recommends the use of prophylaxis for blood clots. More studies will be needed to evaluate the possible mortality benefit or limitation of side effects using this new vasopressor agent. Having an additional vasopressor that works by a different mechanism will hopefully offer advantage in select patient populations.

A flow diagram has also recently been published as the authors' recommendations on hierarchy and dosing of vasopressors as the severity of septic shock increases (Fig. 11.3) [2].

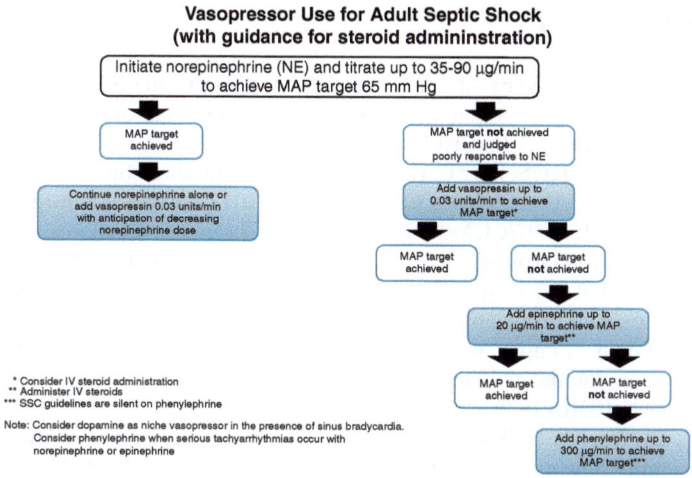

FIGURE 11.3 An example of a vasopressor flow diagram. (Reprinted/adapted with permission from Springer; Dellinger et al. [2])

Review Points

1. Norepinephrine is the first-line vasopressor in septic shock.
2. Low-dose vasopressin and/or epinephrine can be added as second-line agents.
3. Dopamine and phenylephrine are niche vasopressors used in select situations.
4. MAP goal of ≥65 is recommended but must be tailored to the individual patient.
5. Vasopressors should be started early after IV fluid resuscitation when MAP remains low.
6. A peripheral IV above the antecubital fossa may be safe for initial resuscitation.
7. The choice of vasopressor should be selected based on an individual patient's response to treatment and side effects.

References

1. Rhodes A, Evans LE, Alhazzani W, et al. Surviving Sepsis campaign: international guidelines for the management of sepsis and septic shock: 2016. Crit Care Med. 2017;45:486–552.
2. Dellinger RP, Schorr CA, Levy MM. Users' guide to the 2016 surviving sepsis guidelines. Crit Care Med. 2017;45(3):381–5. https://doi.org/10.1097/CCM.0000000000002257.
3. Vieillard-Baron A, Caille V, Charron C, et al. Actual incidence of global left ventricular hypokinesia in adult septic shock. Crit Care Med. 2008;36:1701–6.
4. Martin C, Papazian L, Perrin G, et al. Norepinephrine or dopamine for the treatment of hyperdynamic septic shock? Chest. 1993;103(6):1826–31.
5. De Backer D, Biston P, Devriendt J, et al. Comparison of dopamine and norepinephrine in the treatment of shock. N Engl J Med. 2010;362(9):779–89.
6. Avni T, Lador A, Lev S, et al. Vasopressors for the treatment of septic shock: systematic review and meta-analysis. PLoS One. 2015;10:e0129305.
7. De Backer D, Aldecoa C, Njimi H, et al. Dopamine versus norepinephrine in the treatment of septic shock: a meta-analysis. Crit Care Med. 2012;40:725–30.
8. Myburgh JA, Higgins A, Jovanovska A, et al. CAT study investigators: a comparison of epinephrine and norepinephrine in critically ill patients. Intensive Care Med. 2008;34:2226–34.
9. Landry DW, Levin HR, Gallant EM, et al. Vasopressin deficiency contributes to the vasodilation of septic shock. Circulation. 1997;95:1122–5.
10. Dünser MW, Mayr AJ, Tür A, et al. Ischemic skin lesions as a complication of continuous vasopressin infusion in catecholamine-resistant vasodilatory shock: incidence and risk factors. Crit Care Med. 2003;31:1394–8.
11. Gordon AC, Mason AJ, Thirunavukkarasu N, et al. VANISH investigators: effect of early vasopressin vs norepinephrine on kidney failure in patients with septic shock: the VANISH randomized clinical trial. JAMA. 2016;316:509–18.
12. Bai X, Yu W, Ji W, Lin Z, Tan S, Duan K, et al. Early versus delayed administration of norepinephrine in patients with septic shock. Crit Care. 2014;18:532. https://doi.org/10.1186/s13054-014-0532-y.

13. Beck V, Chateau D, et al. Timing of vasopressor initiation and mortality in septic shock: a cohort study. Crit Care. 2014; 18:R97.
14. Waechter J, Kumar A. Lapinsky et al. interaction between fluids and vasoactive agents on mortality in septic shock: a multicenter, observational study. Crit Care Med. 2014;42(10):2158–68.
15. Dünser MW, Takala J, Ulmer H, Mayr VD, Luckner G, Jochberger S, et al. Arterial blood pressure during early sepsis and outcome. Intensive Care Med. 2009;35:1225–33.
16. Asfar P, Meziani F, Hamel JF, et al. High versus low blood-pressure target in patients with septic shock. N Engl J Med. 2014;370:1583–93.
17. Ricard JD, Salomon L, Boyer A, et al. Central or peripheral catheters for initial venous access of ICU patients: a randomized controlled trial. Crit Care Med. 2013;41(9):2108–15.
18. Cardenas-Garcia J, Schaub KF, et al. Safety of peripheral intravenous administration of vasoactive medication. J Hosp Med. 2015;10:581–5.
19. Loubani OM, Green RS. A systematic review of extravasation and local tissue injury from administration of vasopressors through peripheral intravenous catheters and central venous catheters. J Crit Care. 2015;30(3):653.e9–17.
20. Lakhal K, et al. Noninvasive monitoring of blood pressure in the critically ill: reliability according to the cuff site (arm, thigh, or ankle). Crit Care Med. 2012;40:1207–13.
21. Ribezzo S, Spina E, Di BS, Sanson G. Noninvasive techniques for blood pressure measurement are not a reliable alternative to direct measurement: a randomized crossover trial in ICU. Sci World J. 2014;2014:353628.
22. Scheer B, Perel A, Pfeiffer UJ. Clinical review: complications and risk factors of peripheral arterial catheters used for haemodynamic monitoring in anaesthesia and intensive care medicine. Crit Care. 2002;6:199–204.
23. Daroca-Perez R, Carrascosa M. Digital necrosis: a potential risk of high-dose norepinephrine. Ther Adv Drug Saf. 2017;8(8):259–61.
24. Sharshar T, Blanchard A, Paillard M, et al. Circulating vasopressin levels in septic shock. Crit Care Med. 2003;31:1752–8.
25. Russell JA, Walley KR, Singer J, et al. Vasopressin versus norepinephrine infusion in patients with septic shock. N Engl J Med. 2008;358:877–87.

26. Dünser MW, Mayr AJ, Ulmer H, et al. Arginine vasopressin in advanced vasodilatory shock: a prospective, randomized, controlled study. Circulation. 2003;107:2313–9.
27. Patel BM, Chittock DR, Russell JA, et al. Beneficial effects of short-term vasopressin infusion during severe septic shock. Anesthesiology. 2002;96:576–82.
28. Annane D, Vignon P, Renault A, et al. CATS Study Group: norepinephrine plus dobutamine versus epinephrine alone for management of septic shock A randomised trial. Lancet. 2007;370:676–84.
29. Morelli A, Ertman C, Rehberg S, et al. Phenylephrine versus norepinephrine for initial hemodynamic support of patients with septic shock: a randomized controlled trial. Crit Care. 2008;12:R43.
30. Bellomo R, Chapman M, Finfer S, et al. Low-dose dopamine in patients with early renal dysfunction: a placebo-controlled randomised trial. Lancet. 2000;356:2139–43.
31. Rivers E, Nguyen B, Havstad S, et al. Early goal-directed therapy in the treatment of severe sepsis and septic shock. The New England Journal of Medicine 2001;345(19):1368–77.
32. Khanna A, Shane EW, Wang XS. Angiotensin II for treatment of vasodilatory shock. N Engl J Med. 2017;377:419–30. https://doi.org/10.1056/NEJMoa1704154.
33. López A, Lorente JA, Steingrub J, et al. Multiple-center, randomized, placebo-controlled, double-blind study of the nitric oxide synthase inhibitor 546C88: effect on survival in patients with septic shock. Crit Care Med. 2004;32:21–30.

Chapter 12
Brain Death

Margie Hodges Shaw and David C. Kaufman

Introduction

In 1968, an ad hoc committee of the Harvard Medical School concluded that death of the brain is sufficient criteria for determination of death of the person [1]. The chair of the committee, Henry Beecher, was an anesthesiologist at the Massachusetts General Hospital. Dr. Beecher and his colleagues on the committee were definitive in describing their purpose, namely, to "define irreversible coma as a new criterion for death" [1]. Time and a review of Beecher's archived papers would confirm that the ad hoc committee

M. H. Shaw
Division of Medical Humanities and Bioethics, University of Rochester School of Medicine and Dentistry, Rochester, NY, USA
e-mail: margie_shaw@urmc.rochester.edu
D. C. Kaufman (✉)
Department of Surgery, University of Rochester School of Medicine and Dentistry, Rochester, NY, USA
e-mail: david_kaufman@urmc.rochester.edu

J. A. LaRosa (ed.), *Adult Critical Care Medicine*,
https://doi.org/10.1007/978-3-319-94424-1_12

had indeed been able to define irreversible coma [1], but identifying that status as a single criterion for death is a metaphysical construct, not comprehensible by current applications of the scientific method.

One of the 13 committee members was the 1990 Nobel Laureate Joseph Murray, a surgeon who, in 1954, removed a kidney from a 23-year-old man and transplanted it into his monozygotic twin who was suffering from renal failure. Dr. Murray went on to perform the first cadaveric kidney transplant in 1962 [2]. In their report, deliberately entitled "A Definition of Irreversible Coma," the committee members state that there are two reasons to declare irreversible coma equivalent to death. Firstly, they say, there are burdens on the families and hospitals who care for these comatose patients. Parenthetically, they also state that the burden is great on patients who suffer permanent loss of intellect. They do not describe what burdens a person would suffer if they were permanently comatose, and the record provides no evidence as to what burdens they imagined such a patient could experience. Secondly, they claim that "obsolete criteria for the definition of death can lead to controversy in obtaining organs for transplantation" [1]. Given these facts, it is hard to assert, as many do, that the concept of brain death arose separately from the desire to transplant organs.

Case Presentation

Henry I. Barnard is a 55-year-old man who presents to a hospital in New Jersey to donate a kidney to his daughter who has been struggling with complications from type I diabetes mellitus for over two decades and has been dialysis dependent for 2 years. He flew from Hawaii, where he lives, to New Jersey. There were many airline delays and he was traveling for over 18 h. He did arrive 5 days before the operation, however, and seems well rested the morning of surgery. He undergoes a donor nephrectomy, but during skin closure, he has an acute desaturation with a significant decrease in his end-tidal CO_2. A focused transthoracic echocardiogram reveals a mobile mass in his pulmonary artery, seen on a parasternal short-axis view. On an apical four-chamber view, a severely dilated right ventricle with reduced systolic function, a small but normal left ventricle, and septal flattening are found. Moments later he has pulseless electrical activity (PEA) with sinus tachycardia. Chest compressions are started and epinephrine given. The ECMO team is notified, and he is started on VA-ECMO within 29 min from the time of his PEA arrest. A surgical embolectomy is performed, and he is brought to the intensive care unit where he is weaned from VA-ECMO immediately with stable blood pressures without vasopressor support. Cannulas are removed first thing in the morning.

On postoperative day#1, the nurse informs the physician that Mr. Barnard is not responding to noxious stimuli. On evaluation, he is not on any sedative or narcotic medications and has not received any since the embolectomy 12 h earlier. His pupils are fixed and dilated, and he is breathing at the set rate on the ventilator. The physician confirms the nurse's findings. She learns that no neuromuscular-blocking drugs have been given since the operation and documents that Mr. Barnard has a normal response to train-of-four testing. She documents his temperature at 37 °C. When the physician notifies Mr. Bernard's wife that she will be examining her husband to see if he is brain dead, she screams, "he can't be brain dead," and runs from the waiting room. The doctor begins her examination. She does not notice any response when she applies pressure to his temporomandibular joint. He has no cough or pharyngeal reflexes. Both his corneal and pupillary light reflexes are absent. There is an absence of ocular movements with oculocephalic testing. Finally, an apnea test is performed and is positive. The physician looks at her watch and declares Henry I. Bernard dead at 10:45 AM.

She finds his wife at the bedside of her daughter. They are alone. She explains the results of the testing and states that their husband and father are dead. They tell the doctor that Bernard became a Shintoist shortly after moving to Hawaii and objects to the use of brain criteria in the determination of death.

Assessment and Diagnosis

Mr. Bernard's long plane ride and surgery set him up for a pulmonary embolus. The ECHO findings are confirmatory, and a Trendelenburg procedure (surgical embolectomy) is performed. He is expertly managed after the complication but nevertheless is suffering from a devastating neurologic injury.

Before brain death testing is begun, hypothermia (<36 °C) and hypotension (systolic blood pressure < 100 mmHg) must be corrected. It must also be determined that central nervous system medications and neuromuscular-blocking agents are not contributing to the neurologic findings. Once brain death is suspected, the family should be notified and apprised of the suspicion and need for further testing. All movements must be attributable to spinal cord function. The physician should look for any evidence of brainstem function. The patient cannot have a cough or pharyngeal (a.k.a. gag) reflex. There can be no corneal or pupillary light reflexes. If it is safe to move the patient's neck, they should also be tested for the oculocephalic reflex (doll's eyes). If it is not okay to move the patient's neck, they should be tested for the oculovestibular (cold calorics) reflex. Tympanic membranes must be visualized prior to performing cold calorics. If all these tests are consistent with brain death, an apnea test should be performed. The apnea test is also a test of brainstem function. A rising carbon dioxide level should stimulate the respiratory center in the medulla and cause a respiratory effort. Since a rising carbon dioxide level will increase cerebral blood flow, in someone who potentially has raised intracranial hypertension, it should be the last clinical test performed.

A confirmatory test is not considered necessary but should be performed if any of the standard clinical tests cannot be done. An intracranial Doppler study, an electroencephalogram, and a radionucleotide study are all reasonable options depending on institutional expertise and preference [3].

Once all clinical studies are complete, currently in 49 of the 50 United States, the patient can be declared dead.

Law

There are five sources of law in the United States; constitutional law, statutory law (or legislation), treaties, administrative regulations, and common law (created by court decisions). The laws related to the determination of death are based in common law and codified through legislation. Legal determination of biological death is necessary for criminal law, disposition of property following death, loss of rights of the deceased, the creation of rights for survivors, and the disposition of human remains, including cadaveric transplantation, cremation, and burial. In the United States, state law prescribes how death is determined and, after determination, what can be done with the body and by whom. An advantage of our federalist structure is the ability of states to craft legislation to address specific needs and for states with similar needs to test a variety of solutions. This can also lead to ambiguity and variation in matters of great importance.

Many states enacted laws regulating organ donation before 1967 in response to cadaveric kidney and corneal transplantation. These laws relied upon the then-existing definition of death, the point at which the heart stops beating and respiration ends, and addressed issues around consent and authorization in decision-making. The medicolegal literature in 1967 includes a robust debate about the "brain death problem," the term used to describe the idea proposed by some medical professionals that the cardiorespiratory definition of death attaches the time of death at a point too late for the purposes of heart transplantation [4].

In the 1960s, courts highly valued scientific consensus and testimony of such from the medical establishment. Dr. Beecher anticipated legal challenges to his ideas and considered Harvard legal scholar William J. Curran an essential member of the Ad Hoc Committee. To change the legal definition of death, Curran advised demonstrating a new consensus existed in the medical community that irreversible coma is death. One can argue the report caused the consensus it claimed.

Two years following the release of the report, in 1970, Kansas adopted the first statute that defined death as either the absence of spontaneous respiratory and cardiac functions or the absence of spontaneous brain function [5]. In 1972, Alexander Capron and Leon Kass published "A Statutory Definition for the Standards for Determining Human Death: An Appraisal and a Proposal" [6]. In 1975, the Law and Medicine Committee of the American Bar Association (ABA) drafted the Model Definition of Death Act. By 1979, 25 state legislatures passed related statutes.

The National Conference of Commissioners on Uniform State Laws (NCCUSL) drafts a legislation for the purpose of promoting uniformity of law when desirable. State legislatures may choose to adopt these uniform laws, adopt a modification, or ignore the proposal. In 1978, the NCCUSL created the Uniform Brain Death Act (UBDA) establishing that death is the "irreversible cessation of all functioning of the brain, including the brain stem." The following year, 1979, the American Medical Association (AMA) created its Model Determination of Death Act. In 1980 the NCCUSL replaced the UBDA with the Uniform Determination of Death Act (UDDA) which includes the previous criteria, "irreversible cessation of circulatory and respiratory functions."

Interestingly, in an acknowledgment of the various meanings of death, the NCCUSL does not consider the UDDA to be a definition of death. It expressly limits the scope to the medical determination of biological death. It is a general legal standard that relies on the medical profession to develop and maintain acceptable practices and criteria based on existing medical knowledge, diagnostic tests, and equipment. The NCCUSL also explicitly states that the UDDA is not limited to cases of organ donation and should remain independent from the Uniform Anatomical Gift Act. The AMA approved the UDDA in 1980 and the ABA followed in 1981. In 1981, the US President's Commission for the Study of Ethics Problems in Medicine and Biomedical and Behavioral Research endorsed the UDDA [7].

In 1991, based on the work of the New Jersey (NJ) Commission on Legal and Ethical Problems in the Delivery of Health Care (the New Jersey Bioethics Commission), the NJ legislature enacted the NJ Declaration of Death Act. This Act models the UDDA language while also acknowledging the importance of religion around the concept of death. The Act explicitly denies the physician the ability to determine death based on neurological criteria when the physician "has reason to believe, on the basis of information in the individual's available medical records, or information provided by a member of the individual's family or any other person knowledgeable about the individual's personal religious beliefs that such a declaration would violate the personal religious beliefs of the individual." In such cases, the physician shall only declare death based on the cardiorespiratory criteria described in the Act.

A challenge for current practice is that the UDDA requires "... irreversible cessation of all functions of the entire brain stem...," and medical guidelines measure the cessation of some functions of the brain, while advances in critical care management support comatose patients longer than previously imagined possible. This results in cases where doctors assert certainty in a diagnosis and the family disagrees, and continued medical interventions prevent circulatory death of the loved one, for years. Medical cases like this are a tragedy, for the family and for the medical profession. For example, in 2013, a 13-year-old girl, Jahi McMath, was pronounced dead by neurologic criteria following surgery for sleep apnea, complicated by bleeding and airway obstruction. Her family moved her to New Jersey where she was kept on organ support until she was pronounced dead, 5 years later, using cardiorespiratory criteria. Before her death by cardiorespiratory criteria, a neurologist ascertained that she no longer met death by neurologic criteria, and her family filed a lawsuit in California claiming that she was no longer dead. Legal cases, like the one pursued by Jahi McMath's family could result in a decision concluding that the existing guidelines are insufficient to determine death by neurologic criteria [8]. In the end, the most important question may not be "What is death?" but instead be "What is the role of the doctor in helping patients and loved ones cope with illness and legal death?"

Ethics

Taking care of patients is a moral endeavor, and while ethics is a branch of philosophy, all of us must decide what is right and wrong as we make personal and professional choices. How ought clinicians think about moral issues? Medical school faculty teach the four principles of bioethics (autonomy, beneficence, nonmaleficence, and justice), but the principles alone do not provide a process for resolving disputes. The principles provide language to facilitate communications about conflicts. Often, disagreements occur because of people's preference on different principles in a particular situation. For the sake of illumination, let's say you are caring for a patient following a pancreaticoduodenectomy for pancreatic adenocarcinoma (T3N1M0) who has a pancreaticojejunal leak resulting in adult respiratory distress syndrome and acute kidney injury. The family may weigh autonomy (albeit substituted) the most and argue for withdrawal of life support as what he would have wanted if he understood the circumstances; the surgeon may weigh beneficence the most and argue for continued life support because she believes that is best for the patient; the intensivist may weigh nonmaleficence the most and argue for withdrawal of life support (the same outcome but for a different reason than the family); the nurse may weigh justice the most and argue that we should not use resources when there is so little hope of a good outcome. These kinds of disagreements can occur in any bioethical dilemma. Of note, narrative ethics may facilitate a resolution process; it weighs the principles according to the values of the patient.

In the case of brain death today, however, principlism does not apply. The ad hoc committee redefined death; the medical profession incorporated this diagnosis into their knowledge base and, with the help of the legal profession, created law. Today, if you transplant vital organs from one person to another before the donor is declared dead, it constitutes murder. If you declare the donor dead first, you circumvent the murder problem. Some assert the "dead-donor rule" is necessary for the doctor-patient relationship. Some imagine it reassures donor and donor families of the integrity of the field of transplantation. The transplant community believes this rule is necessary for the expansion of transplantation, something the Harvard framers believed as well. Both of these propositions, along with the history of death declaration, warrant exploration.

Methods for death determination have evolved over time. Hippocratic tradition taught physicians to remove themselves from the care of patients when death was imminent leaving determination of death up to the family or lay practitioners. In ancient Rome, someone would call out a person's name three times, and, if they didn't answer, a finger would be amputated. If they didn't bleed, then they were dead and could be cremated on the funeral pyre. "I am dead" written on a mirror with silver nitrate, an invisible compound, would become visible with putrefaction: Parlor trick or chemical test of death?

The most famous tale of star-crossed lovers, Romeo and Juliet, hinges on the fact that Romeo misdiagnosed Juliet's death. Juliet, obviously the better student, got it right. At the end of *King Lear*, realizing his folly and, holding his dead daughter Cordelia in his hands, the King declares:

> I know when one is dead, and when one lives.
> She is dead as earth. Lend me a looking glass.
> If that her breath will mist or stain the stone, why then she lives.
> -Act V, Scene III

In Elizabethan England, a stone was a mirror, and, although Shakespeare said it more eloquently, the tormented king was hoping for verification of end-tidal carbon dioxide.

The history of death determination does not instill confidence and reveals reasons for public distrust. There was an

English nobleman in the fourteenth century who was so fearful that the doctors of his day would misdiagnosis him as being dead that he left instructions for his executors to leave him unburied in bed for 40 days, and, if they still believed he was dead, then, and only then, they could bury him. Taphephobia was common during the Victorian era. Rendering this fear in 1844, Edgar Allan Poe published *The Premature Burial.* People, more afraid of being buried alive than being dead, would request that their hearts be pierced before burial. Safety coffins included air tubes; strings to animate above ground lanterns, bells, or flags; and spring-loaded lids for those interned in vaults. Academic awards were given to physicians who developed tools to inflict pain to confirm death with enough specificity to qualm the layperson's fears [9].

In what may be an acknowledgment of the history of uncertainty and mistrust, the transplant community is often worried that discussions about death determination and the dead-donor rule will lead to fewer organs for transplantation. Frank discussions could, however, have the opposite effect. Some patients have expressed the desire to donate prior to the determination of death, and some physicians have advocated for "imminent death" donation, a repeal of the dead-donor rule. At the same time, other patients continue to mistrust the medical profession and fear both premature death determination and premature organ retrieval. When we allow patients and families to decide to withdraw life-sustaining treatment, we could also allow patients and families to make the decision for timing of organ retrieval. This approach (respect for autonomy through substituted judgment) would likely increase the donor pool. It would also allow analgesia and sedation to people who meet the current brain death standard as well as people who currently are non-heart-beating donors whose more injured organs are not removed until after the person is pronounced dead by cardiorespiratory criteria. Transplant surgeons sometimes claim that it would be unacceptable to remove an organ from a patient who still has a beating heart. Yet, this is exactly what surgeons do in cases of transplantation following the diagnosis of death by neurologic criteria. The objection appears to be about physician expectations rather than the status of the organs.

In December 2018, the Harvard Brain Death criteria will turn 50 years old [1]. Assuming most students start medical school in their 20s, most doctors today were taught that there are two ways to declare someone dead. Although most people are declared dead utilizing cardiorespiratory criteria and only a few specialists will ever declare someone dead by brain criteria, the phenomenon is accepted as part of the fabric of medicine. However, even though the report succeeded in changing medical practice and the law, the process did not respect the concerns of the public; and the laws, problematically, may not represent an ethical consensus of society. 1968 was a different time than 2018, and it is doubtful that an ad hoc committee of any medical school could have such an influence on the creation of public policy and law today.

Henry Beecher's approach was, at its core, a matter of beneficence. He and his colleagues believed expanding the definition of death was best for society: best for both the donor (who would not regain consciousness) and the recipient (who would benefit from the transplanted organ). It is important to apply ethical principles to the brain death concept and avoid blind acceptance of the dogma because we are fearful of the consequences (a decrease in number of organs to be transplanted). This fear leads to a type of informal logical fallacy. Allowing patients and families access to a wider range of decisions, including donation following a decision to withdraw life support, could lead to more transplantable organs.

In 1968, it was not standard of care or routine medical practice to allow surrogate decision-makers to withdraw life-sustaining treatment from patients. If it had been, one can imagine the ad hoc committee taking a different approach, one that allowed for donation before withdrawal of life-sustaining treatment, once the patient or patient's family made the decision to withdraw treatment. Today, law and medical practice support the right of the patient to make the decision to withdraw life-sustaining treatment. It may be time to consider allowing patients, once they make that decision, to consider whether or not to donate prior to the cessation of life support.

The standard of care changes over time, with advances in technology and scientific understanding. The first heart transplant occurred 8 months before the ad hoc committee published their influential paper, and death determination required the heart had stopped. Christian Bernard may have gotten it right when he let his colleague and brother, Marius Bernard, stop the donor heart with a potassium injection rather than let the organ suffer the ravages of hypoxia. The donor, Denise Durvall, was hemorrhaging after she was hit by a drunk driver while walking across a busy street in Cape Town, South Africa. The cardiac transplant team had stopped breathing for her, and it was, in their minds, a simple choice: stop the heart and transplant a healthy organ or wait for the heart to stop and transplant an injured organ [10].

Patients and surrogate decision-makers have rights not recognized in 1968. It may be time to revisit death determination and organ donation in light of these rights and all the ethical principles (autonomy, beneficence, nonmaleficence, and justice).

Management

Our patient is *legally* dead in all US states except New Jersey. So, in New Jersey, under these circumstances, physicians cannot declare Mr. Barnard brain dead. Physicians can only pronounce Mr. Barnard dead utilizing cardiorespiratory criteria. The physicians must, then, respectfully work with the patient's family (the designated surrogate decision-maker) to determine the wishes of the patient with regard to any treatment decisions. It is critical to consider that while this patient rejects the diagnosis of death by neurologic criteria, that fact does not inform the team about the patient's beliefs about medical treatments that prolong life. The patient may desire life prolonging medical treatments, or he may not. The family provided information about the patient's values with regard to the determination of death. Now, the physician should determine what the family knows about the patient's wishes, values, and beliefs about life and life-sustaining treatment under the current situation and demonstrate respect for those values and beliefs.

References

1. A definition of irreversible coma. JAMA. 1968;205(6):85–8.
2. Dean, C. Joseph E. Murray, transplant doctor and Nobel prize winner, dies at 93. New York Times. 2012, November 27.
3. Wijdicks EFM, Varelas PN, Gronseth GS, Greer DM. Evidence-based guideline update: determining brain death in adults. Neurology. 2010;74:1911–8.
4. Leatherberry WC. Heart transplants: legal problems and the need for new legislation. Case W Res L Rev. 1968;19:1073. Available at: http://scholarlycommons.law.case.edu/caselrev/vol19/iss4/17, citing Ayd, When is a person dead? Med. Sci Apr. 1976 at 33–34; and Fletcher GP. Prolonging life. Wash L Rev. 1967;42:999, 1001.
5. KAN. STAT. ANN. §77–202. 1970.
6. 121 Pa. L. Rev 87. 1972.
7. President's Commission for the Study of Ethical Problems in Medicine and Biomedical and Behavioral Research. Defining death: a report on the medical, legal and ethical issues in the determination of death. Washington, DC: Government Printing Office; 1981.
8. Spears v. Rosen, No. RG15760730. Ca. April 20, 2018.
9. Iverson KV. Dying to know: introduction. In: Iverson KV, editor. Death to dust: what happens to dead bodies? Tuscon: Galen Press, Ltd.; 1994. p. 11–49, 307–364.
10. McRae D. Every second counts. London: G. P. Putnam's Sons; 2006.

Chapter 13
Nutrition Support Therapy During Critical Illness

Jayshil Patel, Ryan T. Hurt, and Manpreet Mundi

Summary of Key Points

1. Critical illness may trigger an exaggerated metabolic stress response, which may lead to uncontrolled catabolism, culminating in a calorie deficit, proteolysis, and anabolic resistance.

J. Patel (✉)
Division of Pulmonary and Critical Care Medicine,
Medical College of Wisconsin, Milwaukee, WI, USA
e-mail: jpatel2@mcw.edu

R. T. Hurt
Division of General Internal Medicine, Mayo Clinic,
Rochester, MN, USA
e-mail: hurt.ryan@mayo.edu

M. Mundi
Division of Endocrinology, Diabetes, Metabolism, and Nutrition,
Mayo Clinic, Rochester, MN, USA
e-mail: mundi.manpreet@mayo.edu

J. A. LaRosa (ed.), *Adult Critical Care Medicine*,
https://doi.org/10.1007/978-3-319-94424-1_13

2. Nutrition support has evolved to nutrition "therapy," which is proactive and enterally delivered to maintain gut integrity, reduce inflammation, and preserve gut immunity.
3. Due to the lack of a consensus definition of malnutrition, the quantity and timing of nutrition support therapy can be guided by identifying "nutritional risk," which is the risk of having a poor outcome due to insufficient nutrition.
4. NUTRIC and NRS-2002 scores can be used to identify nutritional risk in critically ill adults.
5. Critically ill adult patients deemed to be high nutritional risk may benefit from early and aggressive nutrition support therapy.
6. In the absence of contraindications, the enteral route is preferred over the parenteral route.
7. How quickly enteral nutrition should be advanced following initiation is unclear. Enteral nutrition contribution to hyperglycemia, tolerance, and risk for refeeding syndrome should be considered when titrating enteral nutrition to goal.
8. Emerging data suggests parenteral nutrition is a safe and feasible alternative when early enteral nutrition is contraindicated or not tolerated.
9. Critical care survival has improved over the past 30 years. As a consequence, survivors acquire loss of muscle mass leading to reduced physical function and quality of life. Therefore, optimizing protein may be of greater value, as compared to total calories. Observational data suggests protein at doses $\geq$1.2 g/kg/day is associated with improved ICU outcomes.
10. Clinicians should be aware of individual patient-, provider-, and institutional process-related barriers to delivering and optimizing nutrition support therapy.

Case Study

A 75-year-old man with a past medical history of diabetes, hypertension, and alcoholism is brought to the emergency department by his spouse for 3 days of increasing shortness of breath, sputum production, and fever. Last alcohol use was 3 days ago.

Review of systems is positive for 20-lb weight loss over the past 2 months due to poor oral intake. Past surgical and family histories are unremarkable. Social history reveals drinking up to ten beers per day. There is no history of recreational drug use, no recent travel, and no occupational exposures.

Vital signs: temperature 102°F, blood pressure 90/40 mmHg, respiratory rate 28, heart rate 110/min and regular, and oxygen saturation 82% on room air. The body mass index (BMI) is 19.8 (72 inches tall and weighed 150 lbs).

The patient appears anxious and diaphoretic. A jugular venous distention is not visualized. Bitemporal wasting is present. The skin is warm and flushed. Pulses are bounding. There are rhonchi and bronchial breath sounds over the right axillae. The remainder of the examination is unremarkable.

Hematologic studies are significant for elevated white blood cell count to 20,000/hpf. Serum chemistry is significant for potassium 2.9 mmol/L (normal range 3.4–5.1 mmol/L), phosphate 1.5 mg/dL (normal range 2.5–4.5 mg/dL), magnesium 1.0 mg/dL (normal range 1.6–2.6 mg/dL), bicarbonate 18 mmol/L (normal range 22–29 mmol/L), serum creatinine 2.5 mg/dL (normal range 0.50–1.10 mg/dL), and lactic acid 5 mmol/L (normal range 0.5–2.0 mmol/L). Serum albumin level is 2 g/dL (normal range 3.8–5.0 g/dL).

Arterial blood gas shows pH of 7.32, partial pressure carbon dioxide of 40 mmHg, partial pressure oxygen of 80 mmHg, and oxygen saturation of 90% on 10 liters oxygen.

Chest radiograph shows right middle lobe opacity.

Our Diagnoses and Initial Management

1. *Acute hypoxemic respiratory failure secondary to community-acquired pneumonia*

   A. Endotracheal intubation for acute hypoxemic respiratory failure

2. *Sepsis secondary to community-acquired pneumonia*

   A. Intravenous fluid boluses 30 mL/kg for sepsis-related hypotension
   B. Blood and respiratory cultures
   C. Empiric antimicrobial therapy for pneumonia

3. *Acute kidney injury, likely prerenal from hypotension*

   A. Obtain urine electrolytes, creatinine, and microscopy to evaluate for acute tubular necrosis

4. *Lactic acidosis, likely a combination of type A (from hypotension) and B lactic acidosis (from sepsis and thiamin deficiency)*

   A. Intravenous fluid resuscitation
   B. Intravenous thiamine

5. *Chronic alcohol abuse with multiple electrolyte deficiencies*

   A. Monitor for alcohol withdrawal
   B. Supplement magnesium, phosphate, and potassium
   C. Thiamine and folic acid supplementation

What Is the Role of Nutrition in Critical Illness?

The case highlights common conditions (sepsis and respiratory failure) which lead to critical illness. These conditions, along with circulatory shock, trauma, burns, and postoperative states, induce metabolic stress [1]. Metabolic stress may increase activation of neuroendocrine, immune, inflammatory,

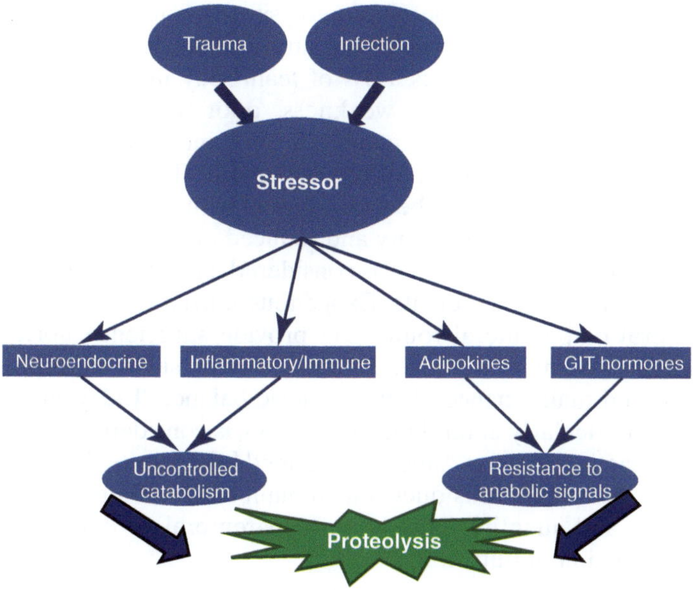

FIGURE 13.1 Triggers such as trauma, infections, respiratory failure, and burns activate the metabolic response to stress which culminates in uncontrolled catabolism and resistance to anabolic signals, leading to proteolysis

adipokine, and gastrointestinal pathways, which can lead to energy substrate use, proteolysis, and anabolic resistance (Fig. 13.1) [2].

First, uncontrolled catabolism leads to a cumulative calorie deficit. This negative energy balance has been associated with development of acute respiratory distress syndrome, renal failure, and pressure sores. Caloric deficits between 4000 and 10,000 kcal have been associated with organ failure and prolonged hospital length of stay [1, 3]. Second, the metabolic stress pathways increase proteolysis and the circulation of muscle-derived amino acids (AA). In one study, the rectus femoris cross-sectional area decreased by 12.5% by day 7 and 17% by day 10 in critically ill patients [4]. Furthermore, critically ill patients are commonly immobilized with muscle disuse. The combination of proteolysis, stress-mediated anabolic resistance, immobilization, and muscle disuse accelerates loss of muscle mass. Loss of lean body mass has been associated with muscle weakness, poor wound healing, mechanical ventilator dependency, and increased risk for nosocomial infection [5, 6]. Among critical illness survivors, loss of muscle mass has been associated with impaired physical functioning and mobility and reduced quality of life [7].

Traditionally, nutrition was considered a form of "support" to mitigate caloric deficits. Exogenous nutrient delivery via enteral or parenteral routes can provide sufficient calories, micronutrients, and antioxidants for energy substrate repletion and maintenance of daily caloric balance. Today, nutrition, particularly enteral nutrition (EN), is considered a form of proactive "therapy" and is prescribed [8]. Despite the paradigm shift, numerous questions remain surrounding optimal timing and quantity, route (enteral, parenteral, or both), and composition of nutrition.

How Much Nutrition Should I Start (If Any)?

How much nutrition should be provided during critical illness? The quantity of early nutrition remains a point of contention. Some experts argue for "less is more," even suggesting a brief period of starvation during the first week of critical illness [9]. Different "less is more" strategies have been recommended: hypocaloric feeding is reducing the nonprotein calories and maintaining optimal protein dose (currently recommended at 1.2–2.0 grams/kg/day), permissive underfeeding is providing 40–60% caloric prescription, and trophic feeding is providing 10–20 mL/h EN to gain the nonnutritional benefits [7]. Hypocaloric and permissive underfeeding have been studied in general critical care patient populations, while trophic feeding has been studied largely in patients with acute respiratory distress syndrome.

The argument for starvation hinges on the concept of preserving autophagy, which serves two important functions. The first is a system of "housekeeping" for cells undergoing oxidative stress to "clean up" unfolded proteins, viruses, and bacteria [7]. The second is to provide a survival mechanism in which amino acids are recycled to make adenosine triphosphate (ATP) for energy and for protein synthesis [7]. Feeding is believed to suppress autophagy, and hence, some experts favor starvation [10]. Opponents suggest the benefit of autophagy may be operative early, peaking at 24 h, and therefore limited, in critical illness. Furthermore, in mild critical illness, autophagy may be beneficial. However, excessive autophagy, as observed in increasing severity of illness, may be detrimental, leading to cellular component degradation and cell death [11]. Identifying the transition point where autophagy converts from a homeostatic mechanism to a pathologic one remains problematic.

Five observational studies [12–16] and three small randomized controlled trials [17–19] (RCT) have shown clinical outcomes are different when underfeeding is compared to full feeding in critically ill patients. Of these, two RCTs showed that underfeeding had lower mortality as compared to full feeding [17, 18]. One RCT showed a worse outcome (greater nosocomial infections) with underfeeding [19]. These studies were methodologically limited, and inferences drawn from (the majority observational) studies should be made with caution.

Four RCTs have shown no differences in outcome between trophic EN versus full EN, hypocaloric EN versus full EN, and permissive underfeeding to full EN [20–23].

Clearly, no two ICU patients are alike. For example, an elderly patient with preexisting malnutrition due to multiple comorbidities admitted with respiratory failure requiring mechanical ventilation intuitively needs greater nutrition than a young athlete admitted after a motor vehicle accident. Identifying which patients will benefit from an aggressive nutrition prescription is key. All the aforementioned studies did not identify which patients would benefit from greater nutrition provision. Based on expert consensus, the 2016 American Society of Parenteral and Enteral Nutrition (ASPEN) and Society of Critical Care Medicine (SCCM) nutrition support guideline recommends determining which

ICU patients would benefit from nutrition therapy by determining nutritional risk [8].

What Is Nutritional Risk?

Malnutrition in the critically ill patient has been difficult to define which has led to a focus on which patients are at nutritional risk. Nutritional risk is the probability of acquiring complications and other forms of adverse outcomes that might have been prevented by timely and adequate nutrition support [24]. Ideally, nutritional risk assesses for preexisting malnutrition and severity of acute illness. Identifying nutritional risk (low or high) may assist in guiding the timing and aggressiveness of nutritional therapy.

How can the components of nutritional risk be identified? Anthropometric variables, such as recent weight loss, recent food intake, and body mass index (BMI) only take into account preexisting nutritional state and do not identify the severity of acute illness. In addition, these measures may be unavailable (e.g., mechanically ventilated and sedated patient) or inaccurate due to recall bias, as they may be self-reported. Furthermore, the "critical care obesity paradox" may disillusion clinicians into believing patients with a BMI >30 kg/m^2 have improved critical care outcomes, as compared to those with a BMI <30 kg/m^2 [25]. However, the BMI does not identify body composition, nor does it distinguish obesity phenotypes, such as sarcopenic ("loss of muscle mass and strength") obesity, which may be more predictive of outcomes. Biomarkers, such as albumin, prealbumin, and transferrin, have been utilized as surrogates for malnutrition; however, this misconception originated from erroneous descriptions of a malnutrition phenotype called kwashiorkor [26]. Albumin and prealbumin are not validated in critical illness for nutritional risk prediction and, overall, are poor measures of adequate nutrient intake and are very nonspecific markers of malnutrition due to their negative acute phase properties (i.e., decreasing during acute illness). Screening tools, such as the Malnutrition Universal Screening Tool, the Short Nutritional Assessment Questionnaire, and the Malnutrition Screening Tool, evaluate nutrition status and do not take into account severity of acute disease.

Over the past decade, scoring systems incorporating variables associated with preexisting nutritional status and acute illness have been developed to determine nutritional risk in critically ill patients. The Nutritional Risk Screening (NRS) 2002 is one such validated scoring system and identifies components of both nutritional status (0–3 points) and acute severity of illness (0–3 points). An additional 1 point is added if the patient is greater than 70 years old. These scores are added together and if the score is ≥3, the patient is at nutritional risk [27].

More recently, Heyland et al. developed and validated (in multiple cohorts) the Nutrition Risk in the Critically ill (NUTRIC) score (Table 13.1) [28]. NUTRIC identified six variables, assigning 0 to 2 points, associated with nutritional risk, including age, Acute Physiology and Chronic Health Evaluation II (APACHE II) and Sequential Organ Failure Assessment (SOFA) scores, number of comorbidities, pre-ICU length of hospital stay, and interleukin-6 level. Realizing not all medical centers can measure or have access to measuring an interleukin-6 level, a modified NUTRIC was developed and validated. A modified NUTRIC score ≥5 is associated with worse clinical outcomes, including mortality and duration of mechanical ventilation, and these patients may benefit from an early aggressive nutrition prescription [29].

In fact, two prospective observational studies suggest patients at nutritional risk, as identified by NUTRIC score, who received early EN had better outcomes than those with low nutritional risk [30, 31]. More recently, observational studies using data from a multinational registry suggest patients with greater nutritional risk (NUTRIC ≥5) had improved outcomes with greater calorie and protein provision [32, 33].

Using validated scoring systems, identifying nutritional risk is prudent in determining which patients may benefit

Table 13.1 The modified NUTRIC score excludes serum interleukin-6 value

Modified NUTRIC score variable	Range	Points
Age in years	<50	0
	50–75	1
	>75	2
APACHE II score	<15	0
	15–19	1
	≥20	2
SOFA score	<6	0
	6–9	1
	≥10	2
Number of comorbidities	0–1	0
	2+	1
Hospitalization days before ICU admission	0–1	0
	1+	1

A total score of ≥5 identifies high nutritional risk
APACHE acute physiology and chronic health evaluation, *ICU* intensive care unit, *SOFA* sequential organ failure assessment

from early and aggressive nutrition therapy and support. Once a patient is risk stratified, how does one determine the optimal route for delivering nutrition?

Should I Start Enteral or Parenteral Nutrition (or Both)?

When a patient is deemed high nutritional risk and, therefore, may benefit from early initiation of nutrition, should they receive nutrition via an enteral route, parenteral route, or both?

Early EN is defined as feeding within 24–48 h, and barring any contraindications to using the gut is recommended over early parenteral nutrition (PN) (Table 13.2) [8]. Meta-analyses comparing EN with PN showed reductions in infectious complications and reduced length of hospital stay with EN [8]. EN, as opposed to PN, provides non-nutritional benefits. EN upholds the functional integrity of the gut and its functions, including maintaining enterocyte mass and function, preserving tight junctions and small bowel villous height, and supporting IgA-producing immunity [34]. Consider the consequences of absent intestinal lumen nutrients: gut contractility would be reduced, and bacteria would

Table 13.2 Recommendations for EN versus PN from major nutrition support guidelines

Guideline	Year	Recommendation for EN vs PN
Canadian Critical Care Practice Guidelines	2013	When considering nutrition support for critically ill patients, we strongly recommend the use of EN over PN.
Society of Critical Care Medicine and American Society of Parenteral and Enteral Nutrition (ASPEN) Guidelines	2016	We recommend that nutrition support therapy in the form of early EN be initiated within 24–48 h in the critically ill patient who is unable to maintain volitional intake.
European Society of Enteral and Parenteral Nutrition (ESPEN) guidelines	2006	All patients who are not expected to be on a full oral diet within 3 days should receive EN. Although there are no data showing improvement in relevant outcome parameters using early EN, the expert committee recommends hemodynamically stable critically ill patients who have a functioning GI tract should be fed early with appropriate amount of EN.

EN enteral nutrition, *GI* gastrointestinal, *PN* parenteral nutrition be more likely to adhere to enterocytes, which would undergo contact-mediated apoptosis and consequently increase enterocyte permeability. Commensal bacteria would sense soluble compounds, such as catecholamines and adenosine, and activate bacterial virulence genes to promote survival. The now dysbiotic bacteria would intercept host signals (via telesensing) to active macrophages and enhance inflammation, promote downstream organ dysfunction, and perpetuate multiple organ failure [35]. Furthermore, using the enteral route provides a conduit for potentially immune-modulating agents and a means for stress ulcer prophylaxis (Table 13.3) [34, 36].

What is the role of PN? Three key questions are answered here: (1) When should exclusive PN be initiated in the critically ill patient with low nutritional risk? (2) When should exclusive PN be initiated for high nutritional risk? (3) When should supplemental PN be used? [37].

According to the 2016 ASPEN/SCCM guidelines, in patients with low nutritional risk, exclusive PN should be withheld for the first 7 days following ICU admission, particularly if early EN is not feasible [8]. In one RCT, exclusive early PN in adult ICU patients with a contraindication to EN showed no benefit [38].

In patients with high nutritional risk and EN is contraindicated, the 2016 ASPEN/SCCM guideline recommends starting PN as soon as possible following ICU admission [8]. Two meta-analyses comparing PN to standard therapy (i.e., no nutrition) in malnourished patients showed reduced complications with PN [39, 40].

In patients with high nutritional risk where EN is unable to meet ˃60% energy targets, supplemental PN is recommended after 7–10 days. Initiating supplemental PN prior to 7–10 days has been shown to be met with worse outcomes (EPANIC trial). Casaer et al. showed increased infectious complications in those patients randomized to receive supplemental PN on ICU day 3, as compared to ICU day 8 [41].

Since publication of the 2016 ASPEN/SCCM guidelines, numerous RCTs have challenged the recommendation sug-

Table 13.3 Nutritional and non-nutritional benefits of early enteral nutrition

Nutritional and non-nutritional benefits of early enteral nutrition
Provision of micro-/macronutrients and antioxidants
Decrease muscle and tissue glycosylation
Increase mitochondrial function
Increase protein synthesis
Maintain lean body mass
Enhance muscle function and mobility
Maintain gut integrity
Decrease gut permeability
Support commensal bacteria
Promote insulin sensitivity
Increase gut absorptive capacity
Increase gut motility and contractility
Reduce inflammation
Attenuate oxidative stress
Reduce gut/lung axis of inflammation
Preserve and enhance immunity
Maintain MALT tissue and increase secretory IgA
Increase anti-inflammatory Th-2 response
Modulate adhesion molecules to decrease macrophage and neutrophil transendothelial migration

Adapted with permission from Ref. [24]
IgA immunoglobulin A, *MALT* mucosal-associated lymphoid tissue, *Th-2* type 2 helper cells

gesting the superiority of early EN over PN in critical illness [42, 43]. Harvey et al. conducted a multicenter pragmatic randomized controlled trial (CALORIES) of adults comparing early EN to PN for up to 5 days and found no significant difference in the primary outcome of all-cause 30-day mortality or secondary outcomes of infectious complications [42]. More recently, Reignier et al. conducted a multicenter pragmatic randomized controlled trial (NUTRICEA-2) of adults comparing early EN to early PN in majority medical ICU patients with predominantly septic shock and found no difference in primary outcome of 28-day mortality. The EN group, as compared to the PN group, had higher cumulative incidences of vomiting, diarrhea, bowel ischemia, and acute colonic pseudo-obstruction [43].

Though CALORIES and NUTRICEA-2 were not powered for non-inferiority, the results of these trials are provocative and suggest early PN can be safely administered, even when early EN is not contraindicated, as in CALORIES, or may be contraindicated (due to shock), as in NUTRICEA-2. Furthermore, NUTRICEA-2 challenges the belief that EN provides non-nutritional benefits. However, it was full-dose EN that was associated with harm, and the benefit of trophic dose EN in shock remains unknown.

When nutrition is started, how fast should it be advanced? With EN, numerous factors must be considered, including initial EN tolerance, hyperglycemia due to endogenous glucose production, and risk for refeeding syndrome [7]. First, patients with high nutritional risk may also be at greater risk for EN intolerance, including vomiting and mesenteric ischemia. Second, metabolic stress leads to hyperglycemia through gluconeogenesis and glycogenolysis. Adding exogenous glucose (via EN or PN) to endogenous glucose production increases hyperglycemia. Refeeding syndrome may be more prevalent than previously thought. According to the United Kingdom NICE guidelines, major risk factors for refeeding syndrome include poor oral intake for greater than the previous 10 days, low BMI (<16 kg/m^2), unintentional weight loss of greater than 15% in the past 3–6 months, or low levels of potassium, phosphate, or magnesium before feeding [44]. These factors should be taken into consideration when advancing nutrition to goal [7].

What Is the Optimal Macronutrient?

Over the past 30 years, a better understanding of critical illness-related disease processes and improvements in management strategies and support systems have increased survival after critical illness [45]. Increased survival has been associated with acquired sarcopenia, impaired physical functioning, and a reduction in overall quality of life [4, 46–49]. ICU-related risk factors for acquired sarcopenia include metabolic stress with anabolic resistance, sedation and immobilization, and inadequate nutrition. Emerging data suggest protein may be the most important component of nutrition support, as opposed to total calories [29, 32, 33, 50, 51].

The 2016 ASPEN/SCCM guideline and recent international protein summit summary paper suggest providing 1.2–2.0 g/kg/day protein for the general critical care patient [8, 52]. The recommendation is based on observational data suggesting improvements in nitrogen balance with at least 1.2 g/kg/day protein [53]. More recently, multiple observational data suggest that achieving protein target during critical illness is associated with improved ICU mortality [32, 33, 54–57]. In one study, Compher et al. demonstrated that each 10% increase in protein intake in high nutritional risk (defined by NUTRIC >5) patients resulted in a decrease in the odds of death by 6.6% in those who remained in the ICU for at least 4 days and 10.1% for those who remained for 12 days [32].

Five randomized controlled trials have compared high versus low protein in critically ill patients [58–62]. These are small studies with low methodologic quality, have heterogeneous populations, and report variable outcomes (such as handgrip strength or change in SOFA score). No study reported morality as a primary outcome. Before widespread implementation of guideline-based recommendations for protein dose can be made, a stronger evidentiary basis in the form of well-designed randomized controlled trials comparing high to low protein is needed.

Unfortunately, a large worldwide international survey suggests critically ill patients around the world receive approximately 55% of prescribed protein (0.7 g/kg/day) [29]. Numerous reasons exist for patients not achieving protein targets. First, patient-related factors, such as nausea and vomiting, limit enteral delivery. Second, provider-related factors such as the perception of intolerance (e.g., what constitutes high gastric residual volume), a belief that greater protein is harmful in various ICU-related conditions such as acute kidney injury, and current calls for permissive underfeeding may inadvertently limit protein provision. Third, process-related factors, such as delays in initiating and advancing nutrition, and ICU-specific barriers, such as withholding or interrupting nutrition for procedures, may limit achieving protein prescription goal [63].

Strategies to increase protein delivery include providing supplemental protein (packets) enterally, using a high-protein enteral formula (newer formulas contain 35–37% of calories from protein), implementing novel enteral feeding strategies (such as volume-based feeding), and using parenteral amino acids (AA) [29].

Our Assessment of Nutritional Risk in Our Patient

Our patient is a 75-year-old man with a past medical history of diabetes, hypertension, and alcoholism admitted for respiratory failure and sepsis secondary to community-acquired pneumonia.

The patient's history of poor oral intake and weight loss suggests pre-hospitalization malnutrition. Age, comorbidities, and severity of current illness leading to critical illness make our patient high nutritional risk (NUTRIC score ≥5), suggesting he may have poor outcomes due to a lack of nutrition or insufficient nutrition. The patient also has major risk factors for refeeding syndrome.

Our Management Strategy for Nutrition in Our Patient

High nutritional risk suggests the patient will benefit from early nutrition. However, the patient's preexisting malnutrition (history of poor oral intake and weight loss) and significant electrolyte depletions put the patient at risk for refeeding syndrome, which may limit early *aggressive* nutrition.

The patient has no reported contraindications for EN, which include hemodynamic instability requiring escalating vasoactive support, vomiting, ileus, active gastrointestinal bleed, and bowel ischemia. Therefore, EN is recommended using a standard (isocaloric) formula with a goal calorie prescription of 25 kcal/kg/day and at least 1.2 g/kg/day protein. EN would be started through a nasogastric tube at an initial rate of 10–20 mL/h and titrated to goal slowly while monitoring for refeeding syndrome. Serum phosphate, potassium, and magnesium should be checked frequently for repletion. Since the protein goal will not be achieved using a trophic EN rate, additional enterally delivered supplemental protein (packets) can be added.

If the patient does not tolerate EN, early exclusive PN has been demonstrated to be safe and efficacious for calorie provision.

References

1. Patel JJ, Hurt RT, McClave SA, Martindale RG. Critical care nutrition: Where's the evidence? Crit Care Clin. 2017;33(2):397–412.
2. Preiser JC, Ichai C, Orban JC, Groeneveld AB. Metabolic response to the stress of critical illness. Br J Anaesth. 2014;113(6):945–54.
3. Dvir D, Cohen J, Singer P. Computerized energy balance and complications in critically ill patients: an observational study. Clin Nutr. 2006;25(1):37–44.
4. Puthucheary ZA, Rawal J, McPhail M, et al. Acute skeletal muscle wasting in critical illness. JAMA. 2013;310(15):1591–600.

5. Hermans G, Van Mechelen H, Clerckx B, et al. Acute outcomes and 1-year mortality of intensive care unit-acquired weakness. A cohort study and propensity-matched analysis. Am J Respir Crit Care Med. 2014;190(4):410–20.
6. Arabi YM, Casaer MP, Chapman M, et al. The intensive care medicine research agenda in nutrition and metabolism. Intensive Care Med. 2017;43:1239.
7. Patel JJ, Martindale RG, McClave SA. Controversies surrounding critical care nutrition: an appraisal of permissive underfeeding, protein, and outcomes. JPEN J Parenter Enteral Nutr. 2017;42:508:148607117721908.
8. McClave SA, Taylor BE, Martindale RG, et al. Guidelines for the provision and assessment of nutrition support therapy in the adult critically ill patient: society of critical care medicine (SCCM) and American society for parenteral and enteral nutrition (A.S.P.E.N.). JPEN J Parenter Enteral Nutr. 2016;40(2):159–211.
9. Marik PE. Is early starvation beneficial for the critically ill patient? Curr Opin Clin Nutr Metab Care. 2016;19(2):155–60.
10. Schetz M, Casaer MP. Van den Berghe G. Does artificial nutrition improve outcome of critical illness? Crit Care. 2013;17(1):302.
11. McClave SA, Weijs PJ. Preservation of autophagy should not direct nutritional therapy. Curr Opin Clin Nutr Metab Care. 2015;18(2):155–61.
12. Ibrahim EH, Mehringer L, Prentice D, et al. Early versus late enteral feeding of mechanically ventilated patients: results of a clinical trial. JPEN J Parenter Enteral Nutr. 2002;26(3):174–81.
13. Krishnan JA, Parce PB, Martinez A, Diette GB, Brower RG. Caloric intake in medical ICU patients: consistency of care with guidelines and relationship to clinical outcomes. Chest. 2003;124(1):297–305.
14. Ash J, Gervasio JM, Zaloga GP. Does the quantity of enteral nutrition affect outcomes in critically ill trauma patients? J Parenter Enter Nutr. 2005;29:S10.
15. Arabi YM, Haddad SH, Tamim HM, et al. Near-target caloric intake in critically ill medical-surgical patients is associated with adverse outcomes. JPEN J Parenter Enteral Nutr. 2010;34(3):280–8.
16. Crosara IC, Melot C, Preiser JC. A J-shaped relationship between caloric intake and survival in critically ill patients. Ann Intensive Care. 2015;5(1):37. 37-015-0079-3. Epub 2015 Nov 5.

17. Braunschweig CA, Sheean PM, Peterson SJ, et al. Intensive nutrition in acute lung injury: a clinical trial (INTACT). JPEN J Parenter Enteral Nutr. 2015;39(1):13–20.
18. Arabi YM, Tamim HM, Dhar GS, et al. Permissive underfeeding and intensive insulin therapy in critically ill patients: a randomized controlled trial. Am J Clin Nutr. 2011;93(3):569–77.
19. Petros S, Horbach M, Seidel F, Weidhase L. Hypocaloric vs normocaloric nutrition in critically ill patients: a prospective randomized pilot trial. JPEN J Parenter Enteral Nutr. 2016;40(2):242–9.
20. Rice TW, Mogan S, Hays MA, Bernard GR, Jensen GL, Wheeler AP. Randomized trial of initial trophic versus full-energy enteral nutrition in mechanically ventilated patients with acute respiratory failure. Crit Care Med. 2011;39(5):967–74.
21. Charles EJ, Petroze RT, Metzger R, et al. Hypocaloric compared with eucaloric nutritional support and its effect on infection rates in a surgical intensive care unit: a randomized controlled trial. Am J Clin Nutr. 2014;100(5):1337–43.
22. National Heart, Lung, and Blood Institute Acute Respiratory Distress Syndrome (ARDS) Clinical Trials Network, Rice TW, Wheeler AP, et al. Initial trophic vs full enteral feeding in patients with acute lung injury: the EDEN randomized trial. JAMA. 2012;307(8):795–803.
23. Arabi Y, Aldawood A, Al-Dorzi H, et al. Permissive underfeeding or standard enteral feeding in high and low nutritional risk critically ill adults: post-hoc analysis of the PermiT trial. Am J Respir Crit Care Med. 2016;195:652. [Epub ahead of print].
24. Patel JJ, Codner P. Controversies in critical care nutrition support. Crit Care Clin. 2016;32(2):173–89.
25. Patel JJ, Rosenthal MD, Miller KR, Codner P, Kiraly L, Martindale RG. The critical care obesity paradox and implications for nutrition support. Curr Gastroenterol Rep. 2016;18(9):45:45-016-0519-8.
26. Kim S, McClave SA, Martindale RG, Miller KR, Hurt RT. Hypoalbuminemia and clinical outcomes: what is the mechanism behind the relationship? Am Surg. 2017;83(11):1220–7.
27. Kondrup J, Johansen N, Plum LM, et al. Incidence of nutritional risk and causes of inadequate nutritional care in hospitals. Clin Nutr. 2002;21(6):461–8.
28. Heyland DK, Dhaliwal R, Jiang X, Day AG. Identifying critically ill patients who benefit the most from nutrition therapy:

the development and initial validation of a novel risk assessment tool. Crit Care. 2011;15(6):R268.
29. Heyland DK, Rooyakers O, Mourtzakis M, Stapleton RD. Proceedings of the 2016 clinical nutrition week research workshop-the optimal dose of protein provided to critically ill patients. JPEN J Parenter Enteral Nutr. 2017;41(2):208–16.
30. Heyland DK, Dhaliwal R, Wang M, Day AG. The prevalence of iatrogenic underfeeding in the nutritionally 'at-risk' critically ill patient: results of an international, multicenter, prospective study. Clin Nutr. 2015;34(4):659–66.
31. Jie B, Jiang ZM, Nolan MT, et al. Impact of nutritional support on clinical outcome in patients at nutritional risk: A multicenter, prospective cohort study in Baltimore and Beijing teaching hospitals. Nutrition. 2010;26(11–12):1088–93.
32. Compher C, Chittams J, Sammarco T, Nicolo M, Heyland DK. Greater protein and energy intake may be associated with improved mortality in higher risk critically ill patients: a multicenter, multinational observational study. Crit Care Med. 2017;45(2):156–63.
33. Nicolo M, Heyland DK, Chittams J, Sammarco T, Compher C. Clinical outcomes related to protein delivery in a critically ill population: a multicenter, multinational observation study. JPEN J Parenter Enteral Nutr. 2016;40(1):45–51.
34. McClave SA, Heyland DK. The physiologic response and associated clinical benefits from provision of early enteral nutrition. Nutr Clin Pract. 2009;24(3):305–15.
35. Krezalek MA, DeFazio J, Zaborina O, Zaborin A, Alverdy JC. The shift of an intestinal "microbiome" to a "pathobiome" governs the course and outcome of sepsis following surgical injury. Shock. 2016;45(5):475–82.
36. El-Kersh K, Jalil B, McClave SA, et al. Enteral nutrition as stress ulcer prophylaxis in critically ill patients: a randomized controlled exploratory study. J Crit Care. 2018;43:108–13.
37. Patel JJ, Lemieux M, McClave SA, Martindale RG, Hurt RT, Heyland DK. Critical care nutrition support best practices: Key differences between Canadian and American guidelines. Nutr Clin Pract. 2017;32(5):633–44.
38. Doig GS, Simpson F, Sweetman EA, et al. Early parenteral nutrition in critically ill patients with short-term relative contraindications to early enteral nutrition: a randomized controlled trial. JAMA. 2013;309(20):2130–8.

39. Braunschweig CL, Levy P, Sheean PM, Wang X. Enteral compared with parenteral nutrition: a meta-analysis. Am J Clin Nutr. 2001;74(4):534–42.
40. Heyland DK, MacDonald S, Keefe L, Drover JW. Total parenteral nutrition in the critically ill patient: a meta-analysis. JAMA. 1998;280(23):2013–9.
41. Casaer MP, Mesotten D, Hermans G, et al. Early versus late parenteral nutrition in critically ill adults. N Engl J Med. 2011;365(6):506–17.
42. Harvey SE, Segaran E, Leonard R. Trial of the route of early nutritional support in critically ill adults. N Engl J Med. 2015;372(5):488–9.
43. Reignier J, Boisrame-Helms J, Brisard L, et al. Enteral versus parenteral early nutrition in ventilated adults with shock: a randomised, controlled, multicentre, open-label, parallel-group study (NUTRIREA-2). Lancet. 2017;391:133.
44. NICE Guideline CG32. Nutrition support for adults: oral nutrition support, enteral tube feeding, and parenteral nutrition. London: Royal College of Surgeons of England; 2006.
45. Villar J, Sulemanji D, Kacmarek RM. The acute respiratory distress syndrome: incidence and mortality, has it changed? Curr Opin Crit Care. 2014;20(1):3–9.
46. Adler J, Malone D. Early mobilization in the intensive care unit: a systematic review. Cardiopulm Phys Ther J. 2012;23(1):5–13.
47. Batt J, dos Santos CC, Cameron JI, Herridge MS. Intensive care unit-acquired weakness: clinical phenotypes and molecular mechanisms. Am J Respir Crit Care Med. 2013;187(3):238–46.
48. Chelluri L, Im KA, Belle SH, et al. Long-term mortality and quality of life after prolonged mechanical ventilation. Crit Care Med. 2004;32(1):61–9.
49. Cuthbertson BH, Roughton S, Jenkinson D, Maclennan G, Vale L. Quality of life in the five years after intensive care: a cohort study. Crit Care. 2010;14(1):R6.
50. Hoffer LJ. Protein requirement in critical illness. Appl Physiol Nutr Metab. 2016;41(5):573–6.
51. Weijs PJ. Protein delivery in critical illness. Curr Opin Crit Care. 2016;22(4):299–302.
52. Hurt RT, McClave SA, Martindale RG, et al. Summary points and consensus recommendations from the international protein summit. Nutr Clin Pract. 2017;32(1_suppl):142S–51S.

53. Ishibashi N, Plank LD, Sando K, Hill GL. Optimal protein requirements during the first 2 weeks after the onset of critical illness. Crit Care Med. 1998;26(9):1529–35.
54. Alberda C, Gramlich L, Jones N, et al. The relationship between nutritional intake and clinical outcomes in critically ill patients: results of an international multicenter observational study. Intensive Care Med. 2009;35(10):1728–37.
55. Weijs PJ, Stapel SN, de Groot SD, et al. Optimal protein and energy nutrition decreases mortality in mechanically ventilated, critically ill patients: a prospective observational cohort study. JPEN J Parenter Enteral Nutr. 2012;36(1):60–8.
56. Allingstrup MJ, Esmailzadeh N, Wilkens Knudsen A, et al. Provision of protein and energy in relation to measured requirements in intensive care patients. Clin Nutr. 2012;31(4):462–8.
57. Weijs PJ, McClave SA. The need to differentiate fear for energy overfeeding from future benefits of protein feeding: so much to gain! Curr Opin Clin Nutr Metab Care. 2016;19(2):116–9.
58. Clifton GL, Robertson CS, Contant CF. Enteral hyperalimentation in head injury. J Neurosurg. 1985;62(2):186–93.
59. Scheinkestel CD, Kar L, Marshall K, et al. Prospective randomized trial to assess caloric and protein needs of critically ill, anuric, ventilated patients requiring continuous renal replacement therapy. Nutrition. 2003;19(11–12):909–16.
60. Rugeles SJ, Rueda JD, Diaz CE, Rosselli D. Hyperproteic hypocaloric enteral nutrition in the critically ill patient: a randomized controlled clinical trial. Indian J Crit Care Med. 2013;17(6):343–9.
61. Doig GS, Simpson F, Bellomo R, et al. Intravenous amino acid therapy for kidney function in critically ill patients: a randomized controlled trial. Intensive Care Med. 2015;41(7):1197–208.
62. Ferrie S, Allman-Farinelli M, Daley M, Smith K. Protein requirements in the critically ill: a randomized controlled trial using parenteral nutrition. JPEN J Parenter Enteral Nutr. 2016;40(6):795–805.
63. Kozeniecki M, McAndrew N, Patel JJ. Process-related barriers to optimizing enteral nutrition in a tertiary medical intensive care unit. Nutr Clin Pract. 2016;31(1):80–5.

Chapter 14
Advanced and Difficult Airway Management in the ICU

Jagroop S. Saran and Joseph W. Dooley

Introduction

Endotracheal intubation in critically ill patients can be difficult and associated with significant morbidity and mortality [1–3]. Patients have underlying life-threatening pathology, may be hypoxemic and hypotensive, and may not tolerate induction and neuromuscular blockers well. Intubations in the ICU may differ vastly from intubations in the operating room which are often elective and performed in a controlled setting by trained anesthesiologists. Incidence of difficult intubation in the ICU as reported in literature ranges from 1% to 23% depending on the definition of the difficult intubation and center [4–7].

J. S. Saran · J. W. Dooley (✉)
Department of Anesthesiology and Perioperative Medicine,
University of Rochester School of Medicine and Dentistry,
Rochester, NY, USA
e-mail: Jagroop_Saran@URMC.rochester.edu;
Joseph_Dooley@URMC.rochester.edu

J. A. LaRosa (ed.), *Adult Critical Care Medicine*,
https://doi.org/10.1007/978-3-319-94424-1_14

The field of airway management has undergone a revolution in the last several decades with the development of vast array of airway devices and algorithms. Supraglottic airways (i.e., laryngeal mask airways) have firmly established their role as a rescue device, and widespread use of indirect laryngoscopy in the form of video laryngoscopes has improved first-time success of endotracheal intubation. In this chapter, we will discuss some of the more advanced airway management techniques that an intensivist may need to utilize in the ICU.

Case Presentation

The patient is a 65-year-old man with a medical history significant for thoracoabdominal aneurysm, coronary artery disease (history of left anterior descending artery stent placed 2 years previously for angina, normal ejection fraction, asymptomatic), chronic obstructive pulmonary disease (no home oxygen, on ipratropium/albuterol combination inhaler, current smoker with a 40-pack year smoking history), and obesity (height 70 inches, weight 125 kg, BMI 39.5 kg/m^2). The thoracoabdominal aneurysm was found incidentally on computed tomography scan of the abdomen obtained 2 years previously on work-up for upper abdominal pain. He was followed with serial ultrasounds and presented for elective repair when the maximum diameter of the aneurysm exceeded 5 cm. Lung isolation was achieved using a 41 French double-lumen endotracheal tube. Intubation was moderately difficult requiring two attempts by an experienced anesthesiologist with only arytenoid cartilage visible during direct laryngoscopy. The total procedure length was 8 hours with an aortic cross clamp time of 90 minutes. Intraoperatively, he received 12 liters of isotonic crystalloid fluid, 8 units of packed red blood cells, 3 units of fresh frozen plasma, and a dose of platelets. The estimated blood loss was 2 liters and the urine output was 3 liters. At the conclusion of the procedure, the patient was left intubated due to the need for ongoing mechanical ventilation in the setting of a prolonged, high blood-loss surgical procedure which required a large-volume administration of crystalloid and blood products intraoperatively. It was also recognized that the patient would likely have an ongoing inflammatory response due to the long aortic cross clamp time. The double-lumen tube was left in place due to concerns for the safety of the patient when replacing the double-lumen tube with a conventional single-lumen endotracheal tube. At that point, the patient had marked facial edema and probable airway edema. As noted previously, the patient was moderately difficult to intubate by an experienced laryngoscopist when he had no edema. The patient was admitted to the ICU, and over the following 16 hours, he required an additional 10 liters of isotonic crystalloid fluid due to a significant systemic inflammatory response. The following morning, he remained obtunded with significant ventilator requirements (fraction of inspired oxygen 60%, PEEP 10 cm H_2O). He had thick secretions that were being inadequately suctioned due to small lumens of the double-lumen tube. On exam, he had severe anasarca with marked edema of the face, lips, tongue, chest/abdominal walls, and extremities. The impression was that he would require mechanical ventilation for a minimum of 7–10 days.

He requires replacement of the double-lumen tube with a conventional single-lumen endotracheal tube due to pulmonary toilet requirements and the need for prolonged mechanical ventilation. What are the options for managing the airway of this patient?

Recognizing the Difficult Airway

It is important to recognize the potential for a difficult airway in order to best prepare for airway management. This should always begin with careful evaluation and planning. Identification of difficult airway management remains challenging, but several patient factors that would suggest potential airway management difficulty include:

TABLE 14.1 Mallampati classification for mouth opening

Mallampati classification	**Visualization**
Class I	Soft palate, fauces, uvula, tonsillar pillars
Class II	Soft palate, fauces, uvula
Class III	Soft palate, uvular base
Class IV	Hard palate only

1. Mallampati Classification of III or IV. Patients with Mallampati Scores of III and IV Are Predictably more Difficult to Intubate than Patients with Mallampati Scores of I or II (Table 14.1).
2. Short thyro-mental distance. A thyro-mental distance less than 3 fingerbreadths (approximately 3 cm) suggests an anteriorly placed larynx that may be difficult to visualize using direct laryngoscopy.
3. Limited mouth opening. Inter-incisor distance of less than 3 fingerbreadths (3 cm) with the mouth fully open.
4. Limited head and neck movement. Neck extension could be limited by disease (arthritis, ankylosing spondylitis, prior fusion) or trauma (neck immobilized to protect against spinal cord trauma).
5. Obesity.
6. Large volume of airway secretions.
7. Blood in the airway.
8. History of difficult intubation. This is the most specific indicator of a difficult airway. Unexpected difficult intubations are often the most difficult to manage since preparations for a difficult intubation have not been made. It is important to question the patient and/or family and scan the medical record to determine if the patient has had a difficult intubation in the past. Similarly, it is important that providers who have encountered difficult intubations adequately document the event and inform the patient and family.

9. Syndromes with associated airway abnormalities (i.e., Pierre Robin, Treacher Collins, Downs, Goldenhar, etc.).
10. Tumors/lesions involving upper airway structures including the tongue, oral cavity, tonsils, larynx, etc.
11. Tumors/lesions involving the trachea.
12. Marked edema of the face, tongue, and/or airway.

Independent Risk Factors for Difficult Mask Ventilation

The ability to predict difficulty of bag-mask ventilation is as important as identifying factors for difficult intubation [8]:

1. Presence of beard
2. BMI > 26 kg/m^2
3. Lack of teeth
4. Age > 55 years
5. History of snoring

Airway Management

The goal of respiratory support is to enable the patient to adequately oxygenate and ventilate. Patients with mild to moderate pulmonary insufficiency may need only supplemental oxygen and an ability to clear secretions on their own to achieve this goal. Patients with respiratory failure either due to general anesthesia or disease often require positive pressure ventilation and supplemental oxygen (mechanical ventilation) to achieve these goals. Most often, an endotracheal tube is placed in order to protect the airway from aspiration while providing optimal mechanical ventilation. Endotracheal tubes enter the patient via the mouth (oral endotracheal tube) or nares (nasal endotracheal tube) or directly into the trachea through the neck (tracheostomy appliance). For the purpose of this chapter, we will refer to the process of securing the airway with an endotracheal tube as airway management.

When placing patients under general anesthesia for surgical procedures, airway management is determined by surgical factors and patient factors. Surgical factors are numerous and include procedure duration, procedure site, positioning, and laparoscopic versus open procedures. Patient factors include the predictors of difficult airway discussed previously as well as comorbid conditions including gastroesophageal reflux disease, esophageal achalasia, and baseline pulmonary disease. For elective operations, patients are usually breathing comfortably and can be preoxygenated. Preoxygenation removes the 79% nitrogen from the functional residual capacity of the lungs which maximizes the amount of time available for intubation. In addition, the option usually exists to cancel the procedure before induction of anesthesia if airway management is deemed too risky or to abort the procedure if attempts to secure the airway after induction are unsuccessful. Consideration can be made for using an alternative means of securing the airway, such as an awake intubation technique with flexible fiber-optic bronchoscopy. There are society guidelines, such as the American Society of Anesthesiologists difficult airway guidelines [9], which help with this decision-making (Fig. 14.1).

In the ICU, the option to abort attempts to secure the airway or to perform an awake intubation is usually not available due to respiratory distress or ventilator dependence. The goal in airway management should always be to not make the respiratory status of the patient worse. While this concept seems to be self-evident, there are often many good arguments to make adequate airway access better. At that point the risks and benefits of changing the airway must be carefully considered.

In the example noted in the case presentation, even a large double-lumen tube (41 French) is difficult to manage long-term. Exact dimensions vary by manufacturer, but each lumen of the 41 French double-lumen tube is small with an inner diameter of 4.6 to 5.4 mm. It has a maximal outer diam-

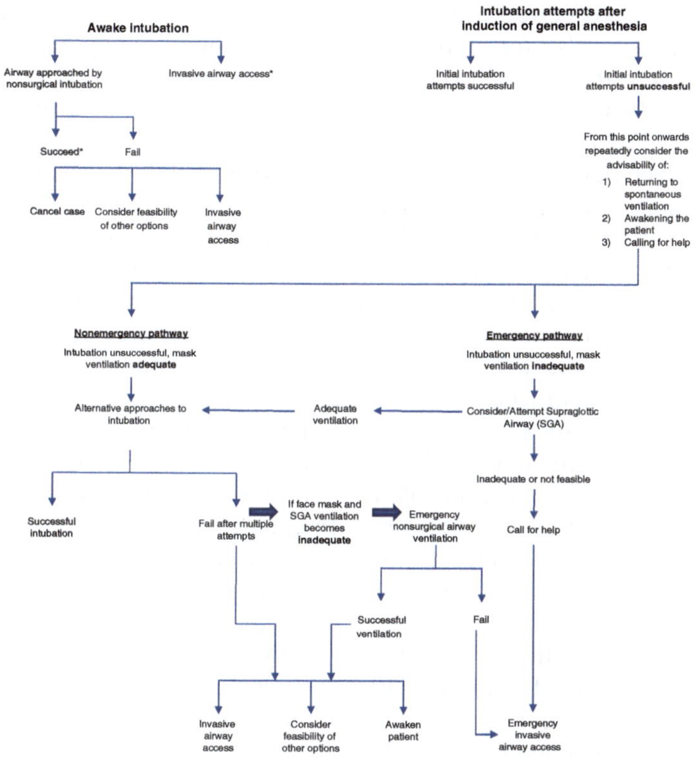

Figure 14.1 Modified from Apfelbaum et al. [9]. Please refer to *Apfelbaum* et al. for more details

eter of 14.3–14.9 mm. A 39 French double-lumen tube has a maximal outer diameter of 14.2–14.4 mm. Compare these dimensions with those of an 8.0 single-lumen endotracheal tube which has an inner diameter of 8.0 mm and an outer diameter of 11 mm. Therefore, it is more difficult to suction secretions from a patient with an appropriately sized double-lumen tube due (39 or 41 French) compared to a patient with a convention, 8.0 single-lumen endotracheal tube. In addition, compared to a single-lumen tube, the larger diameter of the double-lumen tube increases the probability of glottis injury especially when endotracheal intubation is required for a prolonged period of time. Suboptimal pulmonary toilet and increased risk for glottis injury are both good arguments to switch from a 39 French or 41 French double-lumen tube to an 8.0 single-lumen tube. However, exchanging an endotracheal tube in this situation can be challenging and quite risky.

The safest way to manage this airway would have been placing a conventional single-lumen tube preoperatively and isolating the lung using a bronchial blocker. No endotracheal tube exchange would have been required. Unfortunately, lung isolation may be less than ideal for surgical exposure. Also, bronchial blocker placement can sometimes be challenging. Both could preclude using a conventional, single-lumen endotracheal tube for the procedure. Another option would be exchanging the tube in the operating room prior to transfer to the ICU. In this case, the tube would be exchanged in the relatively controlled environment of the operating room by an anesthesiologist with extensive airway expertise with ready availability of a surgeon for a surgical airway. Also, predictably, there would likely be less facial and airway edema immediately postoperatively than 12–24 hours later after an additional large volume of IV fluid. This stresses the importance of communication between the anesthesiology team and ICU team which would have ideally started before the surgical procedure.

As alluded to earlier, airway management outside of the operating room or procedure site tends to be more difficult due to a variety of reasons. Most times, airway management is not elective. The patients usually have not been fasting. In the critical care setting, they tend to have an ileus. They are therefore at increased risk for aspiration. Furthermore, respiratory distress and underlying disease reduce the number of options. The factors noted previously that are associated with difficult intubations are more prevalent in the ICU population than in the general population. Staff of the ICU should be prepared for the urgent need for airway management at all times. This includes having supplemental oxygen, suction, equipment for bag-mask ventilation, laryngoscopes, endotracheal tube sizes in a variety of sizes, endotracheal tube stylets, induction medications, a carbon-dioxide detection device, appropriate monitors, and backup equipment all readily available. Backup equipment could include cricothyroidotomy kits, laryngeal mask airways, video laryngoscopes, airway exchange catheters, and tracheal bougies.

In addition to always being prepared for urgent/emergent airway management, anticipating the need for airway management in the near future is critical. Ideally, airway management is done during normal waking hours when staff members with airway management experience are readily available. Furthermore, if an airway is anticipated to be particularly challenging, surgical backup should be arranged for in advance. If the need for special equipment is expected, that equipment could be obtained in advance.

The general approach to airway management is as follows:

1. The patient is preoxygenated and is monitored with the standard monitors at minimum. This includes ECG, noninvasive blood pressure measurements, and pulse oximetry. Mask assist ventilation is provided if necessary.
2. The patient is induced. Induction agents are determined by the patient's clinical status and are beyond the scope of this chapter. Chemical paralysis will most likely facilitate intubation but should be used with caution. Succinylcholine can lead to hyperkalemic cardiac arrest and is associated with malignant hyperthermia. The risk for hyperkalemia is higher in the ICU population than in the general population. In addition, the risk of being unable to ventilate the patient after paralysis must be considered. The non-depolarizing neuromuscular blocking agents in the past were not immediately reversible. Recently, the FDA has approved sugammadex, a novel drug which binds rocuronium and vecuronium and can rapidly reverse neuromuscular blockade. Sugammadex may not be readily available at all centers.
3. Once induced, there should be multiple options for airway visualization and endotracheal tube placement. For most cases, direct laryngoscopy can be used. If unsuccessful, consideration for a second attempt can be made. Our practice

is to limit attempts by any one individual on the team for any particular method to two. Thereafter, either a different individual should attempt airway placement or a different technique should be used. The intent is to minimize failed intubation attempts and the associated morbidity. Morbidities include injuries associated with hypoxia, injuries to the airway, and worsening airway edema. The different options will be discussed.

4. After placing the airway device, successful placement should be confirmed by checking for end-tidal carbon dioxide. Proper positioning is assessed by auscultation and chest X-ray.

There are a number of devices available to provide adequate oxygenation and ventilation. A secure airway is considered to be a tube positioned in the trachea. Most commonly oral endotracheal tubes or tracheostomy appliances are used to secure the airway. Endotracheal tubes are placed using the following methods:

1. *Direct laryngoscopy*: This is the most commonly used method for endotracheal tube placement. Laryngoscopes are relatively inexpensive but require a significant amount of experience for facile use. Patient positioning is important.
2. *Video laryngoscopy*: Video laryngoscopy has revolutionized airway management. These items vary somewhat by manufacturer. There are some video laryngoscopes which use traditional laryngoscope blades such as Macintosh and Miller blades. This allows trainees to perform traditional direct laryngoscopy or video laryngoscopy while the instructor assesses their performance on a monitor. The instructor can provide verbal feedback and/or indirect assistance with external manipulation of the airway. The GlideScope is a video laryngoscope manufactured by Verathon. The GlideScope blade is curved but has more angulated tip than the Macintosh blade. This may allow for better visualization of an anteriorly positioned larynx than would be possible with a Macintosh or Miller blade. In our experience, successful intubation is more likely achieved

using the rigid, curved, endotracheal tube GlideRite stylet. This is due to the ability to better direct the endotracheal tube tip toward the entrance to the larynx. The GlideRite stylet is also manufactured by Verathon. Video laryngoscopy has greatly reduced the incidence of prolonged intubation attempts at our institution.

3. *Flexible bronchoscopy*: Performance of awake fiber-optic bronchoscopy (Fig. 14.2) is probably the gold standard for a difficult intubation. The airway can be made insensate using topical local anesthesia and/or nerve blocks. Only a moderate amount or no IV sedation is needed. The airway can then be secured with the patient awake and spontaneously breathing, thus eliminating the risk of airway loss while securing the airway. Unfortunately, this method is of little or no use in noncooperative patients or in patients with respiratory distress. Asleep, fiber-optic bronchoscopy can be used but can be less than ideal in patients with marginal oxygenation (high A-a gradient) or in patients with a large volume of secretions.
4. *Lighted stylet*: The lighted stylet (light wand) is a flexible stylet with a very bright light source at its tip (Fig. 14.3). This is an indirect intubation technique where the endotracheal tube is positioned while assessing the brightness of the stylet tip under the skin and is performed with the patient under general anesthesia. This has been very helpful in situations where neck movement needs to be

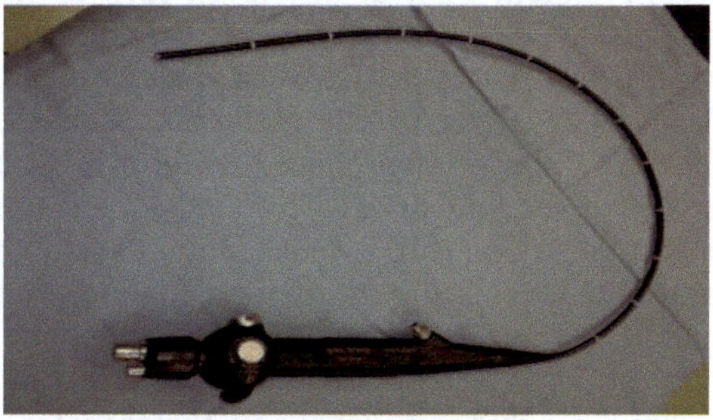

FIGURE 14.2 Karl Storz fiber-optic bronchoscope

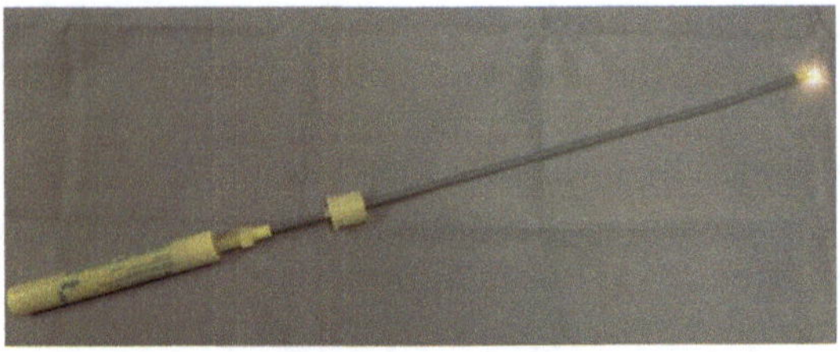

FIGURE 14.3 Light wand lighted stylet by vital signs

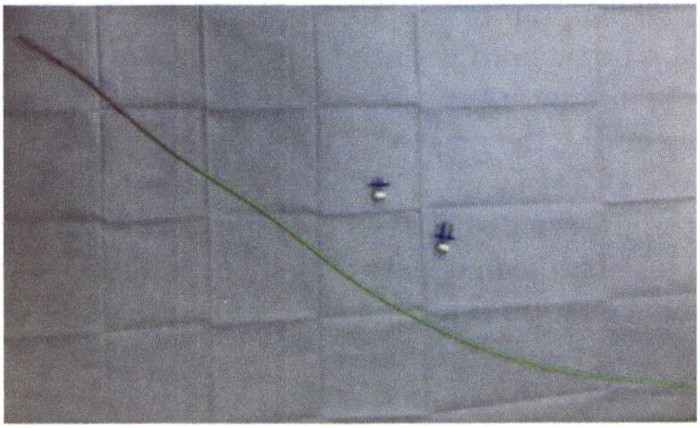

FIGURE 14.4 Cook airway exchange catheter (11 French, 100 cm)

minimized and where movement with coughing could be detrimental. We find this most useful for patients with unstable cervical spine injuries. This technique does require a significant amount of practice. Also a very dark room in required. Ambient light at any level, such as through a shaded window, makes this technique very difficult.

5. *Airway exchange catheter*: Use of an airway exchange catheter (Fig. 14.4) is one of our preferred techniques when replacing an appropriately placed endotracheal tube in a perceived challenging airway. This technique is used if the current tube is damaged, is blocked with secretions, or is inappropriate for the clinical situation. Inappropriate endotracheal tubes include conventional, single-lumen tubes that are too small or double-lumen tubes. Limitations to this technique include an exchange catheter that is too large to pass through the preexisting endotracheal tube or too

small for the replacement endotracheal tube. It is sometimes difficult or impossible to remove an endotracheal tube over an exchange catheter that is too large while keeping the exchange catheter in the trachea. Similarly, if the exchange catheter is too small or not rigid enough, the new endotracheal tube may get snagged on an airway structure, such as a vocal cord, which could leave the patient with no airway. An additional potential complication is airway trauma passing the exchange catheter too deep into the airway. Cook produces a number of airway exchange catheters of varying diameters and lengths. Exchange catheters designed for double-lumen tube replacement have a flexible tip and are relatively rigid. The flexible tip lowers the risk of deep airway trauma. The increased rigidity reduces the risk of displacement of the catheter from the trachea during exchange of the endotracheal tube.

6. *Intubating laryngeal mask airway (LMA)*: Endotracheal tubes can be passed through a conventional LMA or an LMA designed specifically for this purpose. This allows for easier oxygenation and ventilation of the patient between intubation attempts. If the LMA is properly positioned, a relatively small (6–6.5 mm internal diameter) endotracheal tube can then be passed blindly or over a flexible bronchoscope into the trachea through the LMA airway tube. Some LMAs are manufactured specifically for this purpose (Fig. 14.5). Limitations to this technique include the small

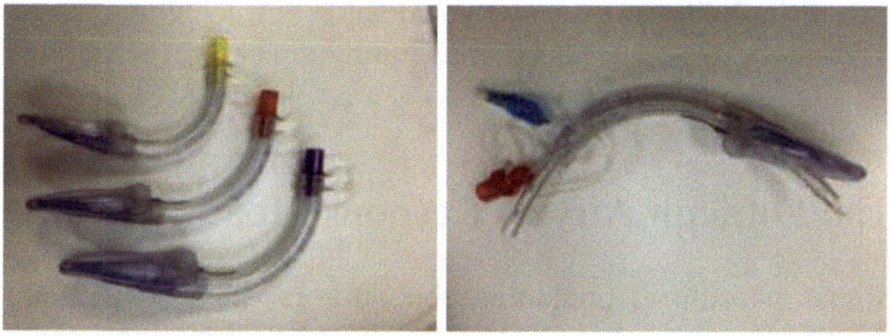

FIGURE 14.5 Disposable air-Q intubating laryngeal mask. Different sizes of the air-Q (left), picture of an endotracheal tube through the inner lumen of the air-Q (right)

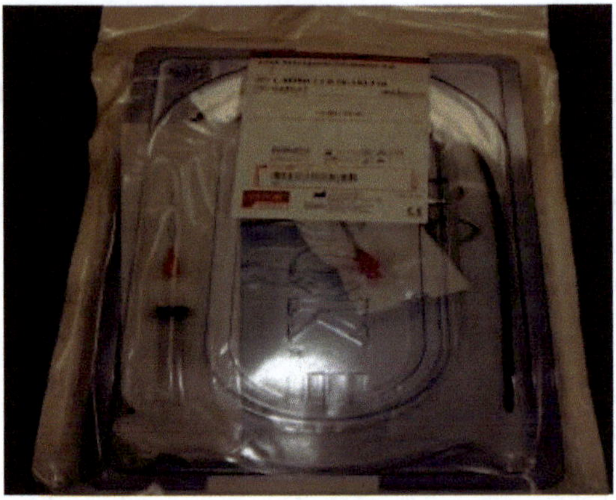

FIGURE 14.6 Cook retrograde intubation set

endotracheal tube size needed to pass through an LMA and the difficulty in properly positioning a laryngeal mask airway in patients with difficult airway anatomy.

7. *Retrograde wire intubation*: This technique requires a percutaneous puncture through the cricothyroid membrane and passing a wire blindly into the hypopharynx, through the pharynx and then out the mouth. An airway exchange catheter is then passed over the wire followed by passing an endotracheal tube into the trachea over the exchange catheter. The most common indications include unstable cervical spine, fracture of the mandible, upper airway mass, and inability to visualize vocal folds due to blood, secretions, or anatomic variations. Commercial kits are available (Fig. 14.6).

The Difficult Airway Response Team

Some institutions, including the authors', have a Difficult Airway Response Team (DART). This multidisciplinary team which includes anesthesiologists, otolaryngologists, trauma surgeons, and emergency medicine physicians is for patients

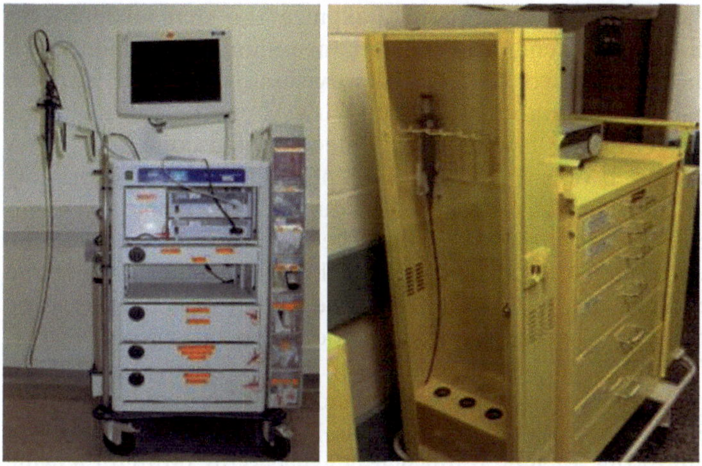

Figure 14.7 University of Rochester Medical Center carts. Mobile Difficult Airway Response Team cart (left), mobile emergency surgical airway cart (right)

with known difficult airways or those who have failed standard attempts at intubation. This team provides around-the-clock coverage in the hospital and has the ability to obtain an emergent surgical airway if needed. At the University of Rochester, this team was developed under the direction of Dr. Zana Borovcanin. Figure 14.7 illustrates two carts that are emergently brought to any DART activation at our institution.

A Reasonable Approach

A reasonable approach to the case presented at the beginning of the chapter is as follows. Using an 11 Fr, 100 cm long soft-tipped Cook catheter specifically designed for double-lumen endotracheal tubes, the 41 French double-lumen endotracheal tube could be replaced with an 8.0 mm inner diameter conventional endotracheal tube. The patient should be ventilated on 100% oxygen for several minutes prior to the exchange attempt to maximize the time available to make the exchange. The exchange should be planned for during the workday with provisions made for surgical backup. In addition, backup airway equipment including conventional laryngoscope, video laryngoscope, and LMA should be on hand. The patient should be appropriately sedated for the procedure. It would be reasonable to chemically paralyze the patient for the procedure to facilitate the exchange. A successful approach for us is performing the endotracheal tube exchange either under direct vision using direct laryngoscopy or using the video laryngoscope. This facilitates passage of the new tube. It also provides for proper laryngoscope position and airway visualization if the exchange catheter unintentionally or intentionally comes out of the trachea. If this were unsuccessful, intubation using direct laryngoscopy, video laryngoscopy, or flexible fiberoptic bronchoscopy could be attempted. The patient could be oxygenated and ventilated between attempts using bag-mask ventilation or a laryngeal mask airway. Intubation through the LMA could also be considered but would require exchange of the small conventional endotracheal tube for a larger tube in the future. Lastly, a surgical airway could be placed if all attempts failed or the patient became hemodynamically unstable or hypoxic. This could include either an emergent open tracheostomy or percutaneous cricothyroidotomy.

Summary

The best approach to management of a difficult airway in the ICU is prevention and adequate preparation. Ideally, the patient comes to the ICU from the operating room with an endotracheal tube that can be used for the duration of the patient's time on mechanical ventilation or until it is replaced with a tracheostomy appliance via a tracheotomy. If a non-intubated patient with a difficult airway has pending respiratory failure, the planning done far in advance of the event is very important. This includes having oxygen, suction, induction medications, endotracheal tubes, airway equipment, and trained personnel ready and available. It is important to have a flexible approach to managing a challenging airway. This includes quickly moving to alternative options if the initial technique is not successful and having a relatively low threshold to proceeding to a surgical airway especially if the patient is unstable.

References

1. Baillard C, Fosse JP, Sebbane M, Chanques G, Vincent F, Courouble P, et al. Noninvasive ventilation improves preoxygenation before intubation of hypoxic patients. Am J Respir Crit Care Med. 2006;174(2):171–7.
2. Jaber S, Amraoui J, Lefrant JY, Arich C, Cohendy R, Landreau L, et al. Clinical practice and risk factors for immediate complications of endotracheal intubation in the intensive care unit: a prospective, multiple-center study. Crit Care Med. 2006;34(9):2355–61.
3. Jaber S, Jung B, Corne P, Sebbane M, Muller L, Chanques G, et al. An intervention to decrease complications related to endotracheal intubation in the intensive care unit: a prospective, multiple-center study. Intensive Care Med. 2010;36(2):248–55.
4. Martin LD, Mhyre JM, Shanks AM, Tremper KK, Kheterpal S. 3,423 emergency tracheal intubations at a university hospital: airway outcomes and complications. Anesthesiology. 2011;114(1):42–8.
5. Heuer JF, Barwing TA, Barwing J, Russo SG, Bleckmann E, Quintel M, et al. Incidence of difficult intubation in intensive care patients: analysis of contributing factors. Anaesth Intensive Care. 2012;40(1):120–7.
6. Simpson GD, Ross MJ, McKeown DW, Ray DC. Tracheal intubation in the critically ill: a multi-centre national study of practice and complications. Br J Anaesth. 2012;108(5):792–9.
7. Le Tacon S, Wolter P, Rusterholtz T, Harlay M, Gayol S, Sauder P, et al. Complications of difficult tracheal intubations in a critical care unit. Ann Fr Anesth Reanim. 2000;19(10):719–24.

8. Langeron O, Masso E, Huraux C, Guggiari M, Bianchi A, Coriat P, et al. Prediction of difficult mask ventilation. Anesthesiology. 2000;92(5):1229–36.
9. Apfelbaum JL, Hagberg CA, Caplan RA, Blitt CD, Connis RT, Nickinovich DG, et al. Practice guidelines for management of the difficult airway: an updated report by the American Society of Anesthesiologists Task Force on Management of the Difficult Airway. Anesthesiology. 2013;118(2):251–70.

Chapter 15
Hemodynamic Monitoring: What's Out There? What's Best for You?

Heath E. Latham

Case Summary

A 68-year-old woman with multiple medical problems presents to the emergency room. She was transported via EMS from her skilled nursing facility with a 1-day history of altered mental status, chest pain, hypotension, and fevers. She was discharged to the skilled nursing facility 4 weeks previously following a 1 week hospital stay for non-ST elevation myocardial infarction (NSTEMI) that required percutaneous coronary intervention with stent placement, as well as acute on chronic renal insufficiency from which her creatinine had returned to her baseline of 2.2 at the time of discharge.

Review of her records reveals a past medical history of chronic respiratory failure requiring 2 liters via nasal cannula, chronic renal insufficiency, anemia of chronic disease,

H. E. Latham
Division of Pulmonary and Critical Care Medicine, Department of Internal Medicine, The University of Kansas Medical Center, Kansas City, KS, USA
e-mail: hlatham@kumc.edu

J. A. LaRosa (ed.), *Adult Critical Care Medicine*,
https://doi.org/10.1007/978-3-319-94424-1_15

congestive heart failure with a reduced ejection fraction of 35% by echo 1 month prior, diabetes mellitus type II with a recent Hgb A1c of 8.2%, and morbid obesity with a BMI of 36 kg/m^2. She is a lifelong non-smoker and recently retired from the food service industry. She is a widow with the death of her husband a year ago. She was living independently previous to her recent hospitalization, but her family was concerned with her ability to care for herself. Her family history is remarkable for cardiac disease in both parents and her brother.

On evaluation in the emergency department, she appears ill and is somnolent but arouses to her name and is able to answer simple questions. She reports feeling fatigued with increased shortness of breath and non-radiating chest discomfort along her sternum with mild nausea. These symptoms were present when she awoke this morning. She was told she had a fever by one of the techs at the nursing facility but denies chills or sweats. She reports taking all her medications which include metoprolol, amlodipine, insulin glargine, insulin aspart, furosemide, atorvastatin, clopidogrel, and aspirin. She denies cough or abdominal pain. She has lower extremity edema which she reports as being chronic and stable.

On examination, the temperature is 38.3 °C, the blood pressure 82/45 mmHg, the pulse 92 beats per minute, the respiratory rate 22 breaths per minute, and the oxygen saturation 95%, while the patient is breathing 8 liters by nasal cannula. Her oral mucosa appears dry and is without lesions. Her body habitus does not allow assessment of JVD. Her heart sounds are distant but normal. There are decreased breath sounds in the bases but no appreciable rales or wheezes. There is dullness to percussion in the bilateral bases. Her abdomen is obese, soft, and without distention or tenderness to palpation. She has 1+ bilateral lower extremity edema to the mid-shins. Her skin is without rash and is warm to the touch peripherally. There are no neurologic deficits.

Laboratory examination is shown in Table 15.1 and is pertinent for a white blood cell count of 16 per mm^3 with a left shift, hemoglobin of 8.4 g/dL, carbon dioxide of 18 mmol/L,

TABLE 15.1 Laboratory data

Variable	Ref. range	Admission	Previous discharge
Hemoglobin (gm/dL)	13.5–16.5	8.4	7.8
Hematocrit (%)	40–50	25.2	23.4
Platelet count (K/uL)	150–400	173	125
White blood cells (K/uL)	4.5–11.0	16.0	7.5
Segmented neutrophils (%)	41–77	72	52
Absolute neutrophil count (K/uL)	1.8–7.0	15.04	4.05
Bands (%)	0–10	22	2
Lymphocytes (%)	24–44	5	40
Monocytes (%)	4–12	1	6
Sodium (mmol/L)	137–147	146	137
Potassium (mmol/L)	3.5–5.1	4.0	3.8
Chloride (mmol/L)	98–110	112	108
CO2 (mmol/L)	21–30	18	23
Blood urea nitrogen (mg/dL)	7–25	64	42
Creatinine (mg/dL)	0.4–1.24	2.90	2.20
Glucose (mg/dL)	70–100	235	184
Albumin (g/dL)	3.5–5.0	3.8	3.1
Calcium (mg/dL)	8.5–10.6	9.8	8.6
Total bilirubin (mg/dL)	0.3–1.2	1.2	0.8
Total protein (mg/dL)	6.0–8.0	7.2	6.5
AST (u/L)	7–40	35	18

(continued)

Table 15.1 (continued)

Variable	Ref. range	Admission	Previous discharge
ALT (u/L)	7–56	42	21
Alk phosphatase (u/L)	25–110	105	80
Lactic acid (mmol/L)	0.5–2.0	3.2	
Troponin I (ng/mL)	0.0–0.05	0.09	
pH-arterial	7.35–7.45	7.34	
pCO2-arterial	35–45	37	
pO2-arterial	80–100	68	

creatinine of 2.9 mg/dL, glucose of 235 mg/dL, and lactic acid of 3.2 mmol/L. Her urinalysis is positive for 2+ glucose, 1+ protein, nitrites, and 2+ leukocytes. Electrocardiogram reveals sinus rhythm with early repolarization and flattening of the T-waves in the lateral leads. A portable chest X-ray reveals small lung volumes with stable small bilateral effusions and cardiomegaly when compared with prior imaging.

Differential Diagnosis

This 68-year-old woman with multiple medical problems including a recent history of NSTEMI with cardiomyopathy presents with shock. Shock is defined as a state of life-threatening acute circulatory failure secondary to one or more of four mechanisms [1, 2]. All categories of shock should be considered time-sensitive medical emergencies requiring focused investigation to identify the etiology and prompt intervention in order to limit the consequences of shock-induced global tissue hypoxia [3]. The three leading considerations for this patient's shock would be distributive shock due to a septic source, obstructive shock due to acute pulmonary embolism (PE) or pericardial tamponade, and cardiogenic shock with her recent history of NSTEMI and coronary stent placement. There are no signs of blood loss or history to support significant volume loss, making hemorrhagic and hypovolemic shock unlikely etiologies for her hypotension.

The clinical picture is most supportive of distributive shock from a septic source. She has four out of four criteria for the systemic inflammatory response syndrome. In particular, she has a leukocytosis with left shift and fever, with findings on the urinalysis concerning for a urinary tract infection. She is warm to the touch peripherally which is most consistent with a distributive form of shock and less consistent with cardiogenic, obstructive, or hypovolemic shock. With her recent history of NSTEMI and stent placement, stent occlusion and cardiogenic shock must be considered. She does report a non-radiating chest pain. Her ECG does have flattening of T-waves, but no acute ST-segment changes that would support a stent occlusion. Her troponin is only mildly elevated and in conjunction with the T-wave changes likely reflects global tissue ischemia as a result of the shock. Additional diagnostic testing of her hemodynamics is important to further evaluate for possible cardiogenic shock as well as obstructive shock.

Obstructive shock from pericardial tamponade or acute PE should be considered but are less likely causes of this patient's shock. It is possible the patient could have a pericardial effusion secondary to a pericarditis as the cause of her chest pain and fever with resultant tamponade causing her shock, but this is less likely compared to septic shock. She does have distant heart sounds, but this is likely related to her morbid obesity and less likely a sign of tamponade. The ECG is without findings of low voltage or electrical alternans. Although a specific finding, the absence of electrical alternans does not rule out the presence of a pericardial effusion or tamponade. In addition, the CXR does not demonstrate abnormalities of the cardiac silhouette suggesting the development of pericardial effusion. Worsening hypoxemia and non-specific chest pain with a relatively unchanged CXR does raise the suspicion of an acute pulmonary embolism as a cause of obstructive shock. She was hospitalized 4 weeks prior which does increase her risk of DVT and PE, but her lower extremity edema is chronic, bilateral, and symmetric without pain.

There are other diagnoses that are more likely which makes DVT and PE less likely in this case. Additional diagnostic noninvasive testing and evaluation of hemodynamics will rule both forms of obstructive shock as a contributing factor.

Treatment and Management I

The treating physician favors the diagnosis of septic shock from a urinary source, and treatment is initiated with appropriate intravenous antibiotics and initial fluid resuscitation per the Surviving Sepsis Guidelines [4]. As the initial fluid bolus is delivered to the patient, additional hemodynamic monitoring should be considered to assess for volume responsiveness to guide further volume resuscitation. Objective assessment for volume responsiveness is critical to the care of shock patients as only 50% of patients in shock benefit from volume challenges [5–8]. Hemodynamic monitoring allows for objective assessment of the cardiovascular system response following volume infusion to improve stroke volume and enhance the delivery of oxygen to tissues in order to meet the metabolic demand which distinguishes fluid responders from non-responders [9, 10]. Depending on institutional resources, monitoring strategies range from simple bedside examination to advanced technologies, although assessment of changes in dynamic variables such as stroke volume is favored over static measures such as CVP or IVC compressibility [4].

Clinical Parameters for Assessing for Volume Responsiveness

For the remainder of this chapter, we will reference the assessment of fluid or volume responsiveness with regard to various hemodynamic monitoring devices or techniques. Evaluating for fluid responsiveness is important to determine whether or not an individual patient is on the ascending portion of the Frank-Starling curve and therefore could benefit from increased cardiac output and oxygen delivery following a fluid bolus [11, 12]. Fluid given to the nonresponsive patient will contribute to third spacing, and a growing body of literature raises concerns of volume overload in the critically ill patient contributing to morbidity and mortality [6, 13–16]. Understanding key clinical principles in which dynamic measures are obtained is essential to ensure any hemodynamic monitoring device or technique is used and interpreted accurately. There are three main principles to consider when assessing for fluid responsiveness: [1] utilizing the heart-lung interaction to evaluate variability indices, [2] direct assessment of stroke volume or a surrogate of stroke volume that is not dependent on the heart-lung interaction, and [3] knowledge of the source of a volume challenge.

Assessment of volume responsiveness utilizing the heart-lung interaction is dependent on the physiologic effects of positive-pressure ventilation on cardiac preload and afterload with resultant breath-to-breath variation in systolic blood pressure, pulse pressure, stoke volume, and arterial flow velocity [17]. During the inspiratory phase of a ventilated breath, the rise in pleural pressure results in a rise in right atrial pressure and impedes filling of the right side of the heart and pulmonary arteries. Simultaneously, there is transient increased filling of the left side of the heart that maximizes stroke volume from the left ventricle at the end of the breath. The impeded filling of the right side of the heart and pulmonary arteries transits the lungs to the left heart over three to four cardiac cycles to produce the stroke volume at the end of the expiratory phase of the respiratory cycle [18, 19]. The more volume deplete the patient, the greater the impact of the positive-pressure ventilation on the right heart filling and the greater the variability in the stroke volume from breath to breath. This variation is the principle by which pulse pressure variation (PPV), systolic pressure variation, (SPV), and stroke volume variation (SVV) are used to determine volume responsiveness (Fig. 15.1) [17, 20, 21]. In order to maximize the accuracy of the heart-lung interaction to predict fluid responsiveness, several parameters must be met. First the patient must be passively ventilated either as the result of paralysis or deep sedation. Second, the tidal volume delivered must be at least

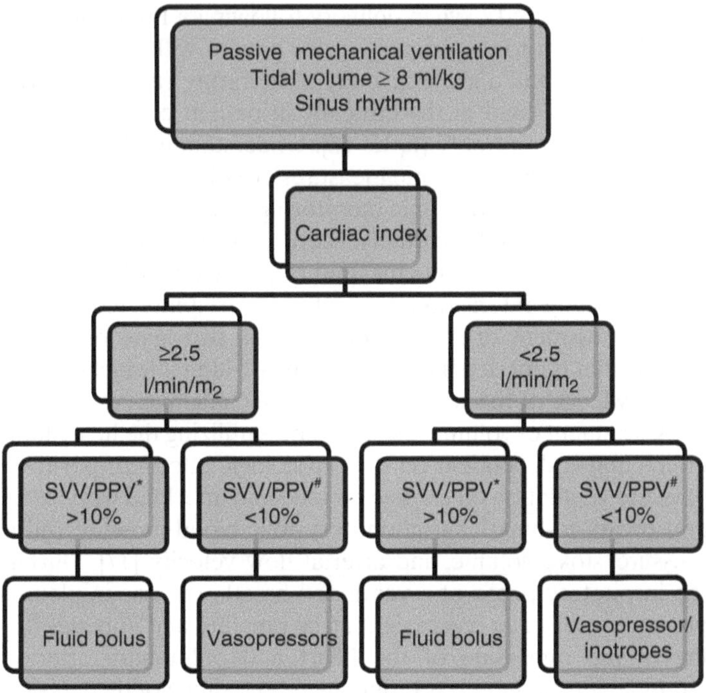

FIGURE 15.1 Resuscitation algorithm for shock based on assessment for breath-to-breath variations in stroke volume (SVV) or pulse pressure (PPV). * indicates volume responder and likely to benefit from additional volume resuscitation. # indicates volume non-responder and unlikely to benefit from additional volume resuscitation

8 mL/kg to optimize the respiratory effect on cardiac physiology [22]. Finally, the patient must be in normal sinus rhythm as an arrhythmia induces variation in the stroke volume regardless of the respiratory cycle. Additional factors such as a heart rate-to-respiratory rate ratio greater than 3.6 and lung compliance greater than 30 ml/cmH_2O are also important to ensure accuracy of any device or technique taking advantage of the heart-lung interaction [23].

Multiple devices and techniques are capable of direct measurement of stroke volume, estimating stroke volume, or measuring a surrogate of stroke volume. Measurement of

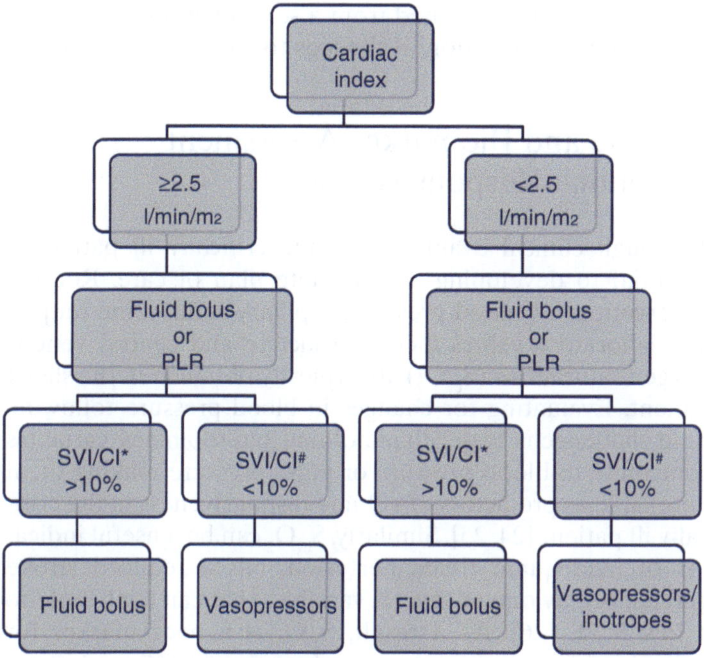

FIGURE 15.2 Resuscitation algorithm for shock based on evaluation of changes in stroke volume (SVI) or cardiac index (CI) following fluid challenge or passive leg raise (PLR). * indicates volume responder and likely to benefit from additional volume resuscitation. # indicates volume non-responder and unlikely to benefit from additional volume resuscitation

stroke volume is not dependent on the heart-lung interaction and can be performed whether or not the patient is passively mechanically ventilated as outlined above or spontaneously breathing with or without mechanical ventilation. The assessment for change in stroke volume is not made breath to breath as with the heart-lung interaction but made following a volume challenge with either 500 mL of crystalloid infused in less than 30 min or by a surrogate of volume challenge with a passive leg raise (PLR) (Fig. 15.2). The PLR serves as a reversible fluid challenge of approximately 350 mL of blood from the lower extremities of a patient that is transitioned from a semi-recumbent position to supine with elevation of the legs to 45° for 3 min [5].

Bedside and Biomarker Assessment of Volume Responsiveness

Thorough clinical evaluation of the critically ill patient is essential to developing an adequate plan of care. Routine observations of blood pressure, capillary refill, urine output, and laboratory values including lactate and central venous oxygen saturations ($S_{cv}O_2$) are typically obtained in the shock patient. Evaluating for changes in blood pressure following fluid challenge is better than nothing, but too many variables contribute to blood pressure or pulse pressure making them unreliable as predictors of volume responsiveness in the critically ill patient [24, 25]. Similarly, $S_{cv}O_2$ can be a useful indicator of inadequate tissue perfusion, but a reduced stroke volume is only one of several variables that can contribute to a low $S_{cv}O_2$ [26]. As a result, $S_{cv}O_2$ is a poor marker for hemodynamic monitoring and volume resuscitation, particularly in the patient presented above with septic shock [27–30]. Lactate may also be an indicator of poor tissue perfusion in shock, but similar to $S_{cv}O_2$, lactate is affected by several other variables [31]. However, lactate-guided resuscitation demonstrated reduced mortality in patients with septic shock compared to other markers of perfusion mentioned above [32–34]. Therefore, if resources are limited to clinical assessment and serial laboratory studies, guided resuscitation via lactate levels is the most evidence-based surrogate of tissue perfusion [4].

End-tidal carbon dioxide ($ETCO_2$) is easily monitored with continuous waveform capnography devices and often available on intubated patients in the ICU. An increase of greater than 5% in the $ETCO_2$ following a PLR or fluid bolus over 30 min in a passively ventilated patient is a reliable predictor of volume responsiveness [35, 36]. However, the use of $ETCO_2$ to predict fluid responsiveness has not been assessed in the non-intubated patient, and thus may not be as applicable to the critically ill population as other devices and techniques described later in this chapter. As the patient presented above is spontaneously breathing, this technique could not be applied even if $ETCO_2$ is monitored.

Central Catheter-Based Hemodynamic Monitoring

Central venous pressure (CVP) can be measured via a pressure transducer connected to any central line with the tip resting at the junction between the superior vena cava and right atrium [7, 37–39]. The CVP may be a marker of right ventricular function, but this static pressure is influenced by multiple factors including vascular tone, intrathoracic pressure, ventricular compliance, and cardiac chamber size making it a poor marker of volume responsiveness [40–44]. Even when evaluating the ability of respiratory variation in the CVP to predict volume responsiveness, the CVP is a poor predictor of fluid responsiveness [45]. In early publications of the Surviving Sepsis Guidelines, fluid resuscitation guided by CVP was recommended in patients such as the one presented in this chapter [46]. Multiple studies evaluating the ability of CVP to predict fluid responsiveness in patients with severe sepsis or septic shock do not support volume resuscitation guided by CVP; and therefore, it is no longer recommended as a hemodynamic monitoring tool for this purpose [3, 4, 47, 48].

Similar to CVP, utilization of the static pressures and volumes obtained via a pulmonary artery (PA) catheter is not reliable to determine fluid responsiveness or guide volume resuscitation in the patient with shock [21, 44, 49, 50]. However, PA catheters are capable of accurately estimating the stroke volume (SV) or cardiac output (CO) and their associated indices [51]. When a PA catheter is in place, changes in the SV or CO following fluid challenges or changes in vasoactive and inotropic medications can be used to guide shock therapy. Patients with acute coronary syndrome or congestive heart failure with cardiogenic shock may benefit from therapy guided by the use of the PA catheter [52–54]. However, cardiac measurements produced by a PA catheter can be obtained by echocardiography as well as other newer technologies, and the use of PA catheters in the cardiac and postsurgical cardiac ICUs is likely to continue to decrease [55–57]. The utilization of the PA catheter in the management of the critically ill patient with hypovolemic shock, septic shock, or acute respiratory distress syndrome does not improve mortality, shorten length of stay, or reduce cost [58–61]. As a result of these studies that do not demonstrate benefit combined with the risk of complication associated with PA catheters, the use of PA catheters has declined substantially throughout intensive care units [57, 62]. Therefore, in the septic patient presented in this chapter, there is no indication to float a PA catheter to assist in the management of her shock.

Ultrasonography

Bedside ultrasonography (US) in the emergency room and the ICU is increasingly used in the critically ill patient as a pluripotential diagnostic tool, and the ability of intensivists and emergency medicine physicians to competently acquire and interpret US images to guide therapy in this patient population has been demonstrated in multiple studies [63–69]. The use of US to assess the shock patient is particularly useful as it allows quick assessment for biventricular size and function, pericardial disease, pulmonary parenchymal abnormalities, or pleural abnormalities such as effusions or pneumothorax [70–75]. In the patient above, bedside thoracic ultrasound reveals a depressed left ventricular function consistent with her known cardiomyopathy. There is no evidence of pericardial effusion or right ventricular dilation or dysfunction. She did not have any parenchymal B-lines along the anterior thoracic wall making pulmonary edema a less likely cause to her acute on chronic hypoxemic respiratory failure and cardiogenic shock an unlikely primary contributor to her shock state on presentation. There are small bilateral effusions consistent with her chest imaging. A quick assessment of her bilateral lower extremities did not reveal any evidence of DVT, and with the normal appearance of her right ventricle, obstructive shock due to pulmonary embolism is essentially ruled out [76]. At this point, the leading consideration of septic shock due to a urinary source is supported by the negative findings on the bedside ultrasound. After the patient is given 30 mL/kg of crystalloid per the Surviving Sepsis Guidelines, she remains in shock, and additional evaluation for fluid responsiveness can be assessed with bedside ultrasound [4].

Point-of-care ultrasound can assess for volume responsiveness via both static and dynamic measures. Echocardiography can measure LV end-diastolic area, RV end-diastolic volume, LV ejection time, and the ratio of pulsed Doppler transmitral flow to mitral annular velocity in early diastole. When these parameters are assessed for change in a passively ventilated patient, they are poor predictors of fluid responsiveness [49, 77–80]. Therefore, the static measures obtained via ultrasonography are no better than the static measures obtained via central catheters discussed above. The diameter of the IVC can be measured via bedside ultrasound and serves as a surrogate of the right atrial pressure [81]. When assessed as a marker of fluid responsiveness, IVC minimum or maximum diameter alone at end expiration in a passively ventilated patient is not an accurate predictor of fluid responsiveness [82].

Dynamic measures obtained via ultrasound are determined via variations in IVC diameter or Doppler-derived changes in arterial blood flow. In a passively ventilated patient, the variation in IVC diameter between end inspiration and end expiration can be used to accurately predict volume responsiveness [82, 83]. This technique to assess for fluid responsiveness has been validated in multiple studies. However, care must be taken to ensure no spontaneous respiratory effort is applied by the patient and tidal volumes are sufficiently above 8 mL/kg to ensure the accuracy of IVC variation to detect fluid responsiveness. Doppler-derived changes in arterial blood flow can be assessed at the LV outflow track, carotid artery, femoral artery, or descending aorta and serve as a surrogate for stroke volume. These measurements are assessed prior to a fluid challenge or passive leg raise and reassessed following the challenge for changes in stroke volume in order to determine fluid responsiveness. When used in this manner, assessment for changes of arterial blood flow via Doppler-derived devices is accurate to predict volume responsiveness [77, 84–89].

Point-of-care ultrasonography is a useful tool for both diagnosis of shock and to monitor treatment response. Additional training is needed to acquire the knowledge and skills for image acquisition and interpretation to allow for the competent application of bedside ultrasonography and Doppler-derived assessments described above. The learning curve is steep but achievable by many learners [68, 90]. As the patient above is spontaneously breathing without the aid of mechanical ventilation, the use of bedside ultrasonography to assess for alterations in breath-to-breath IVC diameter indices is not adequate to determine volume responsiveness. However, Doppler-derived assessment for changes in arterial blood flow at any of the sites mentioned above could be performed before and after volume challenge with crystalloid or a passive leg raise. In this case, a PLR is favored over a volume challenge due to her significant cardiomyopathy and the desire to avoid fluid overload.

Arterial Pressure Waveform Analysis

Multiple devices utilize arterial pressure waveform analysis to estimate stroke volume and therefore cardiac output as well as various other parameters such as PPV, SVV, extravascular lung water index, global end-diastolic volume, pulmonary blood volume, and systemic vascular resistance index.

These measurements are used to determine fluid responsiveness and a patient's systemic and pulmonary vascular compliance and volume status [20, 91, 92]. These devices require the placement of an arterial catheter by which the device utilizes a proprietary algorithm to analyze the pressure waveform on the principle that pulse pressure is directly proportional to SV and inversely related to vascular compliance in order to continuously estimate the stroke volume [93]. Some devices are auto-calibrating while others require dilution methods for calibration [94]. The accuracy of any device utilizing arterial pressure waveform analysis may be affected by over- or under-dampening of the arterial waveform as well as the presence of significant aortic regurgitation.

The FloTrac/Vigileo™ device is an auto-calibrating device that utilizes a standard peripheral arterial catheter to continuously estimate SV/CO via pulse contour analysis. The proprietary algorithm assumes a patient's vascular compliance and elastance based on age, height, sex, and weight. Accuracy of the device is primarily dependent upon whether or not the systemic vascular resistance is being altered by vasoactive agents due to the dependence of the device on algorithmic assumption of vascular compliance [95–97]. Therefore, the device may be less accurate when vasopressors are used.

The lithium dilution cardiac output (LiDCO™) monitor is based on the lithium dilution method to estimate cardiac output. The device requires a standard peripheral arterial catheter and a central venous catheter. A small concentration of lithium chloride is injected intermittently to determine vascular compliance and calibrate the device [98]. This measurement in combination with arterial waveform analysis allows for continuous monitoring of stroke volume and cardiac output. The device must be calibrated at least once daily and if there is a suspected change in vascular compliance. There is an updated version of LiDCO™ named $\text{LiDCO}_{\text{rapid}}$™ that is auto-calibrating similar to the FloTrac/Vigileo™ device and as a result has the same limitations in patients administered vasoactive drugs [99].

The pulse index continuous cardiac output (PiCCO™) monitor is based on the thermodilution method to estimate cardiac output. This device requires a femoral arterial catheter and a central venous catheter. The device is calibrated by standard thermodilution techniques and continuously monitors cardiac output via arterial pressure waveform analysis. As with the other pressure waveform analysis devices, the accuracy of the PiCCO™ device is dependent on the stability of vascular compliance and therefore requires frequent calibration to reliably predict stroke volume [99, 100].

The clinical application of all these devices has been evaluated in multiple settings from the operating room to the intensive care unit with mixed results on the ability of these devices to predict fluid responsiveness and guide care of the critically ill [101–106]. In the patient above, she is likely to require arterial catheter placement for continuous blood pressure monitoring while vasopressors are titrated for optimization of the mean arterial pressure. One of the arterial waveform analysis devices could be utilized for hemodynamic monitoring, but utility of SVV to guide volume management would be inaccurate as the patient is spontaneously breathing. The devices could be used to assess for changes in stroke volume following either PLR or volume challenge to determine fluid responsiveness and guide volume resuscitation while keeping in mind the potential inaccuracy of the device and need for recalibration with changes in vascular compliance as vasoactive drugs are titrated.

Bioreactance

The noninvasive cardiac output monitoring (NICOM™/Starling™) devices utilize bioreactance-based technology to continuously monitor cardiac output. Four electrodes are placed on the anterior thorax, and each electrode injects a high-frequency current into the chest and simultaneously assesses for changes in the time it takes for the current to traverse the thorax, known a phase shift. Phase shift is primarily effected by blood flow through the aorta, and via a proprietary algorithm, the measurement of change in phase shift serves as a surrogate for stroke volume [107]. The device provides hemodynamic parameters of stroke volume, cardiac output, and total peripheral resistance (TPR) which is a measure of vascular tone. Clinical applications have been evaluated in the emergency department, operating room, and ICU to assess the ability of the device to evaluate fluid responsiveness and guide volume management [88, 108–112]. The accuracy of the device is affected when there is significant aortic regurgitation or thoracic aneurysms, the presence of ventricular assist devices or balloon pumps, or excessive cautery in the operating room. Also, electrode adherence to the skin is limited to 72 h or by excessive moisture on the skin.

In the patient presented above, the bioreactance device could be used in the emergency room to assess the baseline hemodynamic parameters. In particular, the SV and CO as well as the total peripheral resistance could be used to assist in diagnosing the cause of shock. One expects the SV and CO to be low in this patient due to the known cardiomyopathy, and the presence of a low TPR would support distributive shock as the major contributor in this case. Then fluid responsiveness could be assessed by evaluating for a change in the stroke volume following a fluid challenge or PLR. Again, PLR would be favored in this patient with cardiomyopathy. If the patient were fluid responsive, then additional fluid boluses should be given until there is no longer evidence of volume responsiveness. If the patient's shock resolved using the bioreactance device, her resuscitation is delivered in a completely noninvasive fashion, even without the need for an arterial catheter.

Fingertip Monitoring Devices

Another form of completely noninvasive hemodynamic monitoring devices are those that utilize technology to assess variations in pulse at the fingertip to estimate cardiac output.

There are three technologies currently available, plethysmographic waveform analysis, estimated continuous cardiac output (esCCO™) monitoring, and ClearSight™ monitoring. Of these technologies, plethysmographic waveform analysis has been around the longest and takes advantage of data derived from a simple pulse oximeter (Masimo Corp., Irvine, CA) to measure the maximal and minimal plethysmographic waveform amplitudes over a given period of time and calculates the percentage of difference between the two, termed pleth variability index (PVI) [113]. In a passively ventilated patient with at least a tidal volume of 8 ml/kg, PVI does predict fluid responsiveness [114–116]. The accuracy of PVI is dependent on adequate peripheral perfusion which may be affected by hypothermia, shock, vasoactive drugs, and the site of measurement [117, 118]. All these limitations can frequently be encountered in the care of a critically ill patient.

The esCCO™ device estimates cardiac output by measuring the pulse wave transit time or time taken for blood from the heart to reach the fingertip which is determined as the time between the peak of the ECG R-wave and the oximeter pulse wave rise point seen at the fingertip of the device. Various studies have reported inconsistent results with most reporting poor reliability, precision, and correlation when compared to established methods of cardiac output monitoring [119–124]. In addition, the esCCO™ device is subject to all the same perfusion limitations listed above.

Finally, the ClearSight™ device continuously measures blood pressure, CO, SVV, and PPV via an inflatable finger cuff. It is subject to the same limitations as the previously discussed fingertip monitoring devices, and as a result the evidence is inconsistent regarding its reliability, especially in patients with poor peripheral perfusion, hypothermia, and peripheral edema [125–127]. As the patient presented above is critically ill with shock, peripheral edema, and likely poor peripheral perfusion due to underlying vascular disease, none of the fingertip monitoring devices are appropriate to use in the assessment of her hemodynamics.

Treatment and Management II

Once the diagnosis of septic shock is determined and the patient is given appropriate antibiotics and a 30 ml/kg infusion of crystalloid, she remains hypotensive with a MAP less than 65. An arterial line is attempted in the radial artery; but due to her peripheral vascular disease, there is difficulty cannulating the artery. Therefore, an arterial pressure waveform device is not able to be used to assess for further fluid responsiveness. Bedside Doppler-derived techniques are appropriate to pursue in this spontaneously breathing patient, but the physician caring for the patient is not trained in assessing stroke volume or surrogates of stroke volume via Doppler-derived techniques. Therefore, volume responsiveness is assessed with a bioreactance device and PLR. The patient demonstrates a 24% improvement in SV following the PLR. Additional fluid boluses of crystalloid are infused over 30 min with assessment for change in SV following each bolus. The patient receives an additional 1.5 liters of crystalloid before she is no longer fluid responsive. Following this resuscitation, her MAP is greater than 65 and her lactic acid improves to 1.8 mmol/L. She does not require initiation of vasopressors, and her oxygen requirement and creatinine return to baseline over the next 48 h.

Conclusion

The care of the critically ill patient in shock is increasingly complex due to the presence of multiple comorbidities, as in the case presented here. There can be multiple potential factors contributing to the shock, and utilization of hemodynamic monitoring devices, when coupled with patient history, physical assessment, standard labs, and diagnostic imaging, is essential to elucidating the shock etiology and guiding volume resuscitation. There is increasing evidence that volume overload may contribute to adverse outcomes, and utilizing the technologies described here, with the knowledge of potential device limitations, will help ensure fluids are delivered in a judicious manner.

References

1. Vincent JL, De Backer D. Circulatory shock. N Engl J Med. 2013;369(18):1726–34.
2. Weil MH, Henning RJ. New concepts in the diagnosis and fluid treatment of circulatory shock. Thirteenth annual Becton, Dickinson and company Oscar Schwidetsky memorial lecture. Anesth Analg. 1979;58(2):124–32.
3. Cecconi M, De Backer D, Antonelli M, Beale R, Bakker J, Hofer C, et al. Consensus on circulatory shock and hemodynamic monitoring. Task force of the European Society of Intensive Care Medicine. Intensive Care Med. 2014;40(12): 1795–815.
4. Rhodes A, Evans LE, Alhazzani W, Levy MM, Antonelli M, Ferrer R, et al. Surviving Sepsis campaign: international guidelines for Management of Sepsis and Septic Shock: 2016. Crit Care Med. 2017;45(3):486–552.
5. Cavallaro F, Sandroni C, Marano C, La Torre G, Mannocci A, De Waure C, et al. Diagnostic accuracy of passive leg raising for prediction of fluid responsiveness in adults: systematic review and meta-analysis of clinical studies. Intensive Care Med. 2010;36(9):1475–83.
6. Latham HE, Bengtson CD, Satterwhite L, Stites M, Subramaniam DP, Chen GJ, et al. Stroke volume guided resuscitation in severe sepsis and septic shock improves outcomes. J Crit Care. 2017;42:42–6.
7. Marik PE, Baram M, Vahid B. Does central venous pressure predict fluid responsiveness? A systematic review of the literature and the tale of seven mares. Chest. 2008;134(1):172–8.
8. Marik PE, Lemson J. Fluid responsiveness: an evolution of our understanding. Br J Anaesth. 2014;112(4):617–20.
9. Hamzaoui O, Monnet X, Teboul JL. Evolving concepts of hemodynamic monitoring for critically ill patients. Indian J Crit Care Med. 2015;19(4):220–6.
10. Monnet X, Julien F, Ait-Hamou N, Lequoy M, Gosset C, Jozwiak M, et al. Lactate and venoarterial carbon dioxide difference/arterial-venous oxygen difference ratio, but not central venous

oxygen saturation, predict increase in oxygen consumption in fluid responders. Crit Care Med. 2013;41(6):1412–20.

11. Marik PE, Monnet X, Teboul JL. Hemodynamic parameters to guide fluid therapy. Ann Intensive Care. 2011;1(1):1.
12. Woodcock TE, Woodcock TM. Revised Starling equation and the glycocalyx model of transvascular fluid exchange: an improved paradigm for prescribing intravenous fluid therapy. Br J Anaesth. 2012;108(3):384–94.
13. Acheampong A, Vincent JL. A positive fluid balance is an independent prognostic factor in patients with sepsis. Crit Care. 2015;19:251.
14. Marik PE, Linde-Zwirble WT, Bittner EA, Sahatjian J, Hansell D. Fluid administration in severe sepsis and septic shock, patterns and outcomes: an analysis of a large national database. Intensive Care Med. 2017;43(5):625–32.
15. Rosenberg AL, Dechert RE, Park PK, Bartlett RH, Network NNA. Review of a large clinical series: association of cumulative fluid balance on outcome in acute lung injury: a retrospective review of the ARDSnet tidal volume study cohort. J Intensive Care Med. 2009;24(1):35–46.
16. Sirvent JM, Ferri C, Baro A, Murcia C, Lorencio C. Fluid balance in sepsis and septic shock as a determining factor of mortality. Am J Emerg Med. 2015;33(2):186–9.
17. Michard F, Teboul JL. Using heart-lung interactions to assess fluid responsiveness during mechanical ventilation. Crit Care. 2000;4(5):282–9.
18. Boyd JH, Forbes J, Nakada TA, Walley KR, Russell JA. Fluid resuscitation in septic shock: a positive fluid balance and elevated central venous pressure are associated with increased mortality. Crit Care Med. 2011;39(2):259–65.
19. Fessler HE, Brower RG, Wise RA, Permutt S. Mechanism of reduced LV afterload by systolic and diastolic positive pleural pressure. J Appl Physiol. 1988;65(3):1244–50.
20. Marik PE, Cavallazzi R, Vasu T, Hirani A. Dynamic changes in arterial waveform derived variables and fluid responsiveness in mechanically ventilated patients: a systematic review of the literature. Crit Care Med. 2009;37(9):2642–7.
21. Michard F, Teboul JL. Predicting fluid responsiveness in ICU patients: a critical analysis of the evidence. Chest. 2002;121(6):2000–8.
22. De Backer D, Heenen S, Piagnerelli M, Koch M, Vincent JL. Pulse pressure variations to predict fluid responsiveness: influence of tidal volume. Intensive Care Med. 2005;31(4):517–23.

23. De Backer D, Taccone FS, Holsten R, Ibrahimi F, Vincent JL. Influence of respiratory rate on stroke volume variation in mechanically ventilated patients. Anesthesiology. 2009;110(5):1092–7.
24. Augusto JF, Teboul JL, Radermacher P, Asfar P. Interpretation of blood pressure signal: physiological bases, clinical relevance, and objectives during shock states. Intens Care Med. 2011;37(3):411–9.
25. Pierrakos C, Velissaris D, Scolletta S, Heenen S, De Backer D, Vincent JL. Can changes in arterial pressure be used to detect changes in cardiac index during fluid challenge in patients with septic shock? Intensive Care Med. 2012;38(3):422–8.
26. Hartog C, Bloos F. Venous oxygen saturation. Best Pract Res Clin Anaesthesiol. 2014;28(4):419–28.
27. Investigators A, Group ACT, Peake SL, Delaney A, Bailey M, Bellomo R, et al. Goal-directed resuscitation for patients with early septic shock. N Engl J Med. 2014;371(16):1496–506.
28. Mouncey PR, Osborn TM, Power GS, Harrison DA, Sadique MZ, Grieve RD, et al. Trial of early, goal-directed resuscitation for septic shock. N Engl J Med. 2015;372(14):1301–11.
29. Pro CI, Yealy DM, Kellum JA, Huang DT, Barnato AE, Weissfeld LA, et al. A randomized trial of protocol-based care for early septic shock. N Engl J Med. 2014;370(18):1683–93.
30. Lyu X, Xu Q, Cai G, Yan J, Yan M. Efficacies of fluid resuscitation as guided by lactate clearance rate and central venous oxygen saturation in patients with septic shock. Zhonghua Yi Xue Za Zhi. 2015;95(7):496–500.
31. Levy B. Lactate and shock state: the metabolic view. Curr Opin Crit Care. 2006;12(4):315–21.
32. Jansen TC, van Bommel J, Schoonderbeek FJ, Sleeswijk Visser SJ, van der Klooster JM, Lima AP, et al. Early lactate-guided therapy in intensive care unit patients: a multicenter, open-label, randomized controlled trial. Am J Respir Crit Care Med. 2010;182(6):752–61.
33. Jones AE, Shapiro NI, Trzeciak S, Arnold RC, Claremont HA, Kline JA, et al. Lactate clearance vs central venous oxygen saturation as goals of early sepsis therapy: a randomized clinical trial. JAMA. 2010;303(8):739–46.
34. Tian HH, Han SS, Lv CJ, Wang T, Li Z, Hao D, et al. The effect of early goal lactate clearance rate on the outcome of septic shock patients with severe pneumonia. Zhongguo wei zhong bing ji jiu

yi xue = Chinese critical care medicine = Zhongguo weizhongbing jijiuyixue. 2012;24(1):42–5.
35. Monge Garcia MI, Gil Cano A, Gracia Romero M, Monterroso Pintado R, Perez Madueno V, Diaz Monrove JC. Non-invasive assessment of fluid responsiveness by changes in partial end-tidal CO2 pressure during a passive leg-raising maneuver. Ann Intensive Care. 2012;2:9.
36. Monnet X, Bataille A, Magalhaes E, Barrois J, Le Corre M, Gosset C, et al. End-tidal carbon dioxide is better than arterial pressure for predicting volume responsiveness by the passive leg raising test. Intensive Care Med. 2013;39(1):93–100.
37. Magder S, Bafaqeeh F. The clinical role of central venous pressure measurements. J Intensive Care Med. 2007;22(1):44–51.
38. Hughes RE, Magovern GJ. The relationship between right atrial pressure and blood volume. AMA Arch Surg. 1959;79(2):238–43.
39. Latham HE, Rawson ST, Dwyer TT, Patel CC, Wick JA, Simpson SQ. Peripherally inserted central catheters are equivalent to centrally inserted catheters in intensive care unit patients for central venous pressure monitoring. J Clin Monit Comput. 2012;26(2):85–90.
40. Godje O, Peyerl M, Seebauer T, Lamm P, Mair H, Reichart B. Central venous pressure, pulmonary capillary wedge pressure and intrathoracic blood volumes as preload indicators in cardiac surgery patients. Eur J Cardiothorac Surg. 1998;13(5):533–9. discussion 9-40
41. Hoeft A, Schorn B, Weyland A, Scholz M, Buhre W, Stepanek E, et al. Bedside assessment of intravascular volume status in patients undergoing coronary bypass surgery. Anesthesiology. 1994;81(1):76–86.
42. Kumar A, Anel R, Bunnell E, Habet K, Zanotti S, Marshall S, et al. Pulmonary artery occlusion pressure and central venous pressure fail to predict ventricular filling volume, cardiac performance, or the response to volume infusion in normal subjects. Crit Care Med. 2004;32(3):691–9.
43. Oohashi S, Endoh H. Does central venous pressure or pulmonary capillary wedge pressure reflect the status of circulating blood volume in patients after extended transthoracic esophagectomy? J Anesth. 2005;19(1):21–5.
44. Wagner JG, Leatherman JW. Right ventricular end-diastolic volume as a predictor of the hemodynamic response to a fluid challenge. Chest. 1998;113(4):1048–54.

45. Heenen S, De Backer D, Vincent JL. How can the response to volume expansion in patients with spontaneous respiratory movements be predicted? Crit Care. 2006;10(4):R102.
46. Dellinger RP, Levy MM, Rhodes A, Annane D, Gerlach H, Opal SM, et al. Surviving sepsis campaign: international guidelines for management of severe sepsis and septic shock: 2012. Crit Care Med. 2013;41(2):580–637.
47. Eskesen TG, Wetterslev M, Perner A. Systematic review including re-analyses of 1148 individual data sets of central venous pressure as a predictor of fluid responsiveness. Intensive Care Med. 2016;42(3):324–32.
48. Osman D, Ridel C, Ray P, Monnet X, Anguel N, Richard C, et al. Cardiac filling pressures are not appropriate to predict hemodynamic response to volume challenge. Crit Care Med. 2007;35(1):64–8.
49. Feissel M, Michard F, Mangin I, Ruyer O, Faller JP, Teboul JL. Respiratory changes in aortic blood velocity as an indicator of fluid responsiveness in ventilated patients with septic shock. Chest. 2001;119(3):867–73.
50. Tavernier B, Makhotine O, Lebuffe G, Dupont J, Scherpereel P. Systolic pressure variation as a guide to fluid therapy in patients with sepsis-induced hypotension. Anesthesiology. 1998;89(6):1313–21.
51. Forrester JS, Ganz W, Diamond G, McHugh T, Chonette DW, Swan HJ. Thermodilution cardiac output determination with a single flow-directed catheter. Am Heart J. 1972;83(3):306–11.
52. Cohen MG, Kelly RV, Kong DF, Menon V, Shah M, Ferreira J, et al. Pulmonary artery catheterization in acute coronary syndromes: insights from the GUSTO IIb and GUSTO III trials. Am J Med. 2005;118(5):482–8.
53. Goldstein JA. Pathophysiology and management of right heart ischemia. J Am Coll Cardiol. 2002;40(5):841–53.
54. Zion MM, Balkin J, Rosenmann D, Goldbourt U, Reicher-Reiss H, Kaplinsky E, et al. Use of pulmonary artery catheters in patients with acute myocardial infarction. Analysis of experience in 5,841 patients in the SPRINT registry. SPRINT study group. Chest. 1990;98(6):1331–5.
55. Oh JK. Echocardiography as a noninvasive swan-Ganz catheter. Circulation. 2005;111(24):3192–4.
56. Thom O, Taylor DM, Wolfe RE, Cade J, Myles P, Krum H, et al. Comparison of a supra-sternal cardiac output monitor

(USCOM) with the pulmonary artery catheter. Br J Anaesth. 2009;103(6):800–4.
57. Wiener RS, Welch HG. Trends in the use of the pulmonary artery catheter in the United States, 1993-2004. JAMA. 2007;298(4):423–9.
58. Connors AF, Speroff T, Dawson NV, Thomas C, Harrell FE, Wagner D, et al. The effectiveness of right heart catheterization in the initial care of critically ill patients. J Am Med Assoc. 1996;276(11):889–97.
59. Rhodes A, Cusack RJ, Newman PJ, Grounds RM, Bennett ED. A randomised, controlled trial of the pulmonary artery catheter in critically ill patients. Intensive Care Med. 2002;28(3):256–64.
60. Richard C, Warszawski J, Anguel N, Deye N, Combes A, Barnoud D, et al. Early use of the pulmonary artery catheter and outcomes in patients with shock and acute respiratory distress syndrome - a randomized controlled trial. J Am Med Assoc. 2003;290(20):2713–20.
61. Wheeler AP, Bernard GR, Thompson BT, Schoenfeld D, Wiedemann HP, deBoisblanc B, et al. Pulmonary-artery versus central venous catheter to guide treatment of acute lung injury. New Engl J Med. 2006;354(21):2213–24.
62. Evans DC, Doraiswamy VA, Prosciak MP, Silviera M, Seamon MJ, Rodriguez Funes V, et al. Complications associated with pulmonary artery catheters: a comprehensive clinical review. Scand J Surg. 2009;98(4):199–208.
63. Manasia AR, Nagaraj HM, Kodali RB, Croft LB, Oropello JM, Kohli-Seth R, et al. Feasibility and potential clinical utility of goal-directed transthoracic echocardiography performed by noncardiologist intensivists using a small hand-carried device (SonoHeart) in critically ill patients. J Cardiothorac Vasc Anesth. 2005;19(2):155–9.
64. Mandavia DP, Hoffner RJ, Mahaney K, Henderson SO. Bedside echocardiography by emergency physicians. Ann Emerg Med. 2001;38(4):377–82.
65. Melamed R, Sprenkle MD, Ulstad VK, Herzog CA, Leatherman JW. Assessment of left ventricular function by intensivists using hand-held echocardiography. Chest. 2009;135(6):1416–20.
66. Pershad J, Myers S, Plouman C, Rosson C, Elam K, Wan J, et al. Bedside limited echocardiography by the emergency physician is accurate during evaluation of the critically ill patient. Pediatrics. 2004;114(6):e667–71.

67. Vignon P, Chastagner C, Francois B, Martaille JF, Normand S, Bonnivard M, et al. Diagnostic ability of hand-held echocardiography in ventilated critically ill patients. Crit Care. 2003;7(5):R84–91.
68. Vignon P, Dugard A, Abraham J, Belcour D, Gondran G, Pepino F, et al. Focused training for goal-oriented hand-held echocardiography performed by noncardiologist residents in the intensive care unit. Intensive Care Med. 2007;33(10):1795–9.
69. Vignon P, Mucke F, Bellec F, Marin B, Croce J, Brouqui T, et al. Basic critical care echocardiography: validation of a curriculum dedicated to noncardiologist residents. Crit Care Med. 2011;39(4):636–42.
70. Husain LF, Hagopian L, Wayman D, Baker WE, Carmody KA. Sonographic diagnosis of pneumothorax. J Emerg Trauma Shock. 2012;5(1):76–81.
71. Lichtenstein DA, Meziere GA. Relevance of lung ultrasound in the diagnosis of acute respiratory failure: the BLUE protocol. Chest. 2008;134(1):117–25.
72. Lichtenstein DA, Meziere GA, Lagoueyte JF, Biderman P, Goldstein I. Gepner a. A-lines and B-lines: lung ultrasound as a bedside tool for predicting pulmonary artery occlusion pressure in the critically ill. Chest. 2009;136(4):1014–20.
73. McLean AS. Echocardiography in shock management. Crit Care. 2016;20:275.
74. Ristic AD, Imazio M, Adler Y, Anastasakis A, Badano LP, Brucato A, et al. Triage strategy for urgent management of cardiac tamponade: a position statement of the European Society of Cardiology Working Group on myocardial and pericardial diseases. Eur Heart J. 2014;35(34):2279–84.
75. Soldati G, Testa A, Sher S, Pignataro G, La Sala M, Silveri NG. Occult traumatic pneumothorax: diagnostic accuracy of lung ultrasonography in the emergency department. Chest. 2008;133(1):204–11.
76. Kory PD, Pellecchia CM, Shiloh AL, Mayo PH, DiBello C, Koenig S. Accuracy of ultrasonography performed by critical care physicians for the diagnosis of DVT. Chest. 2011;139(3):538–42.
77. Lamia B, Ochagavia A, Monnet X, Chemla D, Richard C, Teboul JL. Echocardiographic prediction of volume responsiveness in critically ill patients with spontaneously breathing activity. Intensive Care Med. 2007;33(7):1125–32.
78. Monnet X, Rienzo M, Osman D, Anguel N, Richard C, Pinsky MR, et al. Esophageal Doppler monitoring predicts fluid

responsiveness in critically ill ventilated patients. Intensive Care Med. 2005;31(9):1195–201.
79. Monnet X, Rienzo M, Osman D, Anguel N, Richard C, Pinsky MR, et al. Passive leg raising predicts fluid responsiveness in the critically ill. Crit Care Med. 2006;34(5):1402–7.
80. Solus-Biguenet H, Fleyfel M, Tavernier B, Kipnis E, Onimus J, Robin E, et al. Non-invasive prediction of fluid responsiveness during major hepatic surgery. Br J Anaesth. 2006;97(6):808–16.
81. Brennan JM, Blair JE, Goonewardena S, Ronan A, Shah D, Vasaiwala S, et al. Reappraisal of the use of inferior vena cava for estimating right atrial pressure. J Am Soc Echocardiogr. 2007;20(7):857–61.
82. Feissel M, Michard F, Faller JP, Teboul JL. The respiratory variation in inferior vena cava diameter as a guide to fluid therapy. Intensive Care Med. 2004;30(9):1834–7.
83. Barbier C, Loubieres Y, Schmit C, Hayon J, Ricome JL, Jardin F, et al. Respiratory changes in inferior vena cava diameter are helpful in predicting fluid responsiveness in ventilated septic patients. Intensive Care Med. 2004;30(9):1740–6.
84. Hodgson LE, Forni LG, Venn R, Samuels TL, Wakeling HG. A comparison of the non-invasive ultrasonic cardiac output monitor (USCOM) with the oesophageal Doppler monitor during major abdominal surgery. J Intensive Care Soc. 2016;17(2):103–10.
85. Hodgson LE, Venn R, Forni LG, Samuels TL, Wakeling HG. Measuring the cardiac output in acute emergency admissions: use of the non-invasive ultrasonic cardiac output monitor (USCOM) with determination of the learning curve and inter-rater reliability. J Intensive Care Soc. 2016;17(2):122–8.
86. Mackenzie DC, Khan NA, Blehar D, Glazier S, Chang Y, Stowell CP, et al. Carotid flow time changes with volume status in acute blood loss. Ann Emerg Med. 2015;66(3):277–82 e1.
87. Maizel J, Airapetian N, Lorne E, Tribouilloy C, Massy Z, Slama M. Diagnosis of central hypovolemia by using passive leg raising. Intensive Care Med. 2007;33(7):1133–8.
88. Marik PE, Levitov A, Young A, Andrews L. The use of bioreactance and carotid Doppler to determine volume responsiveness and blood flow redistribution following passive leg raising in hemodynamically unstable patients. Chest. 2013;143(2):364–70.
89. Marquez J, McCurry K, Severyn DA, Pinsky MR. Ability of pulse power, esophageal Doppler, and arterial pulse pressure to estimate rapid changes in stroke volume in humans. Crit Care Med. 2008;36(11):3001–7.

90. Bataille B, Riu B, Ferre F, Moussot PE, Mari A, Brunel E, et al. Integrated use of bedside lung ultrasound and echocardiography in acute respiratory failure: a prospective observational study in ICU. Chest. 2014;146(6):1586–93.
91. Eichhorn V, Goepfert MS, Eulenburg C, Malbrain ML, Reuter DA. Comparison of values in critically ill patients for global end-diastolic volume and extravascular lung water measured by transcardiopulmonary thermodilution: a meta-analysis of the literature. Med Intensiva. 2012;36(7):467–74.
92. Jozwiak M, Teboul JL, Monnet X. Extravascular lung water in critical care: recent advances and clinical applications. Ann Intensive Care. 2015;5(1):38.
93. Wesseling KH, Jansen JR, Settels JJ, Schreuder JJ. Computation of aortic flow from pressure in humans using a nonlinear, three-element model. J Appl Physiol. 1993;74(5):2566–73.
94. Alhashemi JA, Cecconi M, Hofer CK. Cardiac output monitoring: an integrative perspective. Crit Care. 2011;15(2):214.
95. Marque S, Gros A, Chimot L, Gacouin A, Lavoue S, Camus C, et al. Cardiac output monitoring in septic shock: evaluation of the third-generation Flotrac-Vigileo. J Clin Monit Comput. 2013;27(3):273–9.
96. Monnet X, Anguel N, Jozwiak M, Richard C, Teboul JL. Third-generation FloTrac/Vigileo does not reliably track changes in cardiac output induced by norepinephrine in critically ill patients. Br J Anaesth. 2012;108(4):615–22.
97. Suehiro K, Tanaka K, Funao T, Matsuura T, Mori T, Nishikawa K. Systemic vascular resistance has an impact on the reliability of the Vigileo-FloTrac system in measuring cardiac output and tracking cardiac output changes. Br J Anaesth. 2013;111(2):170–7.
98. Linton RA, Band DM, Haire KM. A new method of measuring cardiac output in man using lithium dilution. Br J Anaesth. 1993;71(2):262–6.
99. Bein B, Meybohm P, Cavus E, Renner J, Tonner PH, Steinfath M, et al. The reliability of pulse contour-derived cardiac output during hemorrhage and after vasopressor administration. Anesth Analg. 2007;105(1):107–13.
100. Goedje O, Hoeke K, Lichtwarck-Aschoff M, Faltchauser A, Lamm P, Reichart B. Continuous cardiac output by femoral arterial thermodilution calibrated pulse contour analysis: comparison with pulmonary arterial thermodilution. Crit Care Med. 1999;27(11):2407–12.

101. Benes J, Chytra I, Altmann P, Hluchy M, Kasal E, Svitak R, et al. Intraoperative fluid optimization using stroke volume variation in high risk surgical patients: results of prospective randomized study. Crit Care. 2010;14(3):R118.
102. Cecconi M, Rhodes A. Validation of continuous cardiac output technologies: consensus still awaited. Crit Care. 2009;13(3):159.
103. Gruenewald M, Renner J, Meybohm P, Hocker J, Scholz J, Bein B. Reliability of continuous cardiac output measurement during intra-abdominal hypertension relies on repeated calibrations: an experimental animal study. Crit Care. 2008;12(5):R132.
104. Mowat I, Todman E, Jaggar S. Validation of the LiDCO pulse contour system in patients with impaired left ventricular function. Anaesthesia. 2012;67(2):188; author reply –9
105. Nordstrom J, Hallsjo-Sander C, Shore R, Bjorne H. Stroke volume optimization in elective bowel surgery: a comparison between pulse power wave analysis (LiDCOrapid) and oesophageal Doppler (CardioQ). Br J Anaesth. 2013;110(3):374–80.
106. Renner J, Scholz J, Bein B. Monitoring fluid therapy. Best Pract Res Clin Anaesthesiol. 2009;23(2):159–71.
107. Keren H, Burkhoff D, Squara P. Evaluation of a noninvasive continuous cardiac output monitoring system based on thoracic bioreactance. Am J Physiol Heart Circ Physiol. 2007;293(1):H583–9.
108. Dunham CM, Chirichella TJ, Gruber BS, Ferrari JP, Martin JA, Luchs BA, et al. Emergency department noninvasive (NICOM) cardiac outputs are associated with trauma activation, patient injury severity and host conditions and mortality. J Trauma Acute Care Surg. 2012;73(2):479–85.
109. Garcia X, Simon P, Guyette FX, Ramani R, Alvarez R, Quintero J, et al. Noninvasive assessment of acute dyspnea in the ED. Chest. 2013;144(2):610–5.
110. Kossari N, Hufnagel G, Squara P. Bioreactance: a new tool for cardiac output and thoracic fluid content monitoring during hemodialysis. Hemodial Int. 2009;13(4):512–7.
111. Maurer MM, Burkhoff D, Maybaum S, Franco V, Vittorio TJ, Williams P, et al. A multicenter study of noninvasive cardiac output by bioreactance during symptom-limited exercise. J Card Fail. 2009;15(8):689–99.
112. Waldron NH, Miller TE, Thacker JK, Manchester AK, White WD, Nardiello J, et al. A prospective comparison of a noninvasive cardiac output monitor versus esophageal Doppler monitor

for goal-directed fluid therapy in colorectal surgery patients. Anesth Analg. 2014;118(5):966–75.
113. Cannesson M, Delannoy B, Morand A, Rosamel P, Attof Y, Bastien O, et al. Does the Pleth variability index indicate the respiratory-induced variation in the plethysmogram and arterial pressure waveforms? Anesth Analg. 2008;106(4):1189–94, table of contents
114. Feissel M, Kalakhy R, Banwarth P, Badie J, Pavon A, Faller JP, et al. Plethysmographic variation index predicts fluid responsiveness in ventilated patients in the early phase of septic shock in the emergency department: a pilot study. J Crit Care. 2013;28(5):634–9.
115. Keller G, Cassar E, Desebbe O, Lehot JJ, Cannesson M. Ability of pleth variability index to detect hemodynamic changes induced by passive leg raising in spontaneously breathing volunteers. Crit Care. 2008;12(2):R37.
116. Sandroni C, Cavallaro F, Marano C, Falcone C, De Santis P, Antonelli M. Accuracy of plethysmographic indices as predictors of fluid responsiveness in mechanically ventilated adults: a systematic review and meta-analysis. Intensive Care Med. 2012;38(9):1429–37.
117. Biais M, Cottenceau V, Petit L, Masson F, Cochard JF, Sztark F. Impact of norepinephrine on the relationship between pleth variability index and pulse pressure variations in ICU adult patients. Crit Care. 2011;15(4):R168.
118. Broch O, Bein B, Gruenewald M, Hocker J, Schottler J, Meybohm P, et al. Accuracy of the pleth variability index to predict fluid responsiveness depends on the perfusion index. Acta Anaesthesiol Scand. 2011;55(6):686–93.
119. Bataille B, Bertuit M, Mora M, Mazerolles M, Cocquet P, Masson B, et al. Comparison of esCCO and transthoracic echocardiography for non-invasive measurement of cardiac output intensive care. Br J Anaesth. 2012;109(6):879–86.
120. Biais M, Berthezene R, Petit L, Cottenceau V, Sztark F. Ability of esCCO to track changes in cardiac output. Br J Anaesth. 2015;115(3):403–10.
121. Feissel M, Aho LS, Georgiev S, Tapponnier R, Badie J, Bruyere R, et al. Pulse wave transit time measurements of cardiac output in septic shock patients: a comparison of the estimated continuous cardiac output system with transthoracic echocardiography. PLoS One. 2015;10(6):e0130489.

122. Permpikul C, Leelayuthachai T. Non-invasive estimated continuous cardiac output (escCO) during severe sepsis and septic shock resuscitation. J Med Assoc Thail. 2014;97(Suppl 3):S184–8.
123. Smetkin AA, Hussain A, Fot EV, Zakharov VI, Izotova NN, Yudina AS, et al. Estimated continuous cardiac output based on pulse wave transit time in off-pump coronary artery bypass grafting: a comparison with transpulmonary thermodilution. J Clin Monit Comput. 2017;31(2):361–70.
124. Terada T, Oiwa A, Maemura Y, Robert S, Kessoku S, Ochiai R. Comparison of the ability of two continuous cardiac output monitors to measure trends in cardiac output: estimated continuous cardiac output measured by modified pulse wave transit time and an arterial pulse contour-based cardiac output device. J Clin Monit Comput. 2016;30(5):621–7.
125. Ameloot K, Palmers PJ, Malbrain ML. The accuracy of noninvasive cardiac output and pressure measurements with finger cuff: a concise review. Curr Opin Crit Care. 2015;21(3):232–9.
126. Fischer MO, Coucoravas J, Truong J, Zhu L, Gerard JL, Hanouz JL, et al. Assessment of changes in cardiac index and fluid responsiveness: a comparison of Nexfin and transpulmonary thermodilution. Acta Anaesthesiol Scand. 2013;57(6):704–12.
127. Lansdorp B, Ouweneel D, de Keijzer A, van der Hoeven JG, Lemson J, Pickkers P. Non-invasive measurement of pulse pressure variation and systolic pressure variation using a finger cuff corresponds with intra-arterial measurement. Br J Anaesth. 2011;107(4):540–5.

Chapter 16
Bleeding and Thrombosis in the ICU

Donald S. Houston and Ryan Zarychanski

Part A: Case Presentation

A 34-year-old woman with ulcerative colitis has been receiving treatment with infliximab for 2 years. Her bowel symptoms have been under reasonable control, but a year ago she developed evidence of advanced sclerosing cholangitis. She presents now with cough, rigors, and pleuritic chest pain, and a chest X-ray shows right lower lobe pneumonia. She is admitted to the ICU with hypotension. She remains hypotensive after 2 liters of Ringer's lactate and is started on a

D. S. Houston
Department of Internal Medicine, Section of Medical Oncology and Haematology, University of Manitoba, Winnipeg, MB, Canada

R. Zarychanski (✉)
Department of Internal Medicine, Section of Medical Oncology and Haematology, University of Manitoba, Winnipeg, MB, Canada

Department of Internal Medicine, Section of Critical Care, University of Manitoba, Winnipeg, MB, Canada
e-mail: rzarychanski@cancercare.mb.ca

J. A. LaRosa (ed.), *Adult Critical Care Medicine*,
https://doi.org/10.1007/978-3-319-94424-1_16

norepinephrine infusion. Shortly after the ICU admission, she vomits a basin full of bright red blood.

On exam she has findings of consolidation in the right lung base, her extremities are warm, she is jaundiced, and she has tense ascites and spider nevi. Lactate is 4.3 mmol/L; venous oxygen saturation is 73%.

Her complete blood count shows white blood cells 2.2×10^9/L, hemoglobin 81 g/L, mean corpuscular volume (MCV) 99 fL, platelets 106×10^9/L, international normalized ratio (INR) 2.2, activated partial thromboplastic time (aPTT) 44 s, and fibrinogen 0.9 g/L.

Differential Diagnosis and Assessment

This is a complex patient with multiple factors that may be contributing to her abnormal blood counts and coagulopathy. She has a pertinent background of liver disease, a background of immunosuppression and presents with both sepsis and bleeding. We would consider the differential diagnosis of each of her major issues.

Shock: She appears to have vasopressor-dependent shock. Hypovolemic shock due to her gastrointestinal bleed should be excluded; however, following fluid resuscitation, should her blood pressure remain low, septic shock becomes a strong consideration. She has no cardiac history, is young and well perfused, and has a normal venous oxygen saturation; cardiac or obstructive shock are unlikely. Management of septic shock is beyond the scope of this review.

Prolonged INR: She has multiple possible causes for coagulopathy (see Box 16.1):

- Vitamin K deficiency due to malabsorption related to her biliary tract disease, possibly exacerbated by antibiotics or poor diet if she has been avoiding green vegetables because of her colitis
- Hemodilution
- Synthetic failure due to liver disease
- Disseminated intravascular coagulopathy (DIC) due to sepsis

Box 16.1. Differential Diagnosis of Coagulopathy in Critical Care

- DIC
- Liver failure
- Hemodilution (during massive transfusion)
- Vitamin K deficiency
- Anticoagulants
- Artifactual: heparin contamination of sample, lupus anticoagulant, etc.

Her fibrinogen is low, which shows that the coagulopathy is not solely due to vitamin K deficiency, and moreover it is lower than could readily be entirely explained by hemodilution at this point. The fibrinogen level does not distinguish between the other possibilities, liver failure and DIC. The INR greater than 2.0 with a fibrinogen of 0.9 g/L suggests that multiple coagulation factor deficiencies exist, which can only be corrected with plasma.

With sepsis as a predisposing factor, the findings of thrombocytopenia, a prolonged prothrombin time, and a reduced fibrinogen suggest DIC [1]. A factor VIII level can be useful to distinguish liver disease from DIC, as the FVIII will be elevated in the former and consumed in the latter. Note that the FVIII level is raised in both inflammatory liver disease and in infection, so in this patient even a value in the lower normal range will indicate consumption.

Thrombocytopenia: Multiple factors may contribute to thrombocytopenia in this case:

- Sequestration due to portal hypertension and congestive splenomegaly, consequent to her liver disease
- Deficiency of thrombopoietin due to liver synthetic failure
- Hemodilution
- Sepsis
- DIC

While there are many other potential causes of thrombocytopenia (e.g., immune thrombocytopenia, drug-immune reactions, thrombotic thrombocytopenic purpura (TTP) (see Box 16.2)), Occam's razor suggests they are unlikely to be factors here. If the platelet count deviates strikingly from the clinical trajectory, however, one must be prepared to reconsider a broader differential diagnosis [2].

Box 16.2: Differential Diagnosis of Thrombocytopenia in Critical Care

Common causes

- Sepsis
- Disseminated intravascular coagulation
- Consumption (in major trauma)
- Dilution (with massive transfusion)
- Myelosuppressive chemotherapy
- Mechanical circulatory support devices (e.g., intra-aortic balloon pump, extracorporeal membrane oxygenation)

Less common but important causes of thrombocytopenia that should not be missed:

- Heparin-induced thrombocytopenia
- Hemophagocytic syndrome

Uncommon causes of thrombocytopenia that develop during ICU admission:

- Drug-induced thrombocytopenia (other than heparin or cytotoxic chemotherapy)
- Leukemia, myelodysplasia, aplastic anemia, etc. (unless abnormalities were already present before ICU admission)
- Thrombotic thrombocytopenic purpura
- Immune/idiopathic thrombocytopenia
- Posttransfusion purpura

To the extent that the thrombocytopenia is due to hypersplenism, little can be done; recovery of transfused platelets will be poor because they too will be sequestered (Fig. 16.1).

Thrombocytopenia is highly prevalent in septic shock. Multiple pathophysiological processes may contribute (see Fig. 16.2) [2]. Consideration of these mechanisms suggests hypotheses about treatments that would plausibly be beneficial, but to date no specific treatments are known to improve the thrombocytopenia of sepsis. A recent analysis of the time course of thrombocytopenia in sepsis has illustrated that we cannot expect the platelet count to recover while the patient remains on vasopressors, and indeed the platelet count does not typically start to recover for approximately 2 days after vasopressor infusions stop (see Fig. 16.3) [3].

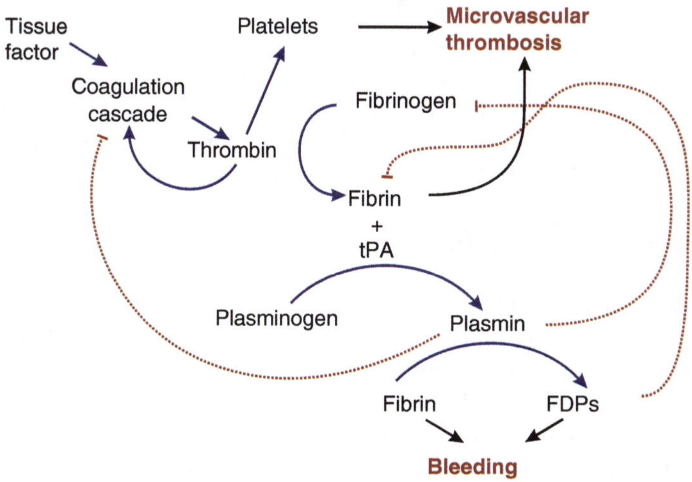

FIGURE 16.1 Pathophysiology of disseminated intravascular coagulation: DIC is a clinical/pathological syndrome of uncontrolled and delocalized thrombin generation followed by uncontrolled plasmin activation, leading both to microvascular (and sometimes macrovascular) thrombosis and to diffuse bleeding

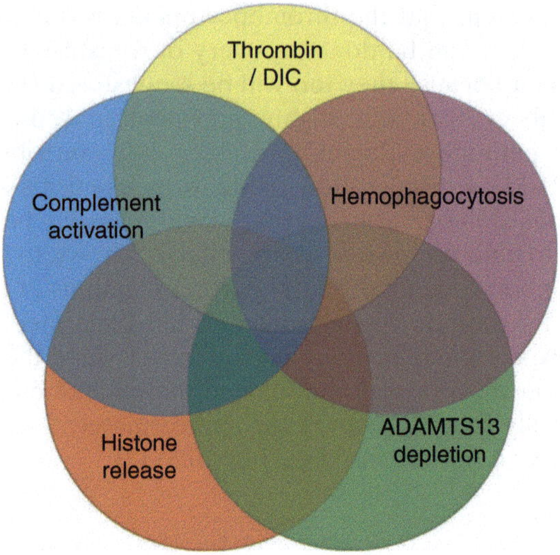

Figure 16.2 Mechanisms of thrombocytopenia in sepsis. Multiple mechanisms have been proposed to contribute to the thrombocytopenia of sepsis. The relative contribution of each potential mechanism may vary among patients and within a given patient over time. DIC, disseminated intravascular coagulation

Management of Bleeding

She is actively bleeding, so the coagulopathy must be corrected. Initial management will be similar regardless of the results of these investigations. Because there may be a component of vitamin K deficiency, empiric replacement with 10 mg of intravenous vitamin K is appropriate, but this should not delay plasma replacement. One liter of plasma should raise her fibrinogen by approximately 1 g/L, will replenish all other coagulation factors, and is expected to decrease her INR, though it will not correct fully. Further replacement should be guided by laboratory testing. Prompt turnaround of conventional hematologic and coagulation tests (platelets, INR, aPTT, fibrinogen) can adequately inform blood product administration. Point-of-care tests (e.g., thromboelastography

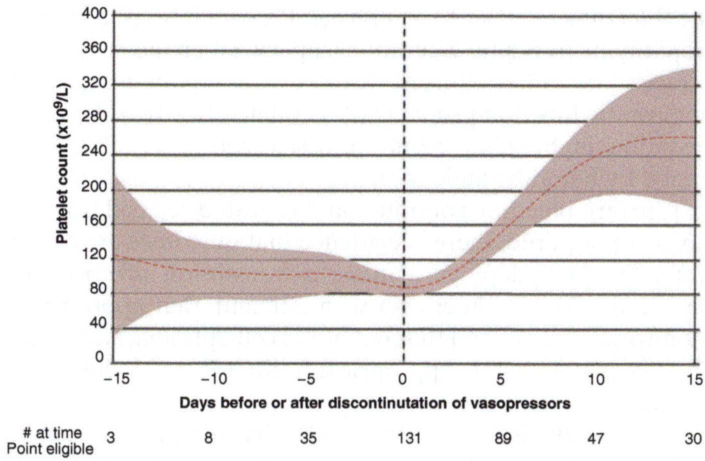

FIGURE 16.3 Time course of thrombocytopenia in septic shock. Mean platelet count (and 95% confidence interval) in patients with septic shock who developed thrombocytopenia after ICU admission. Time axis is anchored to the day that vasopressors were discontinued (day 0). Only data for survivors are included

(TEG) or rotation thromboelastometry (ROTEM)) can also be used to guide blood product transfusion, but have mostly been studied in operative settings or in the management of trauma [4], and have not been conclusively demonstrated to improve clinical outcomes in patients admitted to an ICU. If she has DIC, she will require ongoing replacement until the underlying driver of the DIC (in this case, sepsis) is corrected. A diagnosis of DIC increases her risk of mortality approximately twofold [5]. If the coagulopathy is due to liver failure, the correction achieved with plasma replacement will be transitory. Repeated dosing may be needed, until bleeding is controlled.

While coagulopathy and thrombocytopenia should be corrected (to the extent possible) in a bleeding patient, this should not distract from the need to identify the site of bleeding and achieve local hemostatic control. In this woman, urgent upper endoscopy is required to distinguish whether the bleeding is due to esophageal varices or portal gastropathy or to peptic ulceration, superficial erosions, telangiectasias, or other causes. It is worth commenting that hemostatic function probably plays relatively little role in the cessation of bleeding from varices, which is largely determined by hemodynamic forces.

If severe bleeding continues and repeated red cell transfusions are required, there is evidence that outcomes are better if the hospital deploys a massive transfusion protocol, to ensure that supply keeps up with demand, that appropriate monitoring occurs, and that red blood cells, plasma, and platelets are given in an appropriate ratio to avoid dilutional coagulopathy and thrombocytopenia [6].

Factor VIIa is not recommended. Other than in hemophilia, when studied in randomized trials, it has failed to improve outcomes in coagulopathic bleeding and increases the risk of thrombosis [7]. Prothrombin complex concentrates do not contain all the missing factors (especially Factor V) and, except in the context of warfarin reversal, should not be used. Fibrinogen concentrates may have a role, especially if the patient has volume overload, but we prefer plasma as it is the only product containing all the factors.

Use of tranexamic acid is controversial. The fundamental pathophysiology of DIC is overwhelming activation of coagulation, usually due to delocalized expression tissue factor, and exhaustion of regulatory mechanisms, including tissue factor pathway inhibitor, protein C, and antithrombin (see Fig. 16.1). This leads to widespread thrombin generation and fibrin deposition throughout the microvasculature. Delocalized and excessive plasminogen activation is driven by the excess of fibrin, which then results in fibrinolysis, consumption of clotting factors, and bleeding [1]. Tranexamic acid effectively inhibits plasmin generation and fibrinolysis, and should be effective in reducing bleeding, but since thrombin generation is then unopposed, it risks converting the DIC to a thrombotic phenotype.

In critically ill patients with thrombocytopenia, when platelets should be given is also a matter of clinical judgment, informed by a paucity of high-quality trial data. Although considerable practice variability exists, by extrapolation from practice in the care of hematological malignancies, prophylactic transfusion when the platelet count falls below $10 \times 10^9/L$ is recommended [8, 9]. This extrapolation, however, may not be valid; in patients admitted to medical-surgical ICUs, thrombocytopenia is frequently multifactorial, and may be accompanied by acquired platelet dysfunction, but also increased platelet turnover. For bleeding patients with severe thrombocytopenia, there is consensus that platelet transfusion should be given but little consensus of what the target platelet count should be. Most authorities' suggestions fall in a range between 50 and $100 \times 10^9/L$, depending on the severity or location of bleeding. In practice it is often hard to maintain levels that high with transfusion in such patients. We have provided some suggested target platelet counts previously [2].

For our patient, plasma transfusion certainly takes priority over platelet transfusion unless her platelets fall much more.

Part B: Case Presentation, Continued

The patient described in Part A is treated with broad-spectrum antibiotics to cover respiratory pathogens; the regimen is subsequently tailored when blood and sputum cultures grow *Streptococcus pneumoniae*. Mechanical ventilation is provided because of hypoxia and metabolic acidosis. The patient's coagulopathy improves with plasma. Upper GI endoscopy reveals a bleeding varix that is successfully clipped. She has no further bleeding. Vasopressors are weaned off after 4 days and the patient is extubated on day 5.

On day 6 she develops worsening hypoxemia and tachycardia. A portable chest X-ray shows improvement of her pneumonia. A CT pulmonary angiogram demonstrates bilateral segmental pulmonary emboli.

The patient's hemoglobin is stable at 78 g/L. Platelets are 60 × 10^9/L. They had fallen progressively over the first 4 days after admission but have been stable for the past 2 days. INR is 1.3, and the aPTT is 32 s.

Differential Diagnosis and Assessment

Although the patient is improving, she has a new, life-threatening, thrombotic event. Despite thromboprophylaxis, venous thromboembolism (VTE) has been shown to occur in approximately 6% of patients admitted to general medical-surgical ICUs [10]. Risk factors associated with thrombosis in critically ill patients include [11, 12]:

- Inflammation.
- Immobility.
- Use of vasopressors.
- Presence of central venous catheters.
- Increased body mass index.
- Platelet transfusion.
- Heparin-induced thrombocytopenia (HIT) is not common, occurring in approximately 0.3–0.6% of general medical-surgical ICU patients [10]. The onset of the fall in platelet count due to HIT is characteristically 5–12 days after exposure to heparin and can be associated with venous and sometimes arterial thrombosis due to platelet activation [13].

In this case presented, additional prothrombotic considerations may be present:

- Inflammatory bowel disease has been shown to be an independent risk for thrombosis in epidemiological studies.
- While reduced synthesis of coagulation factor is expected with hepatic dysfunction, the production of endogenous anticoagulant proteins is also reduced. Therefore, patients cannot be assumed to be protected from thrombosis despite elevation in the INR.

Other risk factors for thrombosis in critically ill patients could include [11]:

- Antiphospholipid antibody syndrome
- A personal or family history of venous thromboembolism
- End-stage renal disease
- Mechanical circulatory support
- Microangiopathic hemolytic anemia (e.g., thrombotic thrombocytopenia purpura, DIC)
- Malignancy
- Trauma and major surgery

Our patient has several risk factors for thrombosis, but inflammation, immobility, the presence of a central venous catheter, and recent use of vasopressors are likely the major contributors. Hemorrhage itself adds further risk. The DIC appears to have resolved with treatment of her sepsis. The contribution of inflammatory bowel disease or hepatic dysfunction to her thrombotic propensity is possible. Given the early onset of the fall in platelet count, a fall of less than 50% from baseline, and the presence of an alternate cause of thrombocytopenia (i.e., sepsis), HIT is not suspected [14]. As we've shown above, in sepsis, recovery from thrombocytopenia typically lags behind clinical recovery. Using a 4 T score would help confirm the low pretest risk probability of HIT in this patient.

Management of Thrombosis

A new diagnosis of segmental or main pulmonary artery embolus, or proximal deep venous thrombosis, requires urgent therapeutic anticoagulation. For this patient, we favor the use of intravenous unfractionated heparin, for several reasons:

- It has a short half-life, so it can be interrupted briefly if needed for procedures.
- An antidote (protamine) is available if she has bleeding, for which she remains at elevated risk.
- Its clearance is not altered by renal dysfunction.

The conventional dosing for unfractionated heparin is an 80 units/kg bolus followed by an infusion at 18 units/kg/h to achieve an aPTT of 1.5–2.5× that of the normal baseline. For this patient, we would adhere to this dosing, but given the presence of thrombocytopenia, we would empirically consider reducing the bolus dose by 25%. Prior to the use of therapeutic unfractionated heparin, a baseline aPTT should be obtained. If the baseline aPTT is prolonged, monitoring using anti-Xa levels should be considered. Low molecular weight can also be considered in a stable patient without renal dysfunction and risk factors for hemorrhage and who is not on vasopressor agents; absorption from subcutaneous injections may be impaired during shock [15]. Direct oral anticoagulants (DOACs) are not recommended due to variable gut absorption of oral medications in critical illness and the potential for renal dysfunction.

The presence of thrombocytopenia can complicate the use of therapeutic anticoagulants. While we acknowledge that good studies are lacking, it is commonly accepted that a platelet count of 50×10^9/L or greater permits the use of full-dose anticoagulation. Inferior vena cava (IVC) filters should only be used if full-dose anticoagulation is prohibitively risky; in this case, we would insert a filter only if the heparin infusion had to be stopped, either for bleeding or for a surgical intervention [16]. The patient with a platelet count between 30 and 50×10^9/L who requires therapeutic anticoagulation provides a challenge to the treating intensivist. In that setting, a retrievable IVC filter plus a reduced dose of unfractionated heparin, targeting an aPTT of 45–60 s, could be considered. Prophylactic dose unfractionated heparin plus a retrievable IVC filter may need to be considered for patients with a platelet count less than 30×10^9/L.

Systemic thrombolysis for the treatment of pulmonary embolus is considered only for patients with hypotension due to pulmonary vascular obstruction. In patients with submassive pulmonary embolism, systematic thrombolysis results in earlier hemodynamic improvement but causes increased major bleeding with uncertain difference in mortality [17]. We would be further dissuaded from thrombolysis in this patient because of her recent major hemorrhage.

Outcome

The patient clinically improved on unfractionated heparin. After 5 days of treatment, she was on 2 liters of oxygen via nasal prongs with an oxygen saturation of 98%. Due to concerns regarding oral absorption, on the medical ward, the patient transitioned first to therapeutic LMWH for 4 additional days. Prior to discharge, she was prescribed a direct oral anticoagulant to complete a 3-month course of therapeutic anticoagulation, as is appropriate for a provoked pulmonary embolus.

Key Points

- Multiple causes of both bleeding and thrombosis may coexist in a critically ill patient. Arriving at the causes(s) of each requires the integration of a patient's past history, present illness, and the results of laboratory testing.
- Management of DIC is to treat the underlying disease and to manage either bleeding or thrombosis if present.
- Multiple mechanisms for thrombocytopenia in the ICU can be present. Although drugs are often suspected, they are rarely the cause.
- In septic shock, platelet recovery lags behind clinical recovery.
- Plasma is the product of choice for bleeding in the setting of DIC or liver failure.
- In the setting of acute venous thromboembolism, effective anticoagulation is the priority. An IVC filter should only be used if anticoagulation is contraindicated.

References

1. Thachil J. Disseminated intravascular coagulation: a practical approach. Anesthesiology. 2016;125(1):230–6.
2. Zarychanski R, Houston DS. Assessing thrombocytopenia in the intensive care unit: the past, present, and future. Hematology Am Soc Hematol Educ Program. 2017;2017(1):660–6.
3. Menard CE, Kumar A, Rimmer E, Doucette S. A.F. T, Houston BL, et al. evolution & impact of thrombocytopenia in septic shock. Intens Care Med Exp. 2016;4(Suppl 1):A586.
4. Wikkelso A, Wetterslev J, Moller AM, Afshari A. Thromboelastography (TEG) or thromboelastometry (ROTEM) to monitor haemostatic treatment versus usual care in adults or children with bleeding. Cochrane Database Syst Rev. 2016;8:CD007871.
5. Takemitsu T, Wada H, Hatada T, Ohmori Y, Ishikura K, Takeda T, et al. Prospective evaluation of three different diagnostic criteria for disseminated intravascular coagulation. Thromb Haemost. 2011;105(1):40–4.
6. McDaniel LM, Etchill EW, Raval JS, Neal MD. State of the art: massive transfusion. Transfus Med. 2014;24(3):138–44.
7. Simpson E, Lin Y, Stanworth S, Birchall J, Doree C, Hyde C. Recombinant factor VIIa for the prevention and treatment of bleeding in patients without haemophilia. Cochrane Database Syst Rev. 2012;3:CD005011.
8. Kaufman RM, Djulbegovic B, Gernsheimer T, Kleinman S, Tinmouth AT, Capocelli KE, et al. Platelet transfusion: a clinical practice guideline from the AABB. Ann Intern Med. 2015;162(3):205–13.
9. Rhodes A, Evans LE, Alhazzani W, Levy MM, Antonelli M, Ferrer R, et al. Surviving Sepsis campaign: international guidelines for Management of Sepsis and Septic Shock: 2016. Crit Care Med. 2017;45(3):486–552.
10. Cook D, Meade M, Guyatt G, Walter S, Heels-Ansdell D, Warkentin TE, et al. Dalteparin versus unfractionated heparin in critically ill patients. N Engl J Med. 2011;364(14):1305–14.
11. Cook DJ, Crowther MA, Meade MO, Douketis J, VTEitIW P. Prevalence, incidence, and risk factors for venous thromboembolism in medical-surgical intensive care unit patients. J Crit Care. 2005;20(4):309–13.
12. Lim W, Meade M, Lauzier F, Zarychanski R, Mehta S, Lamontagne F, et al. Failure of anticoagulant thromboprophy-

laxis: risk factors in medical-surgical critically ill patients*. Crit Care Med. 2015;43(2):401–10.
13. Warkentin TE. Heparin-induced thrombocytopenia in critically ill patients. Semin Thromb Hemost. 2015;41(1):49–60.
14. Lo GK, Juhl D, Warkentin TE, Sigouin CS, Eichler P, Greinacher A. Evaluation of pretest clinical score (4 T's) for the diagnosis of heparin-induced thrombocytopenia in two clinical settings. J Thromb Haemost. 2006;4(4):759–65.
15. De Paepe P, Belpaire FM, Buylaert WA. Pharmacokinetic and pharmacodynamic considerations when treating patients with sepsis and septic shock. Clin Pharmacokinet. 2002;41(14):1135–51.
16. Duffett L, Carrier M. Inferior vena cava filters. J Thromb Haemost. 2017;15(1):3–12.
17. Marshall PS, Mathews KS, Siegel MD. Diagnosis and management of life-threatening pulmonary embolism. J Intensive Care Med. 2011;26(5):275–94.

Chapter 17
Diagnosis and Management of Pulmonary Embolism in Pregnancy

Lars-Kristofer N. Peterson

Case Presentation

History of Present Illness (HPI)

A 31-year-old nulliparous female at 41-week gestational age (WGA) with a past medical history of asthma and prior appendectomy presented to obstetric triage for fetal heart rate monitoring. There have been no complications during the course of the pregnancy, and the patient has received all recommended prenatal care. The fetal heart rate monitoring showed the fetus to be in good condition with appropriate heart rate variability and normal motion on ultrasound. Near the conclusion of the monitoring, the patient experiences tachycardia, tachypnea, and complains of dyspnea as well as severe chest pain radiating to her back.

L.-K. N. Peterson
Departments of Medicine and Emergency Medicine, Division of Critical Care Medicine, Cooper University Hospital, Cooper Medical School of Rowan University, Camden, NJ, USA
e-mail: peterson-lars@cooperhealth.edu

J. A. LaRosa (ed.), *Adult Critical Care Medicine*,
https://doi.org/10.1007/978-3-319-94424-1_17

On further history, the patient has noted increasing fatigue but denies breathlessness on exertion or at rest. She denies fever, chills, nausea, vomiting, cough, headache, change in vision, or abdominal pain. She denies leaking of amniotic fluid. The critical care service was consulted to assistance in further diagnosis and management.

Past Medical and Surgical History

Childhood asthma without recurrence in adulthood
Status post appendectomy (12 years old)

Family and Social History

The patient is the only child of two living parents who are healthy, without medical comorbidities. She has never smoked or used illicit drugs and is currently abstinent from alcohol during pregnancy. She has continued to work during pregnancy as an air traffic control manager. She lives with her husband and 3-year-old daughter who are both described as healthy with no recent symptoms. There is a dog in the home which is fully vaccinated.

Physical Examination

Vital Signs Heart Rate (HR), 135; Respiratory Rate (RR), 24; Oxygen Saturation, 96% on room air; Blood Pressure, 110/50; Temperature, 98.6.

General The patient is supine, alert, oriented, with mildly labored breathing.

Head, eyes, ears, nose, throat: Normal oral mucosa, anicteric sclera, no rhinorrhea, tympanic membranes are clear.

Neck Supple, non-tender.

Chest Elevated respiratory rate at 24, no accessory muscle use. The patient is able to speak in full sentences.

Cardiovascular Heart rate 135, regular, no murmur. Radial and dorsalis pedis pulses intact bilaterally.

Abdomen Gravid, non-tender abdomen, fundal height appropriate.

Extremities Bilateral lower extremity pitting edema to mid shin. Hands and feet warm and well perfused.

Neurologic The patient is alert, fully oriented. She has no facial droop, a conjugate gaze, and symmetric pupils. Her gait is normal.

Ancillary Studies

Portable chest X-ray: The trachea is midline, no infiltrates noted, no pneumothorax, normal mediastinal morphology, normal diaphragm, no bony changes. Radiology interpretation is no acute changes.

Differential Diagnosis

The differential diagnosis of a pregnant patient presenting with dyspnea, tachycardia, hypertension, and fatigue with normal chest radiography is challenging. Due to the changes observed in the normal physiology of pregnancy, the findings in this patient may be expected. Or, more worrisome, they may mask underlying serious pathology. Please review Fig. 17.1 to review some of the normal changes in physiology of pregnancy and compare them with the expected changes a clinician might find when diagnosing respiratory or cardiac pathology. As you can see, there is significant overlap in the symptoms and signs observed in normal pregnancy and cardiopulmonary pathology.

Based on the patient's history of presenting illness, medical and surgical history, physical examination, and review of the obtained studies, the leading differential diagnoses include dyspnea of normal pregnancy, asthma, respiratory

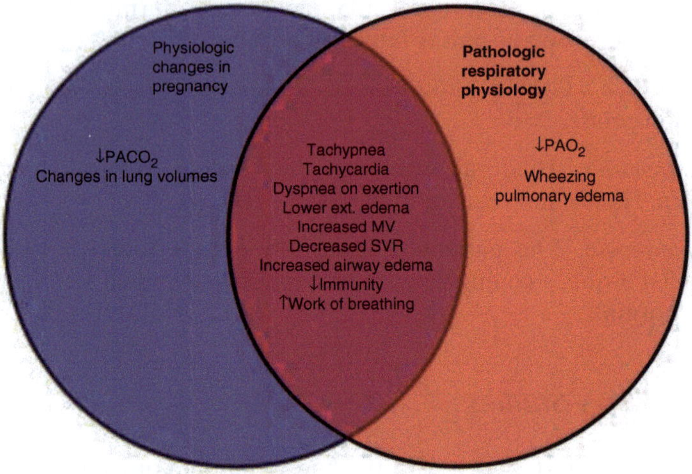

FIGURE 17.1 Overlap in signs and symptoms of respiratory changes in pregnancy and pathologic respiratory states [1–3]. $PaCO_2$ Partial pressure of arterial carbon dioxide, PaO_2 partial pressure of arterial oxygen, MV minute ventilation, SVR systemic vascular resistance

infections, pre-eclampsia, acute coronary and vascular syndromes, peripartum cardiomyopathy, amniotic fluid embolism, and pulmonary embolism [1, 4, 5].

Dyspnea of Normal Pregnancy

The physiology of pregnancy creates increased demand on the respiratory system. This is a result of hormonal factors, increasing metabolic demand over the course of pregnancy and during labor, and changes in maternal abdominal and thoracic anatomy (see Fig. 17.2).

Comparing blood gas values between pregnant patients and nonpregnant patients also demonstrates the changes in respiration which are normal (see Table 17.1). Specifically, pregnant patients experience a respiratory alkalosis compensated by a metabolic acidosis with renal wasting of bicarbonate. When the pregnant patient cannot meet these demands,

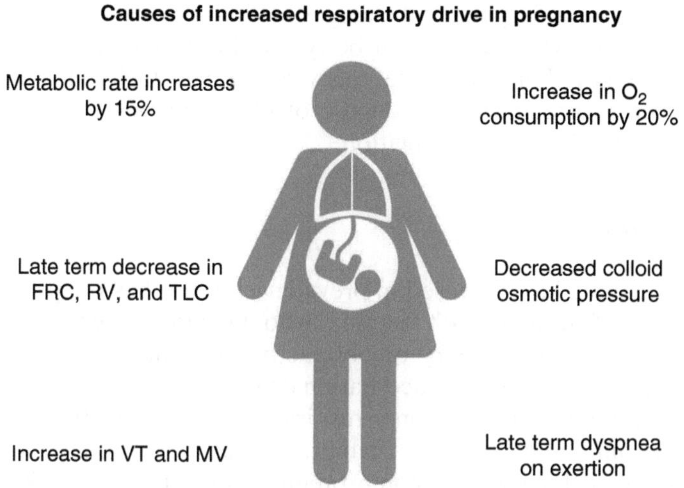

FIGURE 17.2 Causes of increased respiratory drive in pregnancy [2, 6, 7]. FRC Functional reserve capacity, RV residual volume, TLC total lung capacity, VT tidal volume, MV minute ventilation

TABLE 17.1 Arterial blood gas measurements in pregnancy from Hegewald 2011 (used with permission) [47]

Arterial blood gas changes in pregnancy			
ABG measurement	**Nonpregnant**	**First trimester**	**Third trimester**
pH	7.40	7.42–7.46	7.43
PaO_2 (mmHg)	93	105–106	101–106
$PaCO_2$ (mmHg)	37	28–29	26–30
Serum HCO_3 (mEq/L)	23	18	17

the sensation of dyspnea develops. Over the course of gestation, the proportion of patients reporting dyspnea increases, with over 60% of women reporting the symptom in the latter weeks of pregnancy [8]. When considering this diagnosis, it is important that other physical exam findings as well as the clinical history are congruent. In this patient's case, the sensation of dyspnea and changes in vital signs all had a sudden onset which would not be typical in dyspnea of normal pregnancy. Further, while tachycardia and tachypnea are noted in pregnancy, the degree of elevation raises concern requiring further investigation.

Asthma

As asthma has increased in prevalence, so too has the prevalence of women with asthma who become pregnant [9]. Patients with a history of obstructive lung disease such as asthma may have an exacerbation driven by nonadherence to maintenance medications, respiratory tract infections, or environmental irritants. Further, women with poorly controlled asthma who become pregnant are at higher risk of complications such as pre-eclampsia, preterm delivery, and infants small for gestational age [10]. There is significant variability in how pregnancy affects women with asthma. Patient reported data and asthma diaries demonstrate that the proportion of women whose asthma worsened, was unchanged, or improved is grossly equal [11]. In this case, the patient has dyspnea, but lacks some of the other typical clinical features of an asthma exacerbation such as wheezing or cough. The rapidity of unprovoked symptoms is also somewhat inconsistent with an acute asthma exacerbation in a patient whose childhood lung disease has been quiescent.

Pneumonia and Respiratory Infections

Pneumonia is a leading cause of death related to nonobstetric infections in pregnant women [12]. The infectious causes of pneumonia are no different than the nonpregnant population with *Streptococcus pneumoniae* and *Haemophilus influenzae* leading followed by atypical species [13]. Pregnant women are at higher risk to develop pulmonary infections due to alterations in immune response, increased lung water, and increased incidence of aspiration during delivery [13–15].

In pregnant women, influenza represents a special category of respiratory infection. The 2009 H1N1 influenza pandemic disproportionately affected pregnant women and resulted in higher maternal mortality [16]. Pneumonia places the mother and fetus at risk with associated increases in pre-eclampsia, decreased Apgar scores, and low birthweight [17]. In this case, the lack of fever, cough, or radiographic findings as well as the quick development of symptoms makes pneumonia or respiratory infection less likely.

Pre-eclampsia

Pre-eclampsia is characterized as a syndrome of new-onset hypertension (SBP $\geq$ 140, DBP $\geq$ 90) with associated organ dysfunction characterized by either proteinuria, maternal organ dysfunction (new elevation in creatinine, neurologic symptoms, hematologic changes), or uteroplacental dysfunction [18]. The majority of women who present with pre-eclampsia are asymptomatic, but those who present with chest pain or dyspnea are at higher risk for adverse maternal outcomes [19]. In this case, the patient lacks the cardinal feature of hypertension making this diagnosis unlikely.

Acute Coronary and Vascular Syndromes

The majority of pregnant women do not have the traditional risk factors for ischemic cardiac or vascular disease. However, as obesity and advanced maternal age have become more prevalent and more women with chronic medical conditions become pregnant, the rates of coronary heart disease, congenital heart disease, valvular heart disease, and vascular injuries during pregnancy have also increased [20]. Maternal mortality data shows that cardiac causes of death are the most common cause of mortality indirectly related to pregnancy [21]. Unsurprisingly, women who have previously suffered an acute cardiac syndrome (ACS) or have known coronary artery disease are at higher risk of maternal morbidity [22].

Beyond atherosclerotic cardiac ischemia, there are a number of other causes of myocardial infarction such as spontaneous coronary thrombosis, coronary arterial spasm, increased myocardial demand, and anemia [23]. Once evidence of ACS has been established, identifying the underlying cause and then managing the patient appropriately is paramount.

Other causes of acute chest pain and dyspnea include spontaneous coronary artery dissection (SCAD) and aortic dissection. Review of coronary angiogram databases shows SCAD to be on the order of 0.07–1.1% in all patients (not specifically pregnant patients). When truly spontaneous SCAD is separated from SCAD associated with atherosclerotic disease, there is a predominance of female sex (2:1) and a strong association with the peripartum period [24]. Thought leaders have proposed that the true incidence of SCAD related to pregnancy is underestimated [24, 25].

Aortic dissection, while rare, continues to be reported as a cause of pregnancy-related morbidity and mortality [21, 26]. The synthesis of risk factors from pregnancy and the patient (connective tissue diseases, hypertension, etc.) is felt to strengthen the association between aortic dissection and pregnancy. Because it can present with a variety of symptoms (intrathoracic, intra-abdominal, neurologic), aortic dissection is challenging to diagnose. When it does occur, aortic dissection carries a significant burden of maternal and fetal mortality [27].

A hallmark of women who died from acute coronary syndrome and acute vascular injury is that their chest pain and dyspnea were not sufficiently evaluated [21, 28]. Therefore, it is important that the treating clinician respect these disease entities and assess for them when appropriate. Considering this patient, she does not have significant risk factors as she is a non-smoker and not obese and has no cardiac or hypertension history and no familial cardiac history. However, in view of the chest pain with dyspnea and hypoxia, evaluating the patient for coronary ischemia would still be prudent. Similarly, regarding aortic or vascular dissection, she lacks nearly all of the most common risk factors, including any evidence of connective tissue diseases such as Marfan or Ehlers-Danlos syndromes.

Peripartum Cardiomyopathy (PPCM)

PPCM has been recognized since the 19th century and is broadly described as heart failure associated with pregnancy without familial or genetic causes. Research into PPCM has yielded various definitions, the most recent coming in 2010 from the Heart Failure Association of the European Society of Cardiology Working Group on PPCM:

> PPCM is an idiopathic cardiomyopathy presenting with heart failure secondary to left ventricular systolic dysfunction towards the end of pregnancy or in the months following delivery, where no other cause of heart failure is found. It is a diagnosis of exclusion. The left ventricle may not be dilated but the ejection fraction is nearly always reduced below 45% [29].

This definition recognizes that while PPCM tends to occur in the later months of pregnancy, it is not exclusive to that time frame. PPCM has been described in the second trimester and as late as 6 months following delivery. Further it requires that investigations for other causes have been undertaken without result. The reported incidence of PPCM is variable in developed countries with reports of a frequency as high as 1 in 1000 births to 1 in 4000 births (United States, South Africa). Certain locations, namely, Haiti, show a frequency as high as 1 in 300 births [29, 30]. The etiology of PPCM is not well known. It is thought to involve factors secondary to predisposing hemodynamic changes such as pre-eclampsia or hypertension, inflammation, the interaction between gestational hormones and vasculature, as well as genetics [29–31]. Leading risk factors for PPCM include age greater than 30, black race, and preexisting hypertension or pre-eclampsia. The presentation of PPCM is variable in terms of both timing during pregnancy and the nature and severity of symptoms. In general, the symptoms are similar to other causes of heart failure and include bilateral lower extremity swelling, dyspnea, orthopnea, and chest pain [32]. More severe cases may include hypoxia and low output cardiac failure with shock [30]. In the described patient, the time course (sudden, occurring over a few minutes) would be atypical, but this diagnosis warrants investigation given her symptoms, physical findings, as well as age.

Amniotic Fluid Embolism (AFE)

AFE is a feared complication of pregnancy with the hallmarks of acute dyspnea, hypoxia, coagulopathy, hypotension, and shock occurring in the context of labor, delivery, or maternal trauma. Despite being rare, AFE carries a high rate of maternal mortality [33]. Originally, based on identification of amniotic debris within the pulmonary arteries during autopsy, it was thought that the etiology was due to maternal exposure to antigens within the amniotic fluid and obstruction of the pulmonary circulation due to debris [34]. This was challenged following the advent of the pulmonary artery catheter when evidence of fetal amniotic material was identified within the pulmonary circulation but without symptoms consistent with AFE [35]. As further experimental and pathologic data have been obtained, it appears that AFE occurs following disruption of the maternal-fetal barrier with extravasation of fetal and infectious tissue into the maternal circulation. In susceptible patients, this creates a cascade of pro-inflammatory signaling (similar to the systemic inflammatory response syndrome, SIRS) resulting in hemodynamic changes as well as hemostatic changes [35]. This patient has no history of trauma and is not in labor, making AFE unlikely.

Pulmonary Embolism (PE)

Thrombotic pulmonary embolism represents approximately 10% of the maternal mortality burden in the United States [36, 37]. Some countries, such as the United Kingdom, have been successful in reducing the maternal mortality rate due to PE [21]. The reduction in mortality observed is not secondary to a reduction in the rate of venous thromboembolism (VTE). Indeed, the rate of VTE complicating hospitalizations for delivery has increased from 0.81 to 1.39 for every 10,000 births (data from 1998 to 2009) [38].

During the course of pregnancy, the risk for VTE increases and spikes in the immediate postpartum period. The likelihood of VTE returns to baseline approximately 4 weeks following delivery [39]. The VTE risk increases as the components of Virchow's triad (hypercoagulability, venous stasis, and vascular damage) come together with advancing gestational age. In the pregnant patient, the balance of hemostasis favors clot formation as a result of increased prothrombotic factors, decreased inhibitory factors, and impaired blood clot dissolution [40–42]. Blood flow within the venous system slows as a result of venodilation and decreased maternal physical movement [43–46]. During delivery, vascular injury is more likely to occur resulting in activation of the extrinsic clotting pathway. The result of this combination of changes is an increased risk of DVT and PE.

When a PE does occur, the spectrum of signs and symptoms ranges from mild with minimal clinical changes to severe with profound instability and even cardiac arrest. As previously discussed, some of the changes seen in PE (sensation of dyspnea, chest pain, tachycardia, dependent extremity swelling) overlap with physiologic alterations normal in pregnancy. The patient in the clinical vignette has many of the symptoms and signs seen in PE and should undergo further testing to either eliminate or establish this diagnosis.

Diagnosis

The differential diagnosis for the constellation of chest pain, dyspnea, hypoxia, tachycardia, and fatigue in a patient at 41 WGA is broad. The physical exam and history are able to narrow the differential somewhat to include dyspnea of normal pregnancy (a diagnosis of exclusion), acute coronary and vascular syndromes, PPCM, and PE. Additional clinical data can be useful to further assess the patient and come to the correct diagnosis.

Blood and Serum Testing

Arterial Blood Gas (ABG): ABG analysis allows for evaluation of the patient's oxygenation, ventilation, and acid-base status. Certain respiratory diseases may also increase the gradient between the alveolar and arterial oxygen tension, indicating a possible defect in diffusion, ventilation-perfusion (VQ) mismatch, or right-to-left shunting. Unfortunately, ABG is not sensitive nor specific for the leading diagnoses in this case. The maternal ABG differs in significant ways from the ABG obtained from a patient who is not pregnant (see Table 17.1), and it is important to be knowledgeable about the differences.

Two particular areas to monitor in the pregnant patient are oxygenation and appropriate ventilation. Normoxia in a pregnant patient is vital to support fetal oxygenation. In many disease states, an intensivist may be somewhat tolerant of mild degrees of hypoxia. This is not the case in the pregnant patient, and she may require higher degrees of support to maintain appropriate fetal oxygen delivery. Pregnant patients whose $PaCO_2$ "normalizes" may actually be demonstrating respiratory fatigue and possible impending respiratory failure. It should be noted that for many applications, venous blood gas (VBG) testing is an acceptable alternative to ABG, except for assessment of arterial oxygenation [48, 49].

Brain Natriuretic Peptide (BNP): BNP and atrial natriuretic peptide (ANP) are hormones released as a result of myocyte stretch. A rise in these hormones results in vasodilation, inhibition of the renin-angiotensin-aldosterone signaling, and increased natriuresis [50, 51]. Both BNP and N-terminal-proBNP (NT-proBNP, released after cleaving from a BNP precursor) can be measured [52]. BNP is mildly elevated compared to nonpregnant controls during pregnancy but is below the thresholds used in BNP testing [51].

Elevations in BNP are consistent with the diagnosis of PPCM and heart failure [53–56]. BNP also predicts a higher risk for worsened clinical course and outcome in PE [57–59].

Troponin: Troponins are a family of proteins almost exclusively found in cardiac myocytes which can be measured in the serum following cardiac injury. The time course of troponin rise is variable across different assays, but it is usually detectable 2–4 h after injury. Because of this delay, when cardiac injury is otherwise apparent (by history, exam, or echocardiogram), appropriate treatment should begin immediately rather than wait for the result of serial troponin testing. It should also be noted that a number of nonischemic cardiac and noncardiac causes are associated with elevation in troponin [60]. Regarding PE, troponin elevation has been associated with worsened clinical course and outcome [61]. In this patient, because the differential diagnosis includes acute cardiac injury, cardiomyopathy, and pulmonary embolism, initial testing with a troponin assay is warranted to potentially identify a cause of her symptoms as well as to risk stratify her course.

D-Dimer: The use of D-dimer (a product of the breakdown of cross-linked fibrin by plasmin) to diagnose VTE in pregnancy is confounded by the increasing levels of D-dimer noted during gestation [62, 63]. Thought leaders in the diagnosis and management of PE have advocated "trimester-adjusted" D-dimer levels as a way to improve the sensitivity and specificity of D-dimer testing for VTE and reduce the amount of maternal and fetal radiation exposure [64]. This represents an active area of research and practice development, but there are no specialty guidelines supporting this approach.

Electrocardiogram (ECG)

Electrocardiography is perhaps the most common study used to assess adult patients with chest pain, syncope, dyspnea, and hemodynamic and metabolic changes. While there are classic findings of pathology (such as ST segment elevation in myocardial infarction), these are often insensitive and significant disease can be evident with subtle findings. In the case of PPCM, the most common ECG finding is sinus tachycardia and nonspecific changes [30]. Similarly, in PE, the classic finding of $S_1Q_3T_3$ (deep S-wave in I, Q wave in III, inverted T-wave in III) is present in only 12% of patients, and the ECG is normal in 23% of cases [65, 66]. Despite these issues, obtaining an ECG early in the patient's course is advisable as specific changes, when present, can expedite appropriate therapy.

Duplex Ultrasound (US)

Duplex US of the lower extremities is an attractive test in assessing the patient with potential VTE and PE because, unlike CT angiogram or ventilation-perfusion scanning, it does not require ionizing radiation and can be performed by an appropriately trained clinician at the point of care. Most VTE in pregnancy begins in the lower extremities. Provided the patient is experiencing signs or symptoms in the lower extremities, assessment with duplex US is a reasonable place to begin the workup in order to avoid unnecessary radiation [43, 67]. Limitations of duplex US include its dependence on patient habitus and operator expertise. Further, duplex is less sensitive to pelvic vein DVT. If there is significant suspicion for VTE (either DVT or PE), further testing is required.

CT Angiogram (CTA)

CTA of the chest is a useful test to assess for PE, aortic dissection, and other lung pathology. At many hospitals, CTA may be more available than other testing modalities like ventilation-perfusion (VQ) scan or echocardiography, allowing for more rapid diagnosis of PE. In considering radiation, fetal exposure to radiation is lower with CTA than VQ scan. However, maternal radiation exposure is higher than VQ scan [67]. Overall, the American College of Obstetricians and Gynecologists makes this recommendation regarding radiation exposure:

> With few exceptions, radiation exposure through radiography, computed tomography (CT) scan, or nuclear medicine imaging techniques is at a dose much lower than the exposure associated with fetal harm. If these techniques are necessary in addition to ultrasonography or MRI or are more readily available for the diagnosis in question, they should not be withheld from a pregnant patient [68].

There is concern that changes in maternal anatomy and physiology raise the likelihood of nondiagnostic CTAs, in some series significantly [69–71]. The use of intravenous iodinated contrast required in CTA in pregnant or nursing mothers has been investigated and has not been found to be harmful. However, it should only be used when needed [68, 72, 73]. In this patient's case, due to the severity of her pain and consideration of vascular catastrophe, using a CTA to assess for PE and dissection would be reasonable. The use of CTA versus VQ scanning in pregnant patients remains an area of debate.

Ventilation-Perfusion (VQ) Scan

If pulmonary embolism is the leading diagnostic consideration and the patient's chest X-ray is normal, the American Thoracic Society guideline recommends the use of VQ scan over CTA [67]. The Royal College of Obstetricians and Gynaecologists gives CTA and VQ scan equal consideration [74]. The American College of Obstetricians and Gynecologists does not make a recommendation of CTA versus VQ scan, but does note that fetal radiation exposure is low with both [75]. VQ scanning may have a limited availability at some institutions, making a CTA more expedient for diagnosis.

Transthoracic Echocardiogram (TTE)

Echocardiography can be useful in initial diagnosis or, following diagnosis, in risk stratification and prognostication. In assessment for PPCM, pulmonary embolism, and vascular injury, TTE provides significant information. Clinicians with appropriate point-of-care ultrasound (POCUS) echocardiography training can assess global cardiac function and activity, estimate ventricular function, and identify a pericardial effusion [76]. Being able to evaluate these aspects of cardiac function can significantly help in narrowing the differential diagnosis of a patient presenting with dyspnea, chest pain, tachycardia, and hypoxia. More advanced ultrasonographers can examine cardiac function in greater detail including valvular function, evidence of right heart strain, and wall motion abnormalities. It should be noted, however, that 2011 guidelines endorsed by several multispecialty societies recommend against the use of POCUS echocardiography in the diagnosis of PE [77]. Following a diagnosis of PE, echocardiography is useful in assessing right heart function and is part of the definition of submassive PE [77, 78]. TTE has a role to play in the diagnosis of vascular dissection, particularly when CTA is unavailable. Findings of aortic valve dysfunction, pericardial effusion, bicuspid aortic valve, and a proximal aortic intimal flap can indicate an aortic dissection. TTE does not have good sensitivity for dissection, but because it can identify other conditions and potentially reveal impending catastrophe, it is still important in the assessment of the patient with chest pain [79].

Further Diagnostic Patient Data

In this patient, a CTA of the chest was obtained which demonstrated a pulmonary embolism in the right pulmonary artery and no dissection. In addition, an echocardiogram was obtained which showed a mild degree of right heart strain. Her troponin-T was measured as normal, but a BNP was measured as 1000 ng/mL. Taken together with the previously discussed history and clinical data, the patient was diagnosed with a pulmonary embolism.

Treatment and Management

Diagnosis and treatment are not sequential, but rather parallel courses of action. While identifying the underlying cause of the patient's symptoms and hemodynamic changes, the treating clinician must also provide supportive care. Once the underlying cause of the patient's condition has been identified, in this case having a PE, then diagnosis-specific management can begin. Treating PE is an active area of research with standard therapies as the norm and emerging therapies becoming more available.

Standard Therapies

Supportive Critical Care in the Obstetric Patient

When treating a pregnant patient with sudden hemodynamic and respiratory changes, it is vital that the bedside team be familiar with general principles of caring for the critically ill obstetric patient. This topic warrants dedicated review (see References) but the guiding principles will be discussed here [6, 80, 81].

Critical care of the pregnant patient requires a multidisciplinary team working with a systematic mindset. The individual patient's circumstances will direct which specific resources are needed, but broadly speaking the team should involve intensivists, obstetricians with expertise in maternal-fetal medicine, neonatologists, pharmacists, nurses from both critical care and obstetric disciplines, and social work [6]. Further, it is important that the team collaborate and interact *before* a patient-specific crisis to facilitate communication, to preplan logistics, and to discuss common scenarios which require collaboration. The need to transfer a pregnant patient to a higher level of care is governed by gestational age, the threshold of fetal viability of the local institution (and receiving centers), and overall critical care and obstetric capabilities. If there is suspicion for concerning pathology, prioritizing the patient's airway, breathing, and circulation continues to hold true. The patient should be placed on telemetry monitoring and have regular blood pressure and vital signs taken, and IV access should be established. Depending on gestational age, fetal monitoring should also be employed. Guntupalli and colleagues have proposed a five-step approach to conceptualizing critical

TABLE 17.2 Steps to managing critical illness in pregnancy from Guntupalli 2015 (used with permission) [80]

Steps		Rationale
Step 1	Is this a medical or obstetric disorder?	Many obstetric disorders mimic medical disorders
		Treatment of the two differ completely
		Specific treatment available for many medical disorders; drugs of choice may differ in pregnancy
		Delivery may halt progression of most obstetric disorders but only few medical disorders
Step 2	Is there failure of multiple organ systems?	Almost all patients will have organ dysfunction
		Kidney injury, thrombocytopenia, and coagulopathy are commonest
		Support failing organ systems
		Fetal well-being and safety assume importance in selecting treatment options and targets

TABLE 17.2 (continued)

Steps		Rationale
Step 3	Is there a risk to the mother and fetus if pregnancy is continued?	Maternal outcomes are better in some specific disorders if delivery is hastened; these should be identified. Fetal well-being is closely monitored Maternal survival takes precedence over fetal survival
Step 4	If delivery is to be hastened, vaginal delivery or Cesarean section? General or neuraxial anesthesia?	The decision-to-delivery time with mode of delivery and type of anesthesia and their associated risks must be balanced with the benefits
Step 5	What needs to be done to optimize patient for delivery?	Timely achievement of specific targets Hemodynamics, oxygenation, seizure control, thrombocytopenia, and biochemical and coagulation parameters must be optimized to ensure safe delivery

illness in pregnancy which is useful when encountering these difficult scenarios [80] (Table 17.2).

There are idiosyncrasies in caring for the critically ill pregnant patient. In considering airway management, pregnancy predicts a more challenging airway both anatomically and physiologically. This is a result of upper airway edema, decreased functional residual capacity, increased oxygen consumption, and lower tolerance of hypoxia from a maternal and fetal perspective [82]. The maternal Mallampati score worsens during gestation as well as from predelivery to postdelivery [3, 83]. Finally, it is important to respect the increased risk of aspiration in the pregnant population as a result of decreased lower esophageal sphincter tone and delayed gastric emptying and other factors [81, 84]. Because of the importance of appropriate oxygen delivery to the fetus, it is important to maintain a PaO_2 of greater than 70 mmHg (or an oxygen saturation greater than 95%).

When managing the pregnant patient with shock, anatomic and physiologic factors continue to be important to consider. Left lateral positioning is recommended to relieve aortocaval compression, and intravenous access above the diaphragm is preferred in case of compression of the great vessels of the abdomen by the uterus [85]. While dopamine, dobutamine, norepinephrine, and epinephrine have been associated with decreased uterine blood flow, the priority of resuscitation remains with the mother, and these agents should not be withheld if needed. Provided time allows, it is important to focus on positioning and volume expansion prior to initiation of vasoactive agents [6].

The disposition of pregnant patients requires thoughtful consideration. The threshold to admit to an ICU should be lower in pregnant patients as they require closer monitoring and potentially urgent interventions. The maternal and fetal intolerance of hypoxemia necessitates a high degree of respiratory support, and the multidisciplinary nature of critical care lends itself to benefiting the patient. The question of transferring the patient will depend on the patient's condition, the interventions required, the fetal gestational age, and the local gestational age threshold for fetal viability. If at all possible, the patient should be at an institution where both the needs of the mother and fetus can be met.

Anticoagulation

The mainstay of VTE treatment is anticoagulation. As mentioned previously, the balance between thrombosis and thrombolysis is altered in pregnancy to favor clot formation. Anticoagulation mitigates this by preventing further clot formation and tipping the balance to favor endogenous thrombolysis. In the antepartum period, unfractionated heparin (UFH) and low-molecular weight heparin (LMWH) are the favored agents due to their efficacy, reversibility, and lack of teratogenicity. Further neither UFH nor LMWH cross the placenta [75]. The American College of Obstetricians and Gynecologists (ACOG) does not recommend a specific agent, but the American Society of Hematology and the Royal College of Obstetricians and Gynaecologists from the United Kingdom recommend LMWH over UFH [74, 86]. Warfarin and other vitamin K antagonists (VKA) are not recommended during pregnancy (particularly the first trimester) due to teratogenicity [87]. Postpartum, however, warfarin is acceptable as it is not excreted in breast milk [87]. Direct oral anticoagulants such as rivaroxaban or apixaban are not recommended at any time during pregnancy or in breastfeeding mothers due to concerns of placental transmission and excretion in breast milk [88, 89].

The timing of initiation of full anticoagulation is dependent on the patient's risk for VTE and the treating clinician's index of suspicion. In cases with high pretest probability for VTE, empiric anticoagulation while the diagnosis is being investigated is recommended given the potential for rapid deterioration [74, 86, 90]. Certainly, once the diagnosis is established and there are no overt contraindications, therapeutic anticoagulation should begin immediately. The most complicated management of anticoagulation occurs during the peripartum period. Here, concerns of worsening VTE are balanced with needs for neuraxial anesthesia, concern for maternal hemorrhage, and potential need for caesarian section. ACOG suggests consideration of transitioning patients taking LMWH to UFH in the last month of pregnancy, owing to the shorter half-life of UFH. Regarding epidural anesthesia, the American Society of Regional Anesthesia recommends withholding therapeutic LMWH for 24 h prior to placing an epidural catheter [91]. Guidance is less clear in patients using therapeutic UFH, and the recommendation is to assess the risk for bleeding on an individual basis [91]. Anticoagulation is maintained from the time of diagnosis through delivery and should be continued for at least 3 months; including at least 6 weeks postpartum treatment as this is the highest risk period for VTE in mothers [74, 87]. Guidance for prevention of VTE is beyond the scope of this chapter, but further information is available [92, 93].

Massive Pulmonary Embolism

Pulmonary embolisms associated with hemodynamic instability or severe respiratory distress and hypoxia are classified as massive PEs. Massive PE can also present as a cardiac arrest. In addition to standard critical care and anticoagulation described above, massive PE requires emergent clot disruption to relieve right heart strain and improve cardiac and pulmonary physiology. In adults, the recommendation to administer systemic thrombolysis in the setting of massive PE is clear, and meta-analysis has shown an all-cause mortality benefit [94–96]. The most recent American College of Chest Physician guidelines list pregnancy as a relative contraindication for thrombolytic therapy [94]. However, when the life of the mother is at stake, clinicians should consider the emergent use of systemic thrombolytics [43, 97]. The literature base supporting the use of systemic thrombolytics is growing, but remains confined to case reports and small case series [98–101]. Caution should be used when evaluating this literature given the bias toward reporting positive results. The small body of literature limits knowledge regarding maternal and fetal risk following systemic thrombolysis. The chief maternal risk following thrombolysis is major bleeding, including intracranial hemorrhage (ICH). In the general population under 65 years of age, major bleeding complicates thrombolysis for massive PE in approximately 3% of cases.[95]. Studies examining ICH as a result of thrombolysis for pulmonary embolism do not stratify the risk by age (advanced age being the largest risk factor for ICH), but meta-analysis estimates place the incidence at 1.5% of cases. Maternal hemorrhage with thrombolysis has been reported as more frequent, upwards of 8% [102]. However this data was reported in an era where streptokinase was used instead of tissue plasminogen activator (tPA). tPA has been associated with less hemorrhagic complications because it has a higher affinity for plasminogen associated with fibrin; this is more likely to occur at the site of active clot [103]. Regarding fetal risk, the data remains poor, but there is an estimated 6% rate of premature delivery and 6% rate of pregnancy loss [103]. Even though this data was published in 2002, it continues to be cited in the most recent guidelines [97, 104]. Because thrombolysis for submassive PE in the nonpregnant population is an active area of research and controversy, the use of thrombolysis in the absence of hypotension or severe respiratory distress in the pregnant patient is not recommended [97, 105, 106].

Future Directions

Catheter-directed thrombolysis and extracorporeal membrane oxygenation (ECMO) push therapy for massive pulmonary embolism forward. In patients who are not candidates for systemic thrombolysis (such as those with active, life-threatening bleeding or have an absolute contraindication to systemic thrombolytics), catheter-directed therapy may be employed. Further, in cases of massive pulmonary embolism refractory to thrombolysis or in patients for whom thrombolysis is not an option, extracorporeal membrane oxygenation (ECMO) has been used for maternal support.

Catheter-Directed Thrombolysis (CDT)

CDT uses percutaneous vascular technology and interventional techniques to treat PE locally. Through mechanical clot disruption (such as suction, fragmentation, or ultrasound), local delivery of thrombolytics, or a combination of the two, CDT is thought to provide benefits similar to systemic thrombolysis with a lower risk of major bleeding. The disadvantages to CDT include the additional risks of percutaneous vascular access, potential for endovascular damage or perforation, and the additional lead time required to mobilize an interventional radiology or cardiology team to provide the therapy. Further, the specific risks of each modality of CDT vary with technique, equipment, and experience [107]. The studies of CDT are small and often have no pregnant patients in them, or pregnant patients are actively excluded [108, 109]. The only prospective trial of CDT included 59 patients in comparison to the 1775 prospectively studied patients for systemic thrombolysis [95, 109]. However, the results regarding efficacy and safety of CDT in the general population are promising, and registry data shows favorable outcomes compared to systemic thrombolysis [110, 111]. As this technology matures and becomes more readily available, it may become the frontline therapy for massive PE in the pregnant patient.

Extracorporeal Membrane Oxygenation (ECMO)

ECMO can be employed purely for support of oxygenation and ventilation as well as circulatory support. In the venovenous (VV) configuration, deoxygenated blood is removed from the venous system via a central vein, oxygenation and ventilation occur via an oxygenator, and oxygenated blood is returned with relatively low pressure the vena cava for circulation by the heart. When circulatory support is required in addition to oxygenation and ventilation, the centrifugal pump driving the ECMO circuit is adjusted to meet the desired output. Rather than returning to a vein, the blood is returned to an arterial catheter placed proximally for perfusion of the body. This is venoarterial (VA) ECMO. Once only found in highly specialized centers and only implemented in the operating room, ECMO technology has become more portable and cannulation more widely taught. As a result, ECMO can now be initiated in a critical access hospital to stabilize a patient for return to a tertiary center. Internationally, ECMO is being initiated, in selected cases, prehospital for refractory cardiac arrest. In the United States, ECMO use increased by over 400% between 2006 and 2011 and continues to grow [112]. A full overview of ECMO is beyond the scope of this article, but there are further resources available for a more robust review [113, 114]. Case reports discussing ECMO support of pregnant patients had been sporadic until the 2009 H1N1 influenza epidemic when many more patients were placed on ECMO circuits due to ARDS. Several case series were published, and in a meta-analysis including 5 publications (for a total of 39 patients), the overall maternal survival rate for those requiring ECMO for H1N1 influenza was 75% with a 70% fetal survival rate [115]. VA ECMO would be the primary modality for maternal support as a result of cardiogenic shock and respiratory failure from massive pulmonary embolism. Descriptions of maternal and fetal survival following ECMO support for pulmonary embolism are generally favorable, but there is concern for publication bias. The primary complications of ECMO are related to bleeding, due to anatomic factors of cannulation and the required anticoagulation while on circuit. The overall complication rate varies by ECMO modality (VV versus VA) and setting. It is also confounded by differences in reporting. Estimates of significant bleeding complications for ECMO range between 40% and perhaps up to 70% [113]. Because of this, ECMO remains limited to the most serious cases of maternal respiratory and hemodynamic distress.

Case Summary

The patient received therapeutic anticoagulation with LMWH and close monitoring in the ICU. Gradually, her symptoms and vital signs returned to their pre PE baseline. Prior to a planned delivery, she was transitioned to a heparin infusion which was stopped just prior to labor induction to facilitate placement of epidural anesthesia. She delivered a healthy baby girl and was discharged in good condition to home where she completed 3 months of anticoagulation therapy.

References

1. Mehta N, Chen K, Hardy E, Powrie R. Respiratory disease in pregnancy. Best Pract Res Clin Obstet Gynaecol. 2015;29(5):598–611. https://doi.org/10.1016/j.bpobgyn.2015.04.005.
2. Graves CR. Acute pulmonary complications in pregnancy. In: Vincent J-L, editor. Textbook of critical care. 6th ed. Philadelphia: Elsevier; 2011. p. 1187–91.
3. Kodali BS, Chandrasekhar S, Bulich LN, Topulos GP, Datta S. Airway changes during labor and delivery. Anesthesiology. 2008;108(3):357–62. https://doi.org/10.1097/ALN.0b013e31816452d3.
4. Lee S-Y, Chien D-K, Huang C-H, Shih S-C, Lee W-C, Chang W-H. Dyspnea in pregnancy. Taiwan J Obstet Gynecol. 2017;56(4):432–6. https://doi.org/10.1016/j.tjog.2017.04.035.
5. Desai AS, Chutkow WA, Edelman E, Economy KE, Dec GW. Clinical problem-solving. A crisis in late pregnancy. N Engl J Med. 2009;361(23):2271–7. https://doi.org/10.1056/NEJMcps0708258.
6. Lapinsky SE. Critical care medicine in pregnancy. In: Dellinger RP, Parrillo JE, editors. Critical care medicine. 4th ed. Philadelphia: Mosby; 2013. p. 1410–20.
7. Chesnutt AN. Physiology of normal pregnancy. Crit Care Clin. 2004;20(4):609–15. https://doi.org/10.1016/j.ccc.2004.06.001.
8. Milne JA, Howie AD, Pack AI. Dyspnoea during normal pregnancy. Br J Obstet Gynaecol. 1978;85(4):260–3.
9. Hansen C, Joski P, Freiman H, et al. Medication exposure in pregnancy risk evaluation program: the prevalence of asthma medication use during pregnancy. Matern Child Health J. 2012;17(9):1611–21. https://doi.org/10.1007/s10995-012-1173-x.
10. Murphy VE, Namazy JA, Powell H, et al. A meta-analysis of adverse perinatal outcomes in women with asthma. BJOG. 2011;118(11):1314–23. https://doi.org/10.1111/j.1471-0528.2011.03055.x.
11. Schatz M, Harden K, Forsythe A, et al. The course of asthma during pregnancy, post partum, and with successive pregnancies:

a prospective analysis. J Allergy Clin Immunol. 1988;81(3): 509–17.
12. Kaunitz AM, Hughes JM, Grimes DA, Smith JC, Rochat RW, Kafrissen ME. Causes of maternal mortality in the United States. Obstet Gynecol. 1985;65(5):605–12.
13. Brito V, Niederman MS. Pneumonia complicating pregnancy. Clin Chest Med. 2011;32(1):121–32. https://doi.org/10.1016/j.ccm.2010.10.004.
14. Goodnight WH, Soper DE. Pneumonia in pregnancy. Crit Care Med. 2005;33(Supplement):S390–7. https://doi.org/10.1097/01.CCM.0000182483.24836.66.
15. Goodrum LA. Pneumonia in pregnancy. Semin Perinatol. 1997;21(4):276–83.
16. Louie JK, Acosta M, Jamieson DJ, Honein MA, California Pandemic (H1N1) Working Group. Severe 2009 H1N1 influenza in pregnant and postpartum women in California. N Engl J Med. 2010;362(1):27–35. https://doi.org/10.1056/NEJMoa0910444.
17. Chen YH, Keller J, Wang IT, Lin CC, Lin HC. Pneumonia and pregnancy outcomes: a nationwide population-based study. Am J Obstet Gynecol. 2012;207(4):288.e1–7. https://doi.org/10.1016/j.ajog.2012.08.023.
18. Tranquilli AL, Dekker G, Magee L, et al. The classification, diagnosis and management of the hypertensive disorders of pregnancy: a revised statement from the ISSHP. Pregnancy Hypertens Int J Womens Cardiovasc Health. 2014;4(2):97–104. https://doi.org/10.1016/j.preghy.2014.02.001.
19. Dadelszen Von P, Payne B, Li J, Lancet JAT. Prediction of adverse maternal outcomes in pre-eclampsia: development and validation of the fullPIERS model. Lancet. 2011;377(10):219–27. https://doi.org/10.1016/S0140-6736(10)61351-7.
20. Roos-Hesselink JW, Ruys TPE, Stein JI, et al. Outcome of pregnancy in patients with structural or ischaemic heart disease: results of a registry of the European Society of Cardiology. Eur Heart J. 2013;34(9):657–65. https://doi.org/10.1093/eurheartj/ehs270.
21. Cantwell R, Clutton-Brock T, Cooper G, et al. Saving Mothers' lives: reviewing maternal deaths to make motherhood safer: 2006–2008. The Eighth Report of the Confidential Enquiries into Maternal Deaths in the United Kingdom. BJOG. 2011;118(Suppl 1):1–203. https://doi.org/10.1111/j.1471-0528.2010.02847.x.
22. Burchill LJ, Lameijer H, Roos-Hesselink JW, et al. Pregnancy risks in women with pre-existing coronary artery disease, or

following acute coronary syndrome. Heart. 2015;101(7):525–9. https://doi.org/10.1136/heartjnl-2014-306676.
23. El-Deeb M, El-Menyar A, Gehani A, Sulaiman K. Acute coronary syndrome in pregnant women. Expert Rev Cardiovasc Ther. 2014;9(4):505–15. https://doi.org/10.1586/erc.11.19.
24. Kamineni R, Sadhu A, Alpert JS. Spontaneous coronary artery dissection: report of two cases and a 50-year review of the literature. Cardiol Rev. 2002;10(5):279–84. https://doi.org/10.1097/01.CRD.0000028805.70473.72.
25. Tweet MS, Gulati R, Hayes SN. Spontaneous coronary artery dissection. Curr Cardiol Rep. 2016;18(7):60. https://doi.org/10.1007/s11886-016-0737-6.
26. Kamel H, Roman MJ, Pitcher A, Devereux RB. Pregnancy and the risk of aortic dissection or rupture clinical perspective: table. Circulation. 2016;134(7):527–33. https://doi.org/10.1161/CIRCULATIONAHA.116.021594.
27. Zhu J-M, Ma W-G, Peterss S, et al. Aortic dissection in pregnancy: management strategy and outcomes. Ann Thorac Surg. 2017;103(4):1199–206. https://doi.org/10.1016/j.athoracsur.2016.08.089.
28. la Chapelle CF, Schutte JM, Schuitemaker NWE, Steegers EAP, van Roosmalen J, Dutch Maternal Mortality Committee. Maternal mortality attributable to vascular dissection and rupture in the Netherlands: a nationwide confidential enquiry. BJOG. 2012;119(1):86–93. https://doi.org/10.1111/j.1471-0528.2011.03178.x.
29. Sliwa K, Hilfiker-Kleiner D, Petrie MC, et al. Current state of knowledge on aetiology, diagnosis, management, and therapy of peripartum cardiomyopathy: a position statement from the Heart Failure Association of the European Society of Cardiology Working Group on peripartum cardiomyopathy. Eur J Heart Fail. 2014;12(8):767–78. https://doi.org/10.1093/eurjhf/hfq120.
30. Arany Z, Elkayam U. Peripartum cardiomyopathy. Circulation. 2016;133(14):1397–409. https://doi.org/10.1161/CIRCULATIONAHA.115.020491.
31. Elkayam U. Clinical characteristics of peripartum cardiomyopathy in the United States. JAC. 2011;58(7):659–70. https://doi.org/10.1016/j.jacc.2011.03.047.
32. Demakis JG, Rahimtoola SH, Sutton GC, et al. Natural course of peripartum cardiomyopathy. Circulation. 1971;44(6):1053–61.
33. Shamshirsaz AA, Clark SL. Amniotic fluid embolism. Obstet Gynecol Clin N Am. 2016;43(4):779–90. https://doi.org/10.1016/j.ogc.2016.07.001.

34. Steiner PE, Lushbaugh CC. Landmark article, Oct. 1941: Maternal pulmonary embolism by amniotic fluid as a cause of obstetric shock and unexpected deaths in obstetrics. By Paul E. Steiner and C. C. Lushbaugh. JAMA. 1986;255(16):2187–203.
35. Clark SL. Amniotic Fluid Embolism. Obstet Gynecol. 2014;123(2, PART 1):337–48. https://doi.org/10.1097/AOG.0000000000000107.
36. Berg CJ, Callaghan WM, Syverson C, Henderson Z. Pregnancy-related mortality in the United States, 1998 to 2005. Obstet Gynecol. 2010;116(6):1302–9. https://doi.org/10.1097/AOG.0b013e3181fdfb11.
37. Creanga AA, Berg CJ, Syverson C, Seed K, Bruce FC, Callaghan WM. Pregnancy-related mortality in the United States, 2006–2010. Obstet Gynecol. 2015;125(1):5–12. https://doi.org/10.1097/AOG.0000000000000564.
38. Callaghan WM, Creanga AA, Kuklina EV. Severe maternal morbidity among delivery and postpartum hospitalizations in the United States. Obstet Gynecol. 2012;120(5):1029–36. https://doi.org/10.1097/AOG.0b013e31826d60c5.
39. Heit JA, Kobbervig CE, James AH, Petterson TM, Bailey KR, Melton LJ. Trends in the incidence of venous thromboembolism during pregnancy or postpartum: a 30-year population-based study. Ann Intern Med. 2005;143(10):697–706. https://doi.org/10.7326/0003-4819-143-10-200511150-00006.
40. James AH. Pregnancy-associated thrombosis. Hematology Am Soc Hematol Educ Program. 2009;2009(1):277–85. https://doi.org/10.1182/asheducation-2009.1.277.
41. Bremme KA. Haemostatic changes in pregnancy. Best Pract Res Clin Haematol. 2003;16(2):153–68. https://doi.org/10.1053/ybeha.2003.260.
42. Clark P, Brennand J, Conkie JA, McCall F, Greer IA, Walker ID. Activated protein C sensitivity, protein C, protein S and coagulation in normal pregnancy. Thromb Haemost. 1998;79(6):1166–70.
43. Bourjeily G, Paidas M, Khalil H, Rosene-Montella K, Rodger M. Pulmonary embolism in pregnancy. Lancet. 2010;375(9713):500–12. https://doi.org/10.1016/S0140-6736(09)60996-X.
44. Macklon NS, Greer IA, Bowman AW. An ultrasound study of gestational and postural changes in the deep venous system of the leg in pregnancy. Br J Obstet Gynaecol. 1997;104(2):191–7.

45. Macklon NS, Greer IA. The deep venous system in the puerperium: an ultrasound study. Br J Obstet Gynaecol. 1997;104(2):198–200.
46. Renault K, Nørgaard K, Andreasen KR, Secher NJ, Nilas L. Physical activity during pregnancy in obese and normal-weight women as assessed by pedometer. Acta Obstet Gynecol Scand. 2010;89(7):956–61. https://doi.org/10.3109/00016341003792459.
47. Hegewald MJ, Crapo RO. Respiratory physiology in pregnancy. Clin Chest Med. 2011;32(1):1–13–vii. https://doi.org/10.1016/j.ccm.2010.11.001.
48. Malatesha G, Singh NK, Bharija A, Rehani B, Goel A. Comparison of arterial and venous pH, bicarbonate, PCO2 and PO2 in initial emergency department assessment. Emerg Med J. 2007;24(8):569–71. https://doi.org/10.1136/emj.2007.046979.
49. Middleton P, Kelly AM, Brown J, Robertson M. Agreement between arterial and central venous values for pH, bicarbonate, base excess, and lactate. Emerg Med J. 2006;23(8):622–4. https://doi.org/10.1136/emj.2006.035915.
50. Genest J. The atrial natriuretic factor. Br Heart J. 1986;56(4):302–16.
51. Hameed AB, Chan K, Ghamsary M, Elkayam U. Longitudinal changes in the B-type natriuretic peptide levels in normal pregnancy and postpartum. Clin Cardiol. 2009;32(8):E60–2. https://doi.org/10.1002/clc.20391.
52. Kim HN, Januzzi JL. Natriuretic peptide testing in heart failure. Circulation. 2011;123(18):2015–9. https://doi.org/10.1161/CIRCULATIONAHA.110.979500.
53. Silvers SM, Howell JM, Kosowsky JM, Rokos IC, Jagoda AS. Clinical policy: critical issues in the evaluation and management of adult patients presenting to the emergency department with acute heart failure syndromes. Ann Emerg Med. 2007;49(5):627–69. https://doi.org/10.1016/j.annemergmed.2006.10.024.
54. Weber M. Role of B-type natriuretic peptide (BNP) and NT-proBNP in clinical routine. Heart. 2005;92(6):843–9. https://doi.org/10.1136/hrt.2005.071233.
55. Forster O, Hilfiker-Kleiner D, Ansari AA, et al. Reversal of IFN-γ, oxLDL and prolactin serum levels correlate with clinical improvement in patients with peripartum cardiomyopathy. Eur J Heart Fail. 2014;10(9):861–8. https://doi.org/10.1016/j.ejheart.2008.07.005.
56. Gaggin HK, Januzzi JL. Natriuretic peptides in heart failure and acute coronary syndrome. Clin Lab Med. 2014;34(1):43–58–vi. https://doi.org/10.1016/j.cll.2013.11.007.

57. Klok FA, Mos ICM, Huisman MV. Brain-type natriuretic peptide levels in the prediction of adverse outcome in patients with pulmonary embolism. Am J Respir Crit Care Med. 2008;178(4):425–30. https://doi.org/10.1164/rccm.200803-459OC.
58. Verschuren F, Bonnet M, Benoit M-O, et al. The prognostic value of pro-B-type natriuretic peptide in acute pulmonary embolism. Thromb Res. 2013;131(6):e235–9. https://doi.org/10.1016/j.thromres.2013.03.009.
59. Kabrhel C, Okechukwu I, Hariharan P, et al. Factors associated with clinical deterioration shortly after PE. Thorax. 2014;69(9):835–42. https://doi.org/10.1136/thoraxjnl-2013-204762.
60. Hollander JE. Managing Troponin Testing. Ann Emerg Med. 2016;68(6):690–4. https://doi.org/10.1016/j.annemergmed.2016.05.023.
61. Becattini C, Vedovati MC, Agnelli G. Prognostic value of troponins in acute pulmonary embolism: a meta-analysis. Circulation. 2007;116(4):427–33. https://doi.org/10.1161/CIRCULATIONAHA.106.680421.
62. Kline JA. D-dimer concentrations in normal pregnancy: new diagnostic thresholds are needed. Clin Chem. 2005;51(5):825–9. https://doi.org/10.1373/clinchem.2004.044883.
63. Kovac M, Mikovic Z, Rakicevic L, et al. The use of D-dimer with new cutoff can be useful in diagnosis of venous thromboembolism in pregnancy. Eur J Obstet Gynecol Reprod Biol. 2010;148(1):27–30. https://doi.org/10.1016/j.ejogrb.2009.09.005.
64. Orman R. Pulmonary embolism in pregnancy with Jeff Kline. ERCast. http://blog.ercast.org/pulmonary-embolism-in-pregnancy/. Published April 23, 2013. Accessed 6 Jan 2018.
65. Harrigan RA, Jones K. ABC of clinical electrocardiography. Conditions affecting the right side of the heart. BMJ. 2002;324(7347):1201–4.
66. Sreeram N, Cheriex EC, Smeets JL, Gorgels AP, Wellens HJ. Value of the 12-lead electrocardiogram at hospital admission in the diagnosis of pulmonary embolism. AJC. 1994;73(4):298–303.
67. Leung AN, Bull TM, Jaeschke R, et al. An official American Thoracic Society/Society of Thoracic Radiology clinical practice guideline: evaluation of suspected pulmonary embolism in pregnancy. Am J Respir Crit Care Med. 2011;184(10):1200–8. https://doi.org/10.1164/rccm.201108-1575ST.
68. Committee on Obstetric Practice. Committee opinion no. 723: guidelines for diagnostic imaging during pregnancy and lacta-

tion. Obstet Gynecol. 2017;130(4):e210–6. https://doi.org/10.1097/AOG.0000000000002355.
69. Shahir K, Goodman LR, Tali A, Thorsen KM, Hellman RS. Pulmonary embolism in pregnancy: CT pulmonary angiography versus perfusion scanning. Am J Roentgenol. 2010;195(3):W214–20. https://doi.org/10.2214/AJR.09.3506.
70. Cahill AG, Stout MJ, Macones GA, Bhalla S. Diagnosing pulmonary embolism in pregnancy using computed-tomographic angiography or ventilation-perfusion. Obstet Gynecol. 2009;114(1):124–9. https://doi.org/10.1097/AOG.0b013e3181a99def.
71. Ridge CA, McDermott S, Freyne BJ, Brennan DJ, Collins CD, Skehan SJ. Pulmonary embolism in pregnancy: comparison of pulmonary CT angiography and lung scintigraphy. Am J Roentgenol. 2009;193(5):1223–7. https://doi.org/10.2214/AJR.09.2360.
72. Greer IA. The acute management of thrombosis and embolism during pregnancy and the puerperium. London; 2007. p. 1–17.
73. Bourjeily G, Chalhoub M, Phornphutkul C, Alleyne TC, Woodfield CA, Chen KK. Neonatal thyroid function: effect of a single exposure to iodinated contrast medium in utero. Radiology. 2010;256(3):744–50. https://doi.org/10.1148/radiol.10100163.
74. Thompson AJ, Greer IA. Thromboembolic disease in pregnancy and the puerperium: acute management. London: Royal College of Obstetricians & Gynaecologists; 2015. p. 1–32.
75. James A, Committee on Practice Bulletins—Obstetrics. Practice bulletin no. 123: thromboembolism in pregnancy. Obstet Gynecol. 2011;118(3):718–29. https://doi.org/10.1097/AOG.0b013e3182310c4c.
76. Tayal VS, Raio C. Ultrasound guidelines: emergency, point-of-care and clinical ultrasound guidelines in medicine. Ann Emerg Med. 2017;69(5):e27–54. https://doi.org/10.1016/j.annemergmed.2016.08.457.
77. Douglas PS, Garcia MJ, Haines DE, et al. ACCF/ASE/AHA/ASNC/HFSA/HRS/SCAI/SCCM/SCCT/SCMR 2011 appropriate use criteria for echocardiography. JAC. 2011;57(9):1126–66. https://doi.org/10.1016/j.jacc.2010.11.002.
78. Jaff MR, McMurtry MS, Archer SL, et al. Management of massive and submassive pulmonary embolism, iliofemoral deep vein thrombosis, and chronic thromboembolic pulmonary hypertension: a scientific statement from the American Heart Association. Circulation. 2011;123(16):1788–830. https://doi.org/10.1161/CIR.0b013e318214914f.

79. Meredith EL, Masani ND. Echocardiography in the emergency assessment of acute aortic syndromes. Eur J Echocardiogr. 2009;10(1):i31–9. https://doi.org/10.1093/ejechocard/jen251.
80. Guntupalli KK, Hall N, Karnad DR, Bandi V, Belfort M. Critical illness in pregnancy: part I: an approach to a pregnant patient in the ICU and common obstetric disorders. Chest. 2015;148(4):1093–104. https://doi.org/10.1378/chest.14-1998.
81. Guntupalli KK, Karnad DR, Bandi V, Hall N, Belfort M. Critical illness in pregnancy: part II: common medical conditions complicating pregnancy and puerperium. Chest. 2015;148(5):1333–45. https://doi.org/10.1378/chest.14-2365.
82. Munnur U, de Boisblanc B, Suresh MS. Airway problems in pregnancy. Crit Care Med. 2005;33(Supplement):S259–68. https://doi.org/10.1097/01.CCM.0000183502.45419.C9.
83. Pilkington S, Carli F, Dakin MJ, et al. Increase in Mallampati score during pregnancy. Br J Anaesth. 1995;74(6):638–42.
84. Lewin SB, Cheek TG, Deutschman CS. Airway management in the obstetric patient. Crit Care Clin. 2000;16(3):505–13.
85. Jeejeebhoy FM, Zelop CM, Lipman S, et al. Cardiac arrest in pregnancy: a scientific statement from the American Heart Association. Circulation. 2015;132(18):1747–73. https://doi.org/10.1161/CIR.0000000000000300.
86. Rodger M. Evidence base for the management of venous thromboembolism in pregnancy. Hematology Am Soc Hematol Educ Program. 2010;2010(1):173–80. https://doi.org/10.1182/asheducation-2010.1.173.
87. Akgün KM, Crothers K, Pisani M. Epidemiology and management of common pulmonary diseases in older persons. J Gerontol A Biol Sci Med Sci. 2012;67((3):276–91. https://doi.org/10.1093/gerona/glr251.
88. Tang A-W, Greer I. A systematic review on the use of new anticoagulants in pregnancy. Obstet Med. 2013;6(2):64–71. https://doi.org/10.1177/1753495x12472642.
89. Wiesen MHJ, Blaich C, Müller C, Streichert T, Pfister R, Michels G. The direct factor Xa inhibitor rivaroxaban passes into human breast milk. Chest. 2016;150(1):e1–4. https://doi.org/10.1016/j.chest.2016.01.021.
90. Paul D Stein MDF, JWH MS. Prevalence of acute pulmonary embolism among patients in a general hospital and at autopsy. Chest. 2015;108(4):978–81. https://doi.org/10.1378/chest.108.4.978.

91. Horlocker TT, Wedel DJ, Rowlingson JC, et al. Regional anesthesia in the patient receiving antithrombotic or thrombolytic therapy. Reg Anesth Pain Med. 2010;35(1):64–101. https://doi.org/10.1097/AAP.0b013e3181c15c70.
92. James AH. Prevention and treatment of venous thromboembolism in pregnancy. Clin Obstet Gynecol. 2012;55(3):774–87. https://doi.org/10.1097/GRF.0b013e31825cfe7b.
93. Nelson-Piercy C, Maccallum P, Mackillop L. Reducing the risk of venous thromboembolism during pregnancy and the puerperium. 3rd ed: Royal College of Obstetricians and Gynaecologists; 2015. p. 1–40. https://www.rcog.org.uk/globalassets/documents/guidelines/gtg-37b.pdf.
94. Clive Kearon MP, Elie A, Akl MMP, Joseph Ornelas P, et al. Antithrombotic therapy for VTE disease: CHEST guideline. CHEST. 2015:1–122. https://doi.org/10.1016/j.chest.2015.11.026.
95. Chatterjee S, Chakraborty A, Weinberg I, et al. Thrombolysis for pulmonary embolism and risk of all-cause mortality, major bleeding, and intracranial hemorrhage: a meta-analysis. JAMA. 2014;311(23):2414–21. https://doi.org/10.1001/jama.2014.5990.
96. Hao Q, Dong BR, Yue J, Wu T, Liu GJ. Thrombolytic therapy for pulmonary embolism. Cochrane Vascular Group, ed. Cochrane Database Syst Rev. 2015;125(9):CD004437. https://doi.org/10.1002/14651858.CD004437.pub4.
97. Linnemann B, Scholz U, Rott H, et al. Treatment of pregnancy-associated venous thromboembolism – position paper from the Working Group in Women's Health of the Society of Thrombosis and Haemostasis (GTH). Vasa. 2016;45(2):103–18. https://doi.org/10.1024/0301-1526/a000504.
98. Açar G, Şimşek Z, Avci A, et al. Right heart free-floating thrombus in a pregnant woman with massive pulmonary embolism. J Cardiovasc Med. 2015;16:S51–4. https://doi.org/10.2459/JCM.0b013e32834036b4.
99. Lonjaret L, Lairez O, Galinier M, Minville V. Thrombolysis by recombinant tissue plasminogen activator during pregnancy: a case of massive pulmonary embolism. Am J Emerg Med. 2011;29(6):694.e1–2. https://doi.org/10.1016/j.ajem.2010.05.022.
100. Holden EL, Ranu H, Sheth A, Shannon MS, Madden BP. Thrombolysis for massive pulmonary embolism in pregnancy – a report of three cases and follow up over a two year period. Thromb Res. 2011;127(1):58–9. https://doi.org/10.1016/j.thromres.2010.06.003.

101. Raa te GD, Ribbert LSM, Snijder RJ, Biesma DH. Treatment options in massive pulmonary embolism during pregnancy; a case-report and review of literature. Thromb Res. 2009;124(1):1–5. https://doi.org/10.1016/j.thromres.2009.03.001.
102. Turrentine MA, Braems G, Ramirez MM. Use of thrombolytics for the treatment of thromboembolic disease during pregnancy. Obstet Gynecol Surv. 1995;50(7):534–41.
103. Ahearn GS, Hadjiliadis D, Govert JA, Tapson VF. Massive pulmonary embolism during pregnancy successfully treated with recombinant tissue plasminogen activator: a case report and review of treatment options. Arch Intern Med. 2002;162(11):1221–7. https://doi.org/10.1001/archinte.162.11.1221.
104. Regitz-Zagrosek V, Blomstrom Lundqvist C, Borghi C, et al. ESC guidelines on the management of cardiovascular diseases during pregnancy: the task force on the management of cardiovascular diseases during pregnancy of the European Society of Cardiology (ESC). Eur Heart J. 2011;32(24):3147–97. https://doi.org/10.1093/eurheartj/ehr218.
105. Konstantinides SV, Torbicki A, Agnelli G, et al. 2014 ESC guidelines on the diagnosis and management of acute pulmonary embolism. Eur Heart J. 2014;35(43):3033–69–3069a–k. https://doi.org/10.1093/eurheartj/ehu283.
106. Konstantinides SV, Vicaut E, Danays T, et al. Impact of thrombolytic therapy on the long-term outcome of intermediate-risk pulmonary embolism. J Am Coll Cardiol. 2017;69(12):1536–44. https://doi.org/10.1016/j.jacc.2016.12.039.
107. Mostafa A, Briasoulis A, Telila T, Belgrave K, Grines C. Treatment of massive or submassive acute pulmonary embolism with catheter-directed thrombolysis. Am J Cardiol. 2016;117(6):1014–20. https://doi.org/10.1016/j.amjcard.2015.12.041.
108. Kuo WT, Banerjee A, Kim PS, et al. Pulmonary embolism response to fragmentation, embolectomy, and catheter thrombolysis (PERFECT): initial results from a prospective multicenter registry. Chest. 2015;148(3):667–73. https://doi.org/10.1378/chest.15-0119.
109. Kucher N, Boekstegers P, Muller OJ, et al. Randomized, controlled trial of ultrasound-assisted catheter-directed thrombolysis for acute intermediate-risk pulmonary embolism. Circulation. 2014;129(4):479–86. https://doi.org/10.1161/CIRCULATIONAHA.113.005544.
110. Arora S, Panaich SS, Ainani N, et al. Comparison of in-hospital outcomes and readmission rates in acute pulmo-

nary embolism between systemic and catheter-directed thrombolysis (from the National Readmission Database). Am J Cardiol. 2017;120(9):1653–61. https://doi.org/10.1016/j.amjcard.2017.07.066.

111. Kuo WT, Gould MK, Louie JD, Rosenberg JK, Sze DY, Hofmann LV. Catheter-directed therapy for the treatment of massive pulmonary embolism: systematic review and meta-analysis of modern techniques. J Vasc Interv Radiol. 2009;20(11):1431–40. https://doi.org/10.1016/j.jvir.2009.08.002.
112. Sauer CM, Yuh DD, Bonde P. Extracorporeal membrane oxygenation use has increased by 433% in adults in the United States from 2006 to 2011. ASAIO J. 2015;61(1):31–6. https://doi.org/10.1097/MAT.0000000000000160.
113. Squiers JJ, Lima B, DiMaio JM. Contemporary extracorporeal membrane oxygenation therapy in adults: fundamental principles and systematic review of the evidence. J Thorac Cardiovasc Surg. 2016;152(1):20–32. https://doi.org/10.1016/j.jtcvs.2016.02.067.
114. Ventetuolo CE, Muratore CS. Extracorporeal life support in critically ill adults. Am J Respir Crit Care Med. 2014;190(5):497–508. https://doi.org/10.1164/rccm.201404-0736CI.
115. Saad AF, Rahman M, Maybauer DM, et al. Extracorporeal membrane oxygenation in pregnant and postpartum women with H1N1-related acute respiratory distress syndrome. Obstet Gynecol. 2016;127(2):241–7. https://doi.org/10.1097/AOG.0000000000001236.

Chapter 18
Challenges in Oxygenation and Ventilation

Julia West and Caroline M. Quill

Case Part 1

A 44-year-old woman presents to the emergency department with a chief complaint of dyspnea and fever which developed over the course of 3 days. Associated symptoms include rhinorrhea, sore throat, nonproductive cough, noisy breathing, and sensation of chest tightness. On presentation she is most anxious about her breathing which she describes as "difficult." Her past medical history is notable for obesity, HTN, type 2 diabetes, and seasonal allergies. She works in a printing shop, smokes 1/2 PPD of cigarettes, reports occasional social alcohol consumption, and denies any history of drug use. Her family history is notable for breast cancer in her mother and childhood asthma in a sister. Current medications include lisinopril, metformin, atorvastatin, and Tylenol. Vitals show T 39.2 C, HR 116, BP 132/84, RR 28, and SpO2 92%. On exam, she is moderately dyspneic with conversation and appears tired but is alert, with yellow nasal congestion, erythematous posterior OP, 2+ tender cervical LAD bilaterally, tachypneic with decreased air movement bilaterally, diffuse expiratory

J. West · C. M. Quill (✉)
Division of Pulmonary and Critical Care Medicine,
University of Rochester Medical Center, Rochester, NY, USA
e-mail: Caroline_Quill@URMC.Rochester.edu

J. A. LaRosa (ed.), *Adult Critical Care Medicine*,
https://doi.org/10.1007/978-3-319-94424-1_18

wheezing and prolonged exhalation, tachycardic with regular rhythm without murmur, warm and well perfused with flushed appearance, with no peripheral edema. Initial labs are notable for BUN 32, Cr 1.5, WBC 17 with 70% neutrophils, and PLT 480. A VBG shows 7.24/58/40/18, with a lactate of 1.3. PA, and lateral chest X-ray shows mild bilateral perihilar cuffing without focal infiltrate.

Respiratory failure is a common reason for critical care evaluation and ICU admission and invokes a broad differential. Respiratory failure is commonly categorized into four "types" – hypoxemic, hypercapnic, postoperative, and respiratory failure due to shock [1]. There is frequently overlap among the various types of respiratory failure, but it is important to recognize all the contributing etiologies to respiratory failure in each case in order to identify and reverse all pathologies.

This patient presents with dyspnea associated with abnormal ventilation, including wheezing with diminished air movement on exam and acute hypercapnia on venous blood gas: this is a case of type 2 (hypercapnic/ventilatory) respiratory failure. In this case, the clinical exam suggests impaired ventilation, occurring at the level of the small airways. Similar hypercapnic respiratory failure can develop due to impairment in ventilation at any level within the respiratory tract and in some cases can develop in the setting of normal ventilation due instead to an acute ventilation-perfusion (VQ) mismatch such as with acute pulmonary artery obstruction associated with a pulmonary embolism.

The most common causes of type 2 respiratory failure are asthma exacerbation and COPD. In this case, the exam findings indicate a process of diffuse airway narrowing leading to wheezing, most consistent with lower airway bronchoconstriction. Without a prior diagnosis of asthma or COPD and in the setting of risk factors for both (allergies and family history of asthma being risk factors for asthma and tobacco exposure being the major risk factor for COPD), it may be difficult to immediately distinguish between an acute asthma and COPD exacerbation. Her response to therapy and clinical course, and ultimately pulmonary function testing after she has returned to her respiratory baseline, will assist with distinguishing between an underlying diagnosis of asthma and COPD.

If the patient did not have exam findings consistent with diffuse small airway airflow obstruction, the level of concern for alternative diagnoses would rise. Hypoventilation secondary to narcotic substance abuse is an increasingly common etiology of type 2 respiratory failure presenting to the ED as well as onset of type 2 respiratory failure during a hospitalization, and it should be suspected in the setting of decreased respiratory effort and somnolence on exam. This diagnosis is often confirmed by response to a trial of narcan therapy, with improvement in respiratory effort and mental status after narcan often significant enough to avoid intubation for their respiratory failure. Obtundation from other ingestion, injury, or syndrome may present similarly but would be unresponsive to narcan and require additional evaluation for determination of diagnosis and effective management.

Additional life-threatening causes of acute ventilatory dysfunction including pulmonary embolism, acute airway obstruction such as from a foreign body aspiration, acute diaphragm or respiratory muscle weakness, and pneumothorax. For an alert patient with diminished respiratory capability despite apparent good effort, diaphragm injury such as from spinal cord injury and viral or idiopathic phrenic nerve dysfunction can all present with type 2 respiratory failure in the setting of additional associated exam findings. Although many patients presenting with pneumothorax have a clinical history of trauma or predisposing factor such as Marfan syndrome or history of prior spontaneous pneumothorax, an asymmetric pulmonary exam with absent breath sounds on one side of the chest in any patient with acute respiratory changes should raise concern for the possibility of a pneumothorax. In cognitively intact adults, a history of a foreign body aspiration is typically available at the time of presentation; however in a patient with altered cognition, particularly if there is clinical suspicion for risk for aspiration, an asymmetric respiratory exam, upper airway stridor, and occasionally central airway or asymmetric wheezing could be concerning for foreign body aspiration with airway obstruction. If there is clinical uncertainty regarding obstructed airway vs pneumothorax contributing to absent breath sounds on exam, a chest X-ray demonstrating air within the thoracic cavity or hyper-expansion of one side or portion of the lung with or without a radiopaque foreign body can be confirmatory for pneumothorax or foreign body airway obstruction, respectively; if there is a high suspicion for either of these diagnoses in a clinically unstable patient, it is advisable to intervene clinically without waiting for confirmatory imaging, as this may be lifesaving particularly in the case of a tension pneumothorax. Often in the absence of focal exam findings to explain dyspnea with hypercapnia, and especially if a patient reports sudden onset or accompanying chest pain, pulmonary embolism should be considered. If considering pulmonary embolism in your differential, it is helpful to use the Wells criteria to assist with risk-stratifying your patient before choosing to proceed with a diagnostic evaluation for possible PE.

The broad differential for hypercapnic/ventilatory respiratory failure is often narrowed by clinical history and exam, and management may be focused once a thorough clinical evaluation has been completed and the diagnosis is determined. Asthma and COPD exacerbations are clinical diagnoses, and while chest imaging with chest X-ray is often obtained in the evaluation of acute dyspnea, clinical imaging is neither required nor confirmatory for these diagnoses. Chest imaging including chest X-ray, chest CT, or CT angiogram is often obtained in order to exclude an alternative cause for the patient's presentation and is frequently pursued in the absence of clinical history or findings consistent with asthma or COPD. Regardless of the etiology, a blood gas may differentiate between respiratory distress due to difficulty with work of breathing and type 2 respiratory failure associated with insufficient ventilation which would be identified based on respiratory acidosis with elevated PCo_2 and associated acidosis on blood gas. A venous blood sample, preferably a central venous blood sample, is sufficient for the assessment of ventilation, although an arterial blood gas may alternatively be used in a patient with no central access.

Once identified, management of type 2 respiratory failure should be tailored both to the etiology of hypercapnic/hypoventilatory respiratory failure, with, for instance, albuterol, ipratropium, steroids, and magnesium for an asthma exacerbation and to support of the ventilatory distress or impairment associated with the presentation. Respiratory support of ventilation in an alert patient is commonly provided with noninvasive positive pressure ventilation (NIPPV), specifically bi-level positive airway pressure (BIPAP), which provides mechanical assistance with effort of ventilation and which has the benefit of being easy to wean or interrupt in addition to being much more tolerable for many patients than traditional invasive ventilation. In the case of contraindications to NIPPV including a high risk for aspiration (particularly due to altered mental status), physical inability to wear a BIPAP mask due to abnormal facial structure, recent surgery or some overlying skin conditions, patient anxiety or intolerance to BIPAP, or inability to maintain effective ventilation while on BIPAP, the more traditional invasive ventilation with endotracheal intubation and mechanical ventilation may be required. A variety of modes of mechanical ventilation may be successfully used to treat hypercapnic/ventilatory respiratory failure which will not be outlined in depth here, but it is worth recalling that ventilation is determined primarily by tidal volume and respiratory rate [2]. The mainstay of ventilatory support for respiratory failure is volume-cycled, assist-control ventilation, in which providers can optimize expiratory time and enhance patient synchrony with the ventilator. In particular, modes which minimize exhalation such as APRV should be avoided for respiratory failure due to air trapping such as respiratory failure from asthma or COPD.

High-flow nasal cannula has recently come into vogue as a method of providing respiratory support and may be helpful for a patient experiencing type 2 respiratory distress associated with increased work of breathing; however it does not provide as much support as NIPPV with BIPAP, and ventilation cannot be adequately measured or ensured while on HFNC; therefore HFNC is not a preferred method of assisting ventilation in a patient with hypercapnic/hypoventilatory respiratory failure in the acute setting but may be better used as a method for weaning ventilatory support once their acute respiratory failure has been addressed. It is important to note that methods of respiratory support targeting oxygenation, specifically including nasal cannula, ventimask, non-rebreathers, and continuous positive airway pressure (CPAP), are ineffective alone in the management of type 2 respiratory failure as they do not support ventilation and may mask a patient's respiratory decline.

Long-term management for patients experiencing type 2 respiratory failure should include risk-factor modification to minimize the risk of recurrent respiratory failure. This may include intensified medical management of asthma with emphasis on implementation of an effective asthma action plan early in any future asthma exacerbations, or tobacco cessation counseling, medical management of nicotine addiction, and pulmonary rehab for patients with COPD. In some cases patients presenting with apparent acute type 2 respiratory failure may have some degree of untreated chronic hypercapnic respiratory failure to address particularly those with severe COPD or neuromuscular weakness. This should be assessed after they have returned to their previous baseline function but before they are discharged from the hospital, with additional blood gas testing demonstrating chronic hypercapnia. In these cases management with chronic noninvasive ventilatory support such as nocturnal BIPAP, or in severe cases and if maximal support is desired by the patient, tracheostomy, and home chronic ventilation in the case of neuromuscular disease, may be considered. Pulmonary consultation during their hospitalization and outpatient pulmonary clinic follow-up is important for patients who have experienced hypercapnic/hypoventilatory respiratory failure to help modify their disease course and optimize outpatient management in order to avoid recurrence of respiratory failure.

Case Part 2

AD, our 44-year-old patient, does well with BIPAP support and responds to treatment with prednisone and bronchodilator therapy for suspected asthma exacerbation associated with a viral respiratory tract infection and is weaned off of respiratory support and discharged home within a few days. She re-presents to the ED 1 week later complaining of worsening cough productive of thick yellow sputum, dyspnea with minimal exertion, pleuritic chest pain, fatigue, and recurrent fevers. Her medical history and exposures are unchanged. This time, vitals show T 40.3 C, HR 135, BP 92/45, RR 30, and SpO_2 78% on room air which improves to 90% on 50% ventimask. On exam, she is ill appearing, flushed and fatigued, oriented to person and place but not date, with tacky mucous membranes, clear nares, tachypneic and speaking in short sentences with decreased breath sounds in the right lower lung field, diffuse inspiratory crackles and no wheezing, tachycardia with regular rhythm and no murmur, with a soft and non-tender abdomen, and no peripheral edema or extremity tenderness. Labs are notable for BUN 45, Cr 2.7, WBC 17 with 86% neutrophils and 12% bands, and PLT 130. An ABG shows 7.45/24/50/16, with arterial lactate of 2.8. PA, and lateral chest X-ray shows a dense, focal consolidation in the right lower lobe and diffuse fluffy infiltrates scattered throughout all lobes.

Although AD's chief complaint of dyspnea and fever is the same as with her first presentation, her second presentation differs significantly from her prior illness. Her respiratory distress is now associated with hypoxia, and her arterial blood gas demonstrates significant hypoxia, particularly notable as it was obtained while she was on a 50% ventimask, as well as a respiratory alkalosis developing in the setting of increased work of breathing and elevated minute ventilation. In contrast to her first presentation, this is hypoxic, or type 1, respiratory failure. As you will recall, type 2 respiratory failure is hypercapnic/ventilatory respiratory failure and may present with normal or only mild abnormalities in oxygenation, type 3 respiratory failure may be hypoxic but is secondary to postoperative atelectasis, and type 4 respiratory failure is secondary to shock (which is not present here). If she had a concurrent asthma exacerbation leading to hypercapnic respiratory failure in addition to her hypoxic respiratory failure, as many patients with underlying obstructive lung disease do, that could be referred to as a mixed (type 1 and type 2) respiratory failure.

The differential for type 1 or hypoxic respiratory failure is quite broad and includes many infectious and noninfectious processes. AD presents with many symptoms of acute infection including fever, tachycardia, leukocytosis, bandemia, ill appearance, and purulent mucous production with a focal infiltrate on her chest imaging concerning for infectious process including bacterial pneumonia. AD has risk factors for bacterial pneumonia as her recent viral illness places her at risk for development of a secondary bacterial pneumonia during the 1–2 weeks after a viral respiratory illness, as do her recent hospitalization and her suspected underlying lung disease (either asthma or COPD.) In the setting of presentation with sepsis and acute respiratory failure, pneumonia must remain high on the differential until there is diagnostic certainty in a noninfectious source for the respiratory disease. Additional infectious concerns for acute type 1 respiratory failure include viral pneumonia, which can mimic a bacterial process with a focal infiltrate on chest imaging or present with more diffuse interstitial or inflammatory changes, and atypical pneumonias including legionella and mycoplasma which can also present with sepsis, rapid progression, and consolidative lung findings. In cases of more indolent development or the presence of an immunocompromised host, fungal infections including invasive aspergillus, histoplasma and cryptococcal infection, and mycobacterial infections including *Mycobacterium avium complex* and tuberculosis should also be considered. A common pneumonia mimic is aspiration pneumonitis, which may or may not be followed by development of true bacterial aspiration pneumonia and in either case may lead to prolonged and recurrent respiratory distress. There are rare, noninfectious pulmonary processes which may also present in a similar fashion to acute bacterial pneumonia including hypersensitivity pneumonitis and eosinophilic pneumonia; however infectious processes should be comprehensively excluded prior to proceeding with evaluation or treatment for these pulmonary zebras.

Patients presenting with hypoxic respiratory failure without symptoms of acute infection, often with chest imaging concerning for alternative explanations for hypoxia or with illness refractory to treatment for initially suspected infectious process, may exhibit a variety of other structural, obstructive, infiltrative, or alveolar filling processes, or increasingly significantly, inflammatory lung diseases including acute respiratory distress syndrome. Unlike in the case of hypercapnic respiratory failure, chest imaging may be particularly useful in their evaluation and is often necessary in order to prioritize a differential and decide on a rational management approach. Lung masses may be suspected based on chest X-ray imaging and are often best clarified on chest CT imaging, with hypoxic respiratory failure often resulting from post-obstructive pneumonia or atelectasis distal to a solid lung mass associated with airway compression from the mass and/or due to a large volume of lung destroyed by a mass or masses. Absence of lung aeration due to a pleural effusion(s) significant enough to cause hypoxia can be easily visualized with chest X-ray or bedside ultrasound, typically presenting without mediastinal shift, while mucous plugging of medium to large airways leading to hypoxia from associated atelectasis will demonstrate collapsed lobar or peripheral lung regions with absence of aeration and mediastinal shift toward the affected side of the chest. Diagnosis of many less common infiltrative processes such as sarcoidosis, bronchiolitis obliterans, vasculitic lung diseases, or bronchoalveolar carcinoma will rely heavily on unusual imaging findings such as tissue infiltration along airways and diffuse pulmonary nodules as well as clinical suspicion based on the presence of specific risk factors for disease or associated clinical findings, and patients will carry a heavy burden of disease before developing hypoxic respiratory failure. More chronic inflammatory lung diseases are often known based on prior chest imaging, although acute flares of ILD can present with acute inflammatory changes on a background of chronic fibrotic disease. Alveolar filling processes may be focal such as from focal pulmonary bleeding often presenting as hemoptysis with hypoxia, perhaps from a lung mass or a pulmonary AVM or infectious irritation of the airways, or diffuse such as from diffuse alveolar hemorrhage, pulmonary edema including from CHF exacerbations, pulmonary contusions, or drowning injury, or in the case of another pulmonary zebra, pulmonary alveolar proteinosis.

Management of hypoxic respiratory failure relies on treatment or reversal of the underlying process, as well as respiratory support during the course of illness. In the case of a suspected infectious process, early antibiotics targeted to the identified infectious process are a mainstay of therapy. Testing including sputum bacterial culture and gram stain, evaluation for viral respiratory pathogens, and frequently urine antigens for legionella and pneumonia may confirm an infectious etiology although they are often less than 100% sensitive due to sampling error and limitations in detecting all relevant infectious pathogens. Unfortunately, the serum biomarker procalcitonin has not been validated in the diagnosis of infection in the critically ill patient and should not be independently used to guide decisions regarding treatment of possible infectious process, although some data suggest that in a recuperating patient, a declining procalcitonin may be used to assist with decisions regarding completion of shorter rather than longer antibiotic courses. In cases of suspected unusual pulmonary infections where a pathogen has not been identified, additional diagnostic testing may be pursued with bronchoscopy for biologic specimens through bronchoalveolar lavage, bronchial brushings, or transbronchial biopsy.

Diagnostic bronchoscopy, which may be performed by a pulmonary trained physician and by many critical care trained physicians, is typically reserved for cases involving a high suspicion for fungal or other unusual infections, complicated infections occurring in immunocompromised patients, or when there is a high suspicion for a noninfectious process, and it is deemed important to exclude infection before proceeding with immunosuppressive or other involved treatment. Bronchoalveolar lavage may also be diagnostic for diffuse alveolar hemorrhage. Therapeutic bronchoscopy by an interventional pulmonologist may be considered in cases where a pulmonary lesion such as a mass or foreign body is causing respiratory failure due to airway obstruction or for evaluation and treatment of focal airway bleeding contributing to respiratory failure.

The initial goals of respiratory support include both alleviation of hypoxia and support for increased or inadequate work of breathing. In an awake patient without severe distress, CPAP therapy provides a quantifiable and titratable amount of positive end-expiratory pressure which serves to both recruit additional alveolar lung capacity and improve oxygen delivery across the pulmonary alveolar space, while allowing for escalation of the inspired fraction of oxygen up to 100%, and is often used first in the setting of escalating respiratory support in an ICU patient with hypoxic respiratory distress. Many patients requiring some lower levels of positive pressure support may benefit from high-flow nasal cannula which can be delivered at flow rates of up to 50 LPM with FiO_2 approaching 80–90%, and many patients feel less claustrophobic and experience less skin irritation and improved communication with care teams while on HFNC compared with CPAP. HFNC is limited in its ability to deliver PEEP relative to CPAP, and PEEP cannot be quantified while on HFNC. For patients whose oxygen requirement remains high (such as greater than 60%) while on CPAP at escalated levels despite initial treatment to stabilize disease who have unable to tolerate coming off of CPAP even briefly such as for medication administration, who have worsening mental status. Who are at risk for aspiration or emesis. or who have persistent hypoxia or are developing hypercapnic respiratory failure despite addition of BIPAP to support ventilation while receiving PAP therapy, intubation and full mechanical ventilation for definitive control of their respiratory status and high levels of respiratory support should be considered.

Benefits of intubation and full mechanical ventilation include definitive control of oxygenation without periods of interruption of PEEP; definitive control over minute ventilation and airway pressures, often allowing for escalation of PEEP beyond levels at which CPAP may be tolerable; and ability to provide sedation, minimize oxygen consumption by alleviating work of breathing, and if necessary proceed to paralysis for refractory hypoxia. With this approach, the toxicities associated with persistent lung and systemic hyperoxia including lung scarring and chronic respiratory insufficiency and increased mortality may be minimized [3]. Generally acceptable oxygenation goals for an acutely ill patient vary based on the presence of known chronic lung disease such as COPD or interstitial lung disease as well as the severity of illness and relative risk of increased oxygenation support. Goal peripheral oxygen saturations in a patient with COPD are typically >88%, while we often target a goal peripheral saturation of 94–96% corresponding with PaO_2 on ABGs between 70 and 90 in a patient with presumably healthy lung function at baseline. In respiratory failure requiring intubation, arterial blood gas PaO_2 in the 60s may be tolerated if there is increased concern for long-term harm in maintaining FiO_2 greater than 60% or in increasing airway pressures due to risk of barotrauma. Intubation also allows for improved airway clearance compared with CPAP therapy where PEEP is applied without access for endotracheal suctioning of secretions. An important benefit of intubation includes more accurate monitoring and improved control over air flow and airway pressures, beneficial data for which is best established in the setting of ARDS as detailed below.

The most common inflammatory lung disease confounding acute respiratory failure stemming from many sources and independently responsible for acute hypoxic respiratory failure in patients with many initially non-pulmonary ailments, which is a significant contributor to morbidity and mortality in the ICU, is most certainly ARDS, or acute respiratory distress syndrome. ARDS was first described in 1967 [4]; however increasingly robust data has been published on best practices for management of ARDS with a goal of minimizing mortality and pulmonary morbidity for survivors, and it is important for any provider taking care of critically ill patients to be well versed in diagnosis and best-practice management of this process. ARDS is best defined by the Berlin criteria as acute onset (within 7 days) of respiratory inflammatory disease with impaired oxygenation and bilateral pulmonary opacities on chest imaging not better explained by heart failure, attributable to an inflammatory response triggered by an acute medical condition [5]. Specific diagnostic criteria include a calculated ratio of pulmonary arterial oxygen concentration from an arterial blood gas to inspired fraction of oxygen (PaO_2/FiO_2) of less than 300, measured while on a PEEP of 5 or greater. While ARDS can be stratified to mild, moderate, or severe based on PaO_2/FiO_2 ratios of 200–300, 100–200, and <100, practically, consideration for possible ARDS should be given early in any significant acute respiratory illness with respiratory insufficiency or failure. Given the long-term ramifications of lung damage associated with ARDS, any patient suspected to be developing ARDS can be managed under the general principles of ARDS care until ARDS has been excluded. These principles include minimization of barotrauma utilizing sedation combined with low tidal volume ventilation when intubated, avoidance of oxygen toxicity as outlined above, utilization of paralysis and prone positioning to optimize oxygenation while providing supportive care, and adherence to evidence-based limitations on the use of late steroid therapy and benefits of early ECMO in refractory ARDS.

The best data supporting the use of low tidal volume ventilation (LTVV) stems from a study demonstrating dramatically improved mortality and a shorter duration of respiratory failure performed by The Acute Respiratory Distress Syndrome Network and published in the New England Journal of Medicine in 2000 [6]. In this study a tidal volume of 6 ml/kg of ideal body weight or lower was targeted in order to minimize plateau pressures on the ventilator, with a goal of maintaining them below 30. As plateau pressures reflect pressure experienced at the level of the alveoli, this approach acts through reducing repetitive elevation of pressure in the inflamed alveolar and interstitial space. It is important to recognize that plateau pressures can only be adequately measured in a patient who is breathing passively on the ventilator and may be inaccurately measuring low in a patient with very stiff, non-complaint lungs who continues to actively breathe in with a negative inspiratory force while on the ventilator. Plateau pressures should be followed closely after intubation when intubation medications create a window of time with respiratory paralysis, with escalation of sedation as compliance with the ventilator is achieved, and with initiation of paralysis if that is indicated. Given the ability to minimize barotrauma by lowering tidal volumes while maintaining adequate ventilation by concurrently increasing the respiratory rate and accepting permissive hypercapnia and recently published data demonstrating no benefit for high-frequency oscillatory ventilation compared with conventional ventilation in ARDS, there is no longer a role for implementing oscillator-based ventilation for most severe hypoxic respiratory failure in the adult ICU [7].

There are two roles for instituting medical paralysis in the setting of ARDS, and this tool is most effective if implemented early in the course of ARDS. In a patient with profound hypoxia and high oxygen requirements, paralysis with continuous neuromuscular blockade such as with atracurium or cisatracurium infusions can decrease oxygen consumption, thereby improving sustained oxygenation of vital organs while allowing providers to avoid oxygen toxicity (again, with a goal of maintaining an FiO_2 of less than 60%

in the setting of acute lung inflammation). The second, and perhaps most important reason for paralyzing a patient with ARDS for long-term outcomes, is the ability to adequately control ventilation with dedicated attention to maintaining ventilatory compliance and achieving low tidal volume ventilation in an effort to minimize airway pressures and subsequently avoid barotrauma. Best practice is to optimize all other approaches to ARDS ventilatory management including escalated sedation in the first 12–24 h of respiratory failure and then move to paralysis if you are unable to achieve adequate supportive care within 24 h. After implementation, most patients benefit from remaining paralyzed for 2–3 days or longer while allowing time for ARDS to peak, with paralysis lifted when signs of improvement in oxygenation and lung compliance are seen [8].

After paralysis, two additional steps may be helpful for refractory hypoxia. Prone positioning can substantially improve oxygenation in ARDS by shifting the gradient of blood delivery. It should be approached in a methodical manner to minimize risk for extubation or dislodgment of lines during proning and requires adequate staffing to assist with the physical turning of the patient but is otherwise a low-tech intervention with a significant return. To be most effective, the prone position should be maintained for 16 h of the day, with a daily return to supine positioning to allow for attention to skin care and other patient needs. ECMO may also be employed in the setting of ARDS to provide adequate oxygenation and ventilation if a patient fails conventional ventilator strategies; however this should be considered as a bridge through an acute illness, or in rare cases of complex lung disease, a bridge to transplantation, and should not be used in the setting of irreversible lung disease unless transplantation is being actively pursued. In the CESAR study, investigators demonstrated that transfer of patients with severe but potentially reversible respiratory failure despite optimal conventional management to a center with ECMO capabilities improved survival without severe disability [9]. This study did exclude patients who required very high FiO_2

or PEEP for more than 7 days, and given this we would recommend starting discussions regarding potential need for ECMO early in cases of severe ARDS.

There are two strategies for treating ARDS for which there is limited or conflicting data. Flolan, a nebulized form of the vasodilator epoprostenil, can be effectively used to improve oxygen delivery in some patients with ARDS through focused vasodilatation of the pulmonary vasculature. It has a good safety profiles and is worth trying in the setting of refractory hypoxia or high oxygen requirements, but there is as yet no evidence that it improves clinically significant outcomes for patients with ARDS. Contrastingly, there is evidence that initiation of intravenous steroid therapy in ARDS, which had been hypothesized to reduce inflammation and improve long-term pulmonary recovery, significantly increases mortality, risk for infection, and recurrent respiratory failure in patients with ARDS [10]. The evidence of harm is most compelling when steroids were started more than 14 days into an ARDS course, and we therefore strongly advise against the use of steroid therapy for late ARDS and do not recommend routine empiric therapy with steroids for ARDS at any stage based on the current literature.

In cases of type 1 or hypoxic respiratory failure, the importance of attentive supportive care while treating the underlying process cannot be overstated. Although respiratory support with mechanical ventilation can be lifesaving for many of our critical care patients, the downstream complications of positive pressure mechanical ventilation can lead to long-lasting pulmonary dysfunction including weakness and lung scarring. Many patients require substantial time for pulmonary recuperation following cases of severe respiratory failure or prolonged ventilation. Transition from traditional endotracheal intubation to tracheostomy can be considered early for patients who are likely to require a lengthy period of respiratory support and/or prolonged wean off of the ventilator and may help with active rehabilitation. Many patients' oxygen requirement may persist after cases of severe ARDS due to lung scarring, although with time a substantial number of patients discharged on home oxygen may also be able to wean off of this. Patients with any residual pulmonary disease such as an oxygen requirement will also benefit from outpatient pulmonary follow-up after discharge.

AD's second presentation is clinically concerning by history and exam for secondary bacterial pneumonia after a recent viral illness, with severity of illness, degree of hypoxia, and bilateral infiltrates all concerning for development of ARDS in the setting of pneumonia. In her case, she would likely benefit from a lung protective strategy starting with intubation and low tidal volume ventilation with minimization of barotrauma and oxygen toxicity as outlined above.

Summary

Respiratory failure is a heterogeneous diagnosis, and a structured approach involving differentiation into type 1 vs type 2 respiratory failure, a broad differential narrowed based on a thorough clinical evaluation and history as well as response to treatment, and close attention to changes in your patient in response to respiratory support are all critical to successful management of respiratory failure in the ICU. Differentiating between a need for ventilatory support versus enhanced oxygen support can assist with triaging patients in need of critical care evaluation or treatment to the timely support they need. In many cases, the foundation of management of respiratory failure is supportive care while allowing time for treatment or resolution of an underlying pulmonary insult, and this is a critical period during which adherence to best practices in respiratory support can minimize mortality and optimize long-term pulmonary outcomes. There have been many unexpected findings in research into respiratory failure including ARDS, and the importance of following evidence-based recommendations in order to avoid iatrogenic harm while treating respiratory failure cannot be overstated. Exciting new research continues to expand our capabilities in this field and enhance respiratory outcomes for our critically ill patients each year.

References

1. Hall JB, Schmidt GA, Wood LDH. Principles of critical care. 3rd ed. New York: McGraw-Hill, Medical Pub. Division; 2005.
2. West JB, West JB. Pulmonary pathophysiology–the essentials. 5th ed. Baltimore: Williams & Wilkins; 1998.
3. Girardis M, Busani S, Damiani E, Donati A, Rinaldi L, Marudi A, et al. Effect of conservative vs conventional oxygen therapy on mortality among patients in an intensive care unit: the oxygen-ICU randomized clinical trial. JAMA. 2016;316(15):1583–9. https://doi.org/10.1001/jama.2016.11993.
4. Ashbaugh DG, Bigelow DB, Petty TL, Levine BE. Acute respiratory distress in adults. Lancet. 1967;2(7511):319–23.
5. The ARDS Definition Task Force. Acute respiratory distress dyndrome the berlin definition. JAMA. 2012;307(23):2526–33. https://doi.org/10.1001/jama.2012.5669.
6. Acute Respiratory Distress Syndrome N, Brower RG, Matthay MA, Morris A, Schoenfeld D, Thompson BT, et al. Ventilation with lower tidal volumes as compared with traditional tidal volumes for acute lung injury and the acute respiratory distress syndrome. N Engl J Med. 2000;342(18):1301–8. https://doi.org/10.1056/NEJM200005043421801.
7. Lall R, Hamilton P, Young D, Hulme C, Hall P, Shah S, et al. A randomised controlled trial and cost-effectiveness analysis of high-frequency oscillatory ventilation against conventional artificial ventilation for adults with acute respiratory distress syndrome. The OSCAR (OSCillation in ARDS) study. Health Technol Assess. 2015;19(23):1–177, vii. https://doi.org/10.3310/hta19230.
8. Papazian L, Forel JM, Gacouin A, Penot-Ragon C, Perrin G, Loundou A, et al. Neuromuscular blockers in early acute respiratory distress syndrome. N Engl J Med. 2010;363(12):1107–16. https://doi.org/10.1056/NEJMoa1005372.
9. Peek GJ, Mugford M, Tiruvoipati R, Wilson A, Allen E, Thalanany MM, et al. Efficacy and economic assessment of conventional ventilatory support versus extracorporeal membrane oxygenation for severe adult respiratory failure (CESAR): a multicentre randomised controlled trial. Lancet. 2009;374(9698):1351–63. https://doi.org/10.1016/S0140-6736(09)61069-2.
10. Steinberg KP, Hudson LD, Goodman RB, Hough CL, Lanken PN, Hyzy R, et al. Efficacy and safety of corticosteroids for persistent acute respiratory distress syndrome. N Engl J Med. 2006;354(16):1671–84. https://doi.org/10.1056/NEJMoa051693.

Chapter 19
Poisoning and Toxicity: The New Age

Kim Kwai and Patrick Hinfey

Introduction

The approach to the hypotensive, bradycardic patient in the toxicologic setting can be complex, especially when the substance is unknown. The differential diagnosis is broad, but the approach to each patient remains the same.

Case Study

A 63-year-old female with a past medical history of hypertension, dementia, and depression presents to the emergency department with hypotension and bradycardia. The patient was "found down" outside her home by her husband who endorses that she has a history of suicide

K. Kwai (✉)
UC Davis Medical Center, Sacramento, CA, USA

P. Hinfey
Newark Beth Israel Medical Center, Newark, NJ, USA

J. A. LaRosa (ed.), *Adult Critical Care Medicine*,
https://doi.org/10.1007/978-3-319-94424-1_19

attempts in which she intentionally ingested several doses of her medications at once. He does not know her medications. Up until this point in time, the patient was in her usual state of health.

Vital Signs

BP: 70/40, HR 45, rr 15, and SpO2 96%
Fingerstick glucose: 200

Medications: unknown at this time
Past medical history: HTN, dementia, and depression
Past social history: previous history of recreational substance abuse
Past surgical history: none

Physical Exam

General appearance: somnolent, unable to answer questions, and minimally responsive to noxious stimuli.
Head: atraumatic and normocephalic.
Eyes: conjunctivae and corneas clear, 3 mm PERRL brisk, EOM's intact, and sclerae normal.
Ears: external inspection of the ears shows no abnormality.
Nose: normal.
Mouth: mucous membrane moist.
Neck: neck supple, no adenopathy, thyroid symmetric, normal size.
Heart: bradycardic rhythm, regular rate, no gallops, rubs, or murmurs.
Lungs: clear to auscultation and normal respiratory rate.
Abdomen: BS normal, abdomen soft, non-tender, no palpable bladder, no masses or organomegaly.
Skin: skin texture, turgor normal, no rashes or lesions, and axilla WNL.
Neuro: +2 patellar reflexes bilateral symmetrical, no clonus, and no rigidity.
Mental Status: unable to be assessed.
Musculoskeletal: no signs of trauma.

An EKG was obtained and is shown below (Fig. 19.1).

EKG

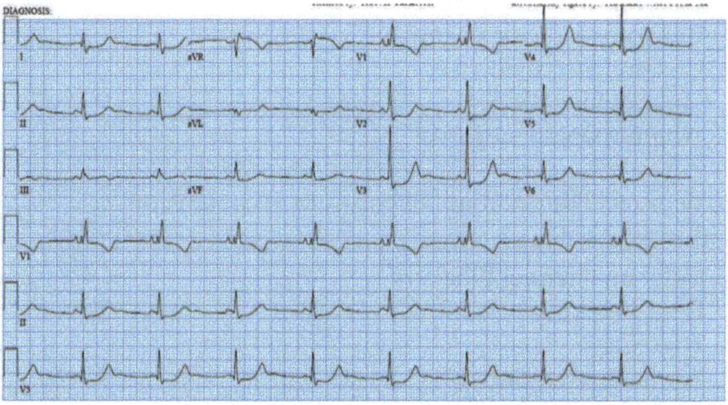

FIGURE 19.1 Sinus bradycardia 53, PR 108, QRS 116, QTc 493

Labwork

WBC 7.3, RBC 4.15, Hgb 12.8, and Hct 38.9
MCV 93.8
PLT 195

Na 128, K 4.9, Cl 110, and CO 20
BUN 15, Cr 1.38, and GFR 48
Glucose 141
Ca 8.6 and Mg 1.4

AST 204, ALT 162, and ALP 96
Protein 5.6, Tbili 0.8, and albumin 3.3
Lipase 45

Digoxin level undetectable

ABG 7.35/30/80/21 on RA

ETOH < 10
APAP < 10
ASA < 4

Urine Drug Screen:

Barbiturates: negative
Benzodiazepines: negative
Cocaine: negative
Opiates: negative
Amphetamine: negative

Toxicologic Differential Diagnosis of Hypotension and Bradycardia

1. Calcium channel blockers
2. Beta-blockers
3. Digoxin
4. Alpha-2 antagonists
5. Opiates
6. Sedative/hypnotics
7. Organophosphates/carbamates/cholinergic drugs

Calcium channel blockers (CCB) are classically divided into two major categories: dihydropyridines and nondihydropyridines. When evaluating an overdose, it can be important to recognize the subtle differences between the two. The nondihydropyridines, such as diltiazem and verapamil, block the myocardial and smooth muscle L-type calcium channels, leading to hypotension and bradycardia through vasodilation and impaired cardiac conduction. Dihydropyridines, such as amlodipine, felodipine, nicardipine, and nifedipine, preferentially block the L-type calcium channels in the vascular smooth muscle, which leads to vasodilation. However, unlike the nondihydropyridines, these drugs do not depress myocardial electrical conduction. Though uncommon, in the setting of an overdose and even at therapeutic doses, the vasodilation may lead to reflex tachycardia [1]. The key point here is that even if a patient presents with profound hypotension and tachycardia, the patient may still have taken a CCB. It is also important to note that many intentional ingestions involve more than one substance, which may alter a patient's "toxidrome," leading to a mixed clinical presentation.

Hyperglycemia may be noted on labwork. Insulin release is mediated by calcium entry into the pancreatic beta cells via L-type calcium channels. CCBs will not only target cardiac and smooth muscle but will also target the cells in the pancreas, blocking insulin release, ultimately leading to elevated blood glucose.

β-blockers (BB) act on the beta-receptors, preventing norepinephrine and epinephrine from binding to the receptor. This leads to decreased production of cAMP in the cardiac myocyte and limits the calcium influx through L-type calcium channels. As with CCBs, this results in myocardial depression and decreased cardiac contractility. Because of the pathophysiologic similarities to CCBs, a BB overdose is generally treated in the same way as a CCB overdose.

Of note, certain beta-blockers have additional concerns from a toxicologic standpoint.

Propranolol works through two different mechanisms: as a beta-receptor antagonist and as a membrane depressant via the sodium channel blockade. This can lead to ventricular tachyarrhythmias [2]. Propranolol is also known to be lipid soluble and can easily cross the blood-brain barrier, increasing risk for CNS depression and seizure [3].

Sotalol is a type III antiarrhythmic well established in literature to prolong the QT interval and can lead to torsades de pointes [4].

Hypoglycemia may or may not be observed in an overdose. It has been described in children and diabetics, though is less in adults. It is classically thought that hypoglycemia is facilitated through the blunting of sympathetic hypoglycemic symptoms, such as tremors, sweats, and tachycardia [5].

Digoxin

Digoxin is a cardiac glycoside that has been used in the treatment of atrial fibrillation and heart failure. It increases contractility by increasing cytosolic calcium. Digoxin and other cardiac glycosides bind and block the Na+/K+ ATPase transporter on the extracellular membrane, leading to decreased Na + transport out of the cell and decreased K+ into the cell. The increased concentration of intracellular Na + allows for extracellular Na + to be pumped into the cell via the Na+/Ca2+ channel, while intracellular Ca2+ is pumped out. The increased calcium leads to further Ca2+ release from the sarcoplasmic reticulum during systole, increasing cardiac contractility.

It is worth noting that while we are discussing the hypotensive, bradycardic patient, digoxin toxicity can cause any type of change in both heart rate and cardiac rhythm. EKG findings can include PVCs, sinus bradycardia, atrial fibrillation, and ventricular tachycardias [6].

The clinical appearance of a patient with a digoxin overdose generally begins with GI symptoms – nausea, vomiting, and abdominal pain. Severe toxicity can lead to CNS symptoms – somnolence, confusion, lethargy, headache, and hallucination. Classically, patients have also described "yellow halos" in their fields of vision [7].

Potassium must be monitored in an overdose. As digoxin blocks the Na+/K+ pump, extracellular potassium increases. Hyperkalemia will further hyperpolarize myocardial conduction tissue and increases AV nodal block. The degree of hyperkalemia is a prognostic indicator of mortality [8].

In the undifferentiated hypotensive, bradycardic patient, a serum digoxin should be obtained; however, levels may be falsely elevated depending on when the last dose of digoxin was taken. After peak absorption, digoxin is then redistributed into the body stores. Blood concentrations taken prematurely (<6 h after last dose) are difficult to interpret and will not reflect complete redistribution levels. Because levels may be falsely elevated, it is important to assess how the patient clinically appears.

The indications for giving the antidote, digoxin-specific antibody fragments (digibind/digifab), are based on the patient's clinical picture and the following:

1. Cardiac arrest
2. Hemodynamic instability

3. Any life-threatening dysrhythmia
4. K+ > 5.0 in acute toxicity
5. Serum digoxin level > 10 nmol/L measured more than 6 h after ingestion in an acute ingestion regardless of symptoms
6. Acute ingestion of >10 mg in an adult (4 mg in a child)
7. Ingestion of non-pharmaceutical cardiac glycoside (e.g., as found in plants like foxglove and oleander, animals like the *Bufo* species toad, herbal preparations and traditional cultural medicines like *Chan Su*)

For elevated digoxin levels <10 nmol/L, treating with antidote must be weighed against the clinical picture and the patient's need for digoxin [9]. If the patient is not severely ill, ascertain why the patient was started on digoxin. Once the antidote has been given, digoxin levels can no longer be accurately measured until the digibind-digoxin complex has been eliminated. Digoxin assays are unable to accurately measure digoxin levels for 3 weeks, rendering it difficult to restart patient on therapy and properly dose the patient [10]. Also consider the high medical cost of the antidote.

Calculating the dose of digifab needed is unreliable if time of ingestion is unknown as measured serum digoxin level may not reflect the steady-state (postdistibutional) serum concentration.

Treatment is as follows [11]:

Acute toxicity:

- Known dose:
  - Dose (number of vials) = total ingested (mg) × 0.8 (bioavailability of tablet preparation) ÷ 0.5 of digitalis bound/vial
- Unknown dose:
  - Give five vials initially if the patient is hemodynamically stable
  - Give ten vials initially if the patient is hemodynamically unstable

- Repeat doses of five ampoules should be given every 30 min until reversal of digoxin toxicity is achieved
- In cardiac arrest give 20 vials (760 mg)

Chronic digoxin toxicity:

- Known level: number of vials required = (serum digoxin concentration – ng/L × (weight – kg) ÷ 100
- Empiric dosing: give one to three vials, can be re-dosed after 30 min and titrated to clinically effect.

Note that if a patient is ill due to ingestion of non-pharmaceutical cardiac glycoside (found in plants and animals), the digoxin level should not be used to estimate dosing. Treat with empiric dosing.

Alpha-2 Agonists

Clonidine, *tizanidine*, *guanfacine*, *methyldopa*, and *dexmedetomidine* are centrally acting alpha-2 adrenergic agonists. They reduce sympathetic outflow to the CNS, leading to a decrease in blood pressure, heart rate, and vascular tone. In an overdose, these agents can cause a prolonged CNS depression and, occasionally, hypothermia. Note that alpha agonism will lead to pinpoint/constricted pupils, often leading to the misdiagnosis of an opioid toxicity. Respiratory rate may be depressed, but unlike in an opiate toxicity, this generally responds well to external stimuli (auditory or tactile).

Naloxone has been used in high doses (4–10 mg) for reversal with variable response [12]. The mechanism behind increased blood pressure, heart rate, and level of arousal after naloxone is not well defined but is thought to relate to the modulation of CNS sympathetic outflow by endogenous CNS opioids [13].

The following substances may cause bradycardia and occasionally hypotension and can be peripherally regarded when thinking about the hypotensive, bradycardic patient. When considering the hypotensive, bradycardic patient, CCBs, BBs, alpha-2 agonists, and digoxin should be first on the differential diagnosis.

Opioids

Although uncommon, narcotics can cause varying degrees of hypotension (generally orthostatic) and bradycardia. *Methadone* in particular has been shown to have calcium channel antagonism [14, 15].

Sedative/Hypnotics

Benzodiazepines, *barbiturates*, *baclofen*, *GHB*, *sodium oxybate*, *and carisoprodol (SOMA)* are all examples of sedative-hypnotics that can lead to hypotension and bradycardia.

Though their exact mechanisms vary, simplistically, these medications involve agonism of the GABA-A or GABA-B receptor and can clinically present as decreased mental status, respiratory depression, and bradycardia.

Flumazenil has been used for iatrogenic and pediatric benzodiazepine overdoses. It is generally not recommended to give flumazenil in an adult who potentially is benzodiazepine-dependent due to the precipitation of withdrawal. Benzodiazepine withdrawal is not benign and can lead to seizures, hypertension, tachycardia, hallucinations, psychosis, and coma. Once flumazenil is administered, the specific binding site for benzodiazepines is blocked. Should the patient experience seizures, the patient will not be able to respond to benzodiazepines [16]. It is worth noting that barbiturates, while also GABA-A agonists, bind to a separate site on the GABA receptor and could potentially be used in a seizing patient unresponsive to benzodiazepines.

GHB is a GABA-B agonist that has historically been abused by bodybuilders for its supposed anabolic properties. It is also known to be used as a recreational substance or for facilitation of physical/sexual assault. Ingestion can cause deep sedation, bradycardia, and coma, sometimes requiring intubation. The classic presentation is of a patient who presents comatose and is intubated for airway protection. Ninety minutes later, the patient abruptly awakens and self-extubates [17].

Organophosphates/Carbamates

Organophosphates and carbamates are compounds often found in insecticides and agents of warfare.

In the body, acetylcholine is a neurotransmitter that functions in multiple ways. It is used at the neuromuscular junction to activate skeletal muscles, used as a neurotransmitter in the autonomic nervous system, and also used as a neurotransmitter in the CNS in both the parasympathetic and sympathetic nervous system.

Organophosphates and carbamates inhibit the enzyme cholinesterase, which is the enzyme breakdown acetylcholine. This leads to an excess of acetylcholine at nerve synapses and neuromuscular junctions, which results in overexcitation of acetylcholine receptors. This is better known as a cholinergic crisis, which can manifest as nausea, headache, shortness of breath, rhinorrhea, salivation, diaphoresis, confusion, bronchorrhea, muscle fasciculations, seizure, diarrhea, paralysis, and coma.

Because acetylcholine functions as a neurotransmitter for both the sympathetic and parasympathetic nervous systems, a patient with a severe overdose may present with autonomic instability. Parasympathetic stimulation commonly predominates, which manifests as hypotension, bradycardia, and miosis. A patient may have a mixed picture as the sympathetic stimulation leads to tachycardia, hypertension, and mydriasis [18].

There are also *cholinergic agents* to keep in mind, such as *donezepil (Aricept)*, *physostigmine*, *neostigmine*, *rivastigmine*, *and galantamine*.

Depending on type and route of exposure, treatment involves decontamination (skin and mucous membranes) and provider protection with chemical-protective clothing.

Atropine addresses the life-threatening muscarinic symptoms including bradycardia, hypotension, bronchorrhea, and bronchospasm. It should be given in escalating doses, starting at 2–5 mg IV, and titrated every 5–10 min until patient's secretions and clinical picture improve.

Pralidoxime is used in the setting of an organophosphate (OP) overdose to reactivate cholinesterase enzymes; however, based on route of exposure, type of OP (some organophosphates may quickly irreversibly bind to cholinesterase), this may or may not be helpful in an overdose. It is most helpful in an OP overdose when given as early as possible. It is not typically given with carbamates.

Pralidoxime should be given as a loading dose (30–50 mg/kg, total of 1–2 g in adults) over 30 min, followed by a continuous infusion of 8–20 mg/kg/h (up to 650 mg/h) [19].

Plants, Herbs, and Animals

As providers are exposed to different cultures, it is worth briefly noting that there are many plants (e.g., oleander, foxglove), traditional medicinal preparations (e.g., aconite in Chinese herbal preparations), and diet (e.g., shellfish poisoning/toxic fish poisonings) that can cause hypotension and bradycardia [20, 21]. Obtaining a comprehensive history may be crucial to identifying the patient's source of exposure once the patient has been stabilized.

Management of the Acutely Ill, Hypotensive, Bradycardic Patient

1. Establish and *maintain the patient's airway*.
2. Place patient on *cardiac monitor* and place *pacer pads*.
3. Obtain adequate *intravenous access*. Establish central access if anticipating need for multiple pressors, large amounts of fluid, and high concentration solutions like D20W.
4. Send CBC, BMP, LFTs, ETOH, ASA, and APAP. If undifferentiated, it is reasonable to add a digoxin level.
5. If patient presents within *1–2 h after ingestion*, consider aggressive *early decontamination*. For example, in the

case of CCB/BB overdose, the severity of toxicity can be profound, and the benefit to decontamination is great:

(a) If the patient is *alert* and able to maintain an airway, consider giving *activated charcoal.*
(b) If patient is *intubated*, consider giving *activated charcoal and performing gastric lavage.*
(c) If the patient has taken sustained release tablets or if bezoar formation is suspected, whole bowel irrigation may also be considered. Note that a negative CT does not rule out a bezoar [22].

6. Assess volume status:

(a) Bedside US can be utilized to assess ejection fraction, ventricular wall movement, and IVC collapsibility.
(b) Give *IV fluid bolus in the absence of fluid overload.*

7. *Atropine*

(a) Inhibits the effects of vagal stimulation, which can temporarily reverse AV nodal blocks, leading to an increased electrical conduction and increased heart rate.
(b) Given the relative ease of access to atropine, it is a reasonable medication to try. In severe antihypertensive overdose, however, it is usually not successful.
(c) *Dose: 0.5 mg–1 mg IV q 3–5 min; max 3 mg total.*

8. *Intravenous calcium*

(a) If the patient is known to have taken a CCB, the theory behind giving intravenous calcium is competitive antagonism and peripheral vascoconstriction. Note that calcium chloride contains three times the amount and has potential to be venosclerotic.
(b) If the patient is known to have taken digoxin, it may be prudent to avoid giving calcium; however, this stems from older animal models that showed an increase in digoxin toxicity when calcium was given.

The theory behind this being calcium may lead to an irreversible noncontractile state, due to impaired diastolic relaxation from calcium-troponin C binding. The human evidence for developing cardiac tetany or a "stone heart" is poor [23]. IV calcium should not be withheld from a critical patient if it may prove beneficial.

(c) *Dose: calcium chloride 1 g IV or calcium gluconate 3 g IV with goal serum calcium 12-13 mg/dL.*

9. *Pressors*

   (a) *Norepinephrine/epinephrine*

      - In regard to *dopamine*: dopamine receptor selectivity is poor, and its mechanism of action is indirect and less predictable than that of norepinephrine. Dopamine preferentially binds to dopamine receptors which may cause hypotension at low doses. It then converted to NE and stimulates the release of NE. If a patient is already on NE, adding dopamine does not necessarily confer increased pressor support. Additionally, the 2016 Cochrane review of vasopressors for hypotensive shock noted increased arrhythmogenicity with dopamine.

   (b) *Vasopressin* does not act on adrenergic receptors and may be added if there is no response to norepinephrine/epinephrine.

   (c) In a patient with poor cardiac contractility, also consider dobutamine and phosphodiesterase III inhibitors (inamrinone, milrinone, and enoximone).

10. Give *antidote* if indicated

   (a) *Digifab* for digoxin (see above digoxin section for dosing)

   (b) *Naloxone*

      - 4–10 mg IV for clonidine

11. *Glucagon*

    (a) A reasonable therapy to start, especially if suspecting a beta-blocker overdose.
    (b) Glucagon stimulates adenyl cyclase via G proteins, resulting in increased intracellular cyclic AMP which in turn leads to stimulation of muscle contraction, resulting in positive inotropic and chronotropic effects, similar to beta-agonists [24].
    (c) *Dose: 5–10 mg IV bolus and watch for response within 5 min.* Glucagon may be re-dosed. If clinical response is noted, patient should immediately be started on a *glucagon infusion at response dose per hour.*
    (d) Note that glucagon may cause nausea and emesis, which may compromise the patient's airway.

12. *High-dose insulin euglycemia therapy (HIET)*

    (a) Pathophysiology

        - The myocardium uses free fatty acids for energy but in a shock state will use insulin. In a CCB overdose, patients become hyperglycemic and insulin resistant. The heart enters a metabolic stress state but is unable to utilize glucose. Without the needed energy, myocardial depression and hypotension ensue [25]. HIET promotes uptake of glucose and facilitates oxidation and clearance of metabolic "stress state" by-products, including lactic acid and end products of glycolysis [26].
        - Insulin has also been shown to provide inotropy as demonstrated in animal studies [27].

    (b) Labwork

        - Frequent glucose checks are necessary, and serial electrolytes need to be monitored. Hypokalemia due to insulin-mediated intracellular shifting can be supplemented with IV potassium; however, it is important to remember that patient's total body potassium is not depleted. When HIE is stopped, potassium will shift out of the cells.

(c) *Dosing*

- Start insulin as soon as possible as it will take time to see clinical effect (approximately 20–30 min). Bridge with pressors as needed.
- *Bolus 1 IU/kg insulin with or without 25 g dextrose bolus*

  1. Avoid insulin bolus if glucose <150
  2. Avoid dextrose bolus if glucose >400

- *Start 1–2 IU/kg/h drip with goal blood glucose of 100–250*

  1. Perform glucose checks q30 minutes until blood glucose is stable, and then space to 1–2 h
  2. Check potassium levels q1 hour, and replete when K < 2.5 mEq/L

(d) Goals of treatment

- Therapy should be guided by patient's hemodynamic status. A *HR > 50 and MAP > 65* is a reasonable goal.
- HIET is stopped after vasopressors have been weaned. The approach to cessation of HIET is not well defined as some physicians advocate a slow taper, while others advocate for abruptly cessation to allow for self-tapering of insulin from insulin release of body lipid stores [28].
- We recommend weaning insulin infusion 0.5 U/kg/h every 2–4 h once vasopressors have been stopped. Closely monitor glucose and electrolytes during the weaning process and for 24 h after discontinuation of insulin infusion.

If the above steps have not led to adequate control of the patient's clinical presentation, consider the following:

13. Other pressors

    (a) Methylene blue

        - The suspected mechanism of action of methylene blue is inhibition of the enzyme nitric oxide synthase, which ultimately prevents the smooth muscle dilation [29].
        - This will turn the patient blue and will interfere with colorimetric lab testing like CO-oximetry and also lead to inaccurate readings on pulse oximeter [30].

    (b) Hydroxocobalamin

        - The suspected mechanism of action is the sequestration and subsequent depletion of nitric oxide in vascular endothelium preventing vasodilation [31].
        - It changes colors of body fluid to a dark-wine color, which can interfere with colorimetric methods used in laboratory measurements such as aspartate aminotransferase, total bilirubin, creatinine, magnesium, and serum iron [32]. It also may interfere with CO-oximetry testing of carboxyhemoglobin, methemoglobin, and oxyhemoglobin.
        - Depending on the hemodialysis machine, hydroxocobalamin may trigger the blood leak alarm on a dialysis circuit due to its color. When it crosses the semipermeable membrane, some machines have been known to terminate dialysis because it interprets the presence of hydroxocobalamin as in the dialysate [33].

14. *Lipid emulsion therapy*

    (a) The exact mechanism for intralipid therapy is not completely understood, but it is thought that once intralipid is circulation, the emulsion extracts lipophilic drugs, preventing them from distributing into the serum [34]. The evidence of lipid emulsion therapy comes from the treatment of local anesthetics, such as lidocaine and bupivacaine; however, further investigation is underway to assess benefit in other lipophilic medications.

(b) Medications that are thought to have had some benefit include amlodipine, verapamil, bupropion, carvedilol, cyclic antidepressants, diphenhydramine, flecainide, metoprolol, organophosphates, propranolol, quetiapine, and timolol [35, 36].

(c) *Pitfall:* It is important to draw labs such as ABG, CBC, electrolytes, triglycerides, and serum drug concentrations prior to dosing as intralipid will interfere with these lab tests once administered.

(d) *Note:* It is contraindicated in use in patients with severe egg or soybean allergy.

(e) Using intralipid is not without risk:

- Hypertriglyceridemia, acute pancreatitis, cholestasis, and increased risk of infection have been described [37].
- Fat overload syndrome is a well-known complication of intravenous lipid emulsion therapy, directly relating to the rate of administration of infusion. As this is a relatively novel therapy, the upper limits of infusion rates and dose are not defined. The syndrome is characterized by headaches, fever, anemia, jaundice, hepatosplenomegaly, respiratory distress, ARDS, and DIC [38].

(f) *Dose: 1.5 mL/kg as an initial bolus followed by 0.25 mL/kg/min for 30–60 min.*

(g) If considering extracorporeal membrane oxygenation (ECMO), note that intralipid may potentially create problems, including clogging and cracking in an ECMO circuit [39]. To this point, if a patient is already actively receiving ECMO, it may not be salient to start intralipid. Conversely, failed intralipid therapy should not stop a provider from starting ECMO.

15. Nonpharmacologic therapies [40]
    (a) Temporary cardiac pacing can be considered but usually unsuccessful in treating the severely ill, poisoned patient.
    (b) *Dialysis:* antihypertensive agents are poorly dialyzed, though some studies have shown that atenolol, acebutolol, and sotalol may have some clearance through dialysis [41]. This may or may not translate to better clinical outcomes and should only be considered if pharmacologic therapies have been exhausted.
    (c) *Intra-aortic balloon pump/left ventricular assist device/VA ECMO*
        - Mobilize these therapies early if the patient is severely ill.

Case Conclusion

The patient's husband was able to find his wife's medication list, which included diltiazem. The patient received IV fluids, atropine, pressors, and glucagon (with no effect) and ultimately was placed on HIET with full recovery.

Key Points

- The undifferentiated toxicologic hypotensive bradycardic patient has a wide differential diagnosis. Obtaining a comprehensive history is important and may help further guide management, but in the critically ill patient, starting the algorithm may help attain hemodynamic stability.
- Given the elevated morbidity and mortality of calcium channel and beta-blocker overdoses, consider early aggressive decontamination.
- In the undifferentiated patient, a digoxin level should strongly be considered.

- Not all calcium channel blockers and beta-blockers are equivalent. In addition to hypotension and bradycardia, consider seizures and tachyarrhythmias in propranolol; consider QTc prolongation in sotalol.
- In a severely ill patient, a single agent is not likely to help. Starting multiple therapies, e.g., IV fluids + IV calcium + pressors + glucagon + high-dose insulin, is more likely to be successful in stabilizing the patient.
- Insulin *needs* to be started at and is most effective at high doses (1–2 IU/kg) with frequent monitoring of electrolytes and glucose.
- Consider intralipid therapy if all other pharmacologic therapies have failed.
- Mobilize dialysis/IABP/LVAD/VA ECMO early in a critical patient.

References

1. Stanek EJ, Nelson CE, DeNofrio D. Amlodipine overdose. Ann Pharmacother. 1997;31(7–8):853–6. [PubMed].
2. Craig CR, Stitzel RE. Modern pharmacology with clinical applications. 6th ed; Lippincott Williams & Wilkins, Philideplphia: 2004. p. 182–4.
3. Wang DW, Mistry AM, Kahlig KM, Kearney JA, Xiang J, George AL Jr. Propranolol blocks cardiac and neuronal voltage-gated sodium channels. Front Pharmacol. 2010;1:144.
4. MacNeil DJ. The side effect profile of class III antiarrhythmic drugs; focus on d,l-sotalol. Am J Cardiol. 1997;80:90G–8G.
5. Mani BK, Osborne-Lawrence S, Vijayaraghavan P, Hepler C, Zigman JM. β1-Adrenergic receptor deficiency in ghrelin-expressing cells causes hypoglycemia in susceptible individuals. J Clin Investig. 2016;126:3467–78. https://doi.org/10.1172/JCI86270.
6. Smith TW, Antman EM, Friedman PL, et al. Digitalis glycosides: mechanisms and manifestations of toxicity. Part I. Prog Cardiovasc Dis. 1984;26:413.

7. Lawrenson JG, Kelly C, Lawrenson AL, Birch J. Acquired colour vision deficiency in patients receiving digoxin maintenance therapy. Br J Ophthalmol. 2002;86:1259–61.
8. Manini AF, Nelson LS, Hoffman RS. Prognostic utility of serum potassium in chronic digoxin toxicity: a case-control study. Am J Cardiovasc Drugs. 2011;11:173–8.
9. DigiFab [product monograph]. Ottawa: Canadian Pharmacists Association; Available: www.e-cps.ca.
10. McMillin GA, Owen WE, Lambert TL, De BK, Frank EL, Bach PR, et al. Comparable effects of DIGIBIND and DigiFab in thirteen digoxin immunoassays. Clin Chem. 2002;48(9):1580–4. PubMed PMID: 12194938.
11. Kearney TE. Digoxin-specific antibodies. In: Poisoning & drug overdose. 7th ed; BTG, a UK pharmaceutical company. 2017.
12. Bamshad MJ, Wasserman GS. Pediatric clonidine intoxications. Vet Hum Toxicol. 1990;32:220–3.
13. Seger D. Clonidine toxicity revisited. Clin Toxicol. 2002;40:145–55.
14. Alinejad S, Kazemi T, Zamani N, Hoffman RS, Mehrpour O. A systematic review of the cardiotoxicity of methadone. EXCLI J. 2015;14:577–600.
15. Seyler DE, Borowitz JL, Maickel RP. Calcium channel blockade by certain opioids. Fundam Appl Toxicol. 1983;3:536–42.
16. Mintzer MZ, Griffiths RR. Flumazenil-precipitated withdrawal in healthy volunteers following repeated diazepam exposure. Psychopharmacology. 2005;178:259–67.
17. Roberts T, Thompson J. Illegal substances in anaesthetic and intensive care practices. Contin Educ Anaesth Crit Care Pain Adv Access. 2012;16(3):226–229.
18. Waseem M, Perry C, Bomann S. Cholinergic crisis after rodenticide poisoning. West J Emerg Med. 2010;11(5):524–7.
19. Vohra R. Organophosphorus and carbamate insecticides. In: Poisoning & drug overdose. 7th ed;Lange, New York: 2017.
20. Ito S, Nakazato Y, Ohga A. Further evidence for the involvement of Na+ channels in the release of adrenal catecholamine: the effect of scorpion venom and grayanotoxin I. Br J Pharmacol. 1981;72(1):61–7.
21. Chan TYK. Aconite poisoning. Clin Toxicol. 2009;47:279–85. https://doi.org/10.1080/15563650902904407.
22. Lung D. Venlafaxine pharmacobezoar causing intestinal ischemia requiring emergent hemicolectomy. J Med Toxicol. 2011;7:232–5.
23. Erickson CP, Olson KR. Case files of the medical toxicology fellowship of the California poison control system-San Francisco:

calcium plus digoxin-more taboo than toxic? J Med Toxicol. 2008;4(1):33–9.
24. Bailey B. Glucagon in beta-blocker and calcium channel blocker overdoses: a systematic review. J Toxicol Clin Toxicol. 2003;41(5):595–602. Review. PubMed PMID: 14514004.
25. Kerns W II. Management of beta-adrenergic blocker and calcium channel antagonist toxicity. Emerg Med Clin North Am. 2007;25(2):309–31.
26. Kline JA, Raymond RM, Leonova ED, Williams TC, Watts JA. Insulin improves heart function and metabolism during nonischemic cardiogenic shock in awake canines. Cardiovasc Res. 1997;34:289–98. https://doi.org/10.1016/S0008-6363(97)00022-9.
27. Das UN. Insulin: an endogenous cardioprotector. Curr Opin Crit Care. 2003;9(5):375–83.
28. Yuan TH, Kerns WP, Tomaszewski CA, Ford MD, Kline JA. Insulin-glucose as adjunctive therapy of severe calcium channel antagonist poisoning. J Toxicol Clin Toxicol. 1999;37:463–74. https://doi.org/10.1081/CLT-100102437.
29. Jang DH, Nelson LS, Hoffman RS. Methylene blue for distributive shock: a potential new use of an old antidote. J Med Toxicol. 2013;9(3):242–9. https://doi.org/10.1007/s13181-013-0298-7.
30. Gourlaine H, Buneaux F, Borron W, Gouget B, Levillain P. Interference of methylene blue with CO-oximetry of hemoglobin derivatives. Clin Chem. 1997;43:1078–80.
31. Roderique JD, Van Dyck K, Holman B, Tang D, Chui B, Spiess BD. The use of high-dose hydroxocobalamin for vasoplegic syndrome. Ann Thorac Surg. 2014;97:1785–6.
32. Fueyo L, Robles J, Aguilar I. Hemolysis index to detect degree of hydroxocobalamin interference with common laboratory tests. J Clin Lab Anal. 2017;31.
33. Sutter M, Tereshchenko N, Rafii R, et al. Hemodialysis complications of hydroxocobalamin: a case report. J Med Toxicol. 2010;6:165–7.
34. Ciechanowicz S, Patil V. Lipid emulsion for local anesthetic systemic toxicity. Anesthesiol Res Pract. 2012;2012:11. https://doi.org/10.1155/2012/131784.131784.
35. Cave G, Harvey M. Intravenous lipid emulsion as antidote beyond local anesthetic toxicity: a systematic review. Acad Emerg Med. 2009;16:815–24.
36. Armenian P, French D, Smollin C, Olson K, Wu AHB. Prolonged absorption from sustained-release verapamil preparation with

documentation of serum levels and their response to intralipids. Clin Toxicol. 2010;48(6):646.
37. Mirtallo JM, et al. State of the art review: intravenous fat emulsions: current applications, safety profile, and clinical implications. Ann Pharmacother. 2010;44:688–700.
38. Hayes BD, Gosselin S, Calello DP, et al. Systematic review of clinical adverse events reported after acute intravenous lipid emulsion administration. Clin Toxicol. 2016;54:365–404.
39. Lee HM, Archer JR, Dargan PI, Wood DM. What are the adverse effects associated with the combined use of intravenous lipid emulsion and extracorporeal membrane oxygenation in the poisoned patient? Clin Toxicol (Phila). 2015;53:145–50.
40. St-Onge M, Dubé PA, Gosselin S. Treatment for calcium channel blocker poisoning: a systematic review. Clin Toxicol. 2014;52:926–44.
41. Weir MA, Dixon SN, Fleet JL, Roberts MA, Hackam DG, Oliver MJ, et al. b-Blocker dialyzability and mortality in older patients receiving hemodialysis. J Am Soc Nephrol. 2015;26:987–96.

Index

J. A. LaRosa (ed.), *Adult Critical Care Medicine*,
https://doi.org/10.1007/978-3-319-94424-1

V

MIX
Papier aus verantwortungsvollen Quellen
Paper from responsible sources
FSC® C105338

If you have any concerns about our products,
you can contact us on
ProductSafety@springernature.com

In case Publisher is established outside the EU,
the EU authorized representative is:
Springer Nature Customer Service Center GmbH
Europaplatz 3, 69115 Heidelberg, Germany

Printed by Libri Plureos GmbH
in Hamburg, Germany